Algorithms in Differential Diagnosis

How to Approach Common Presenting Complaints in Adult Patients, for Medical Students and Junior Doctors

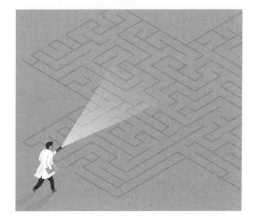

Algorithms in Differential Diagnosis

How to Approach Common Presenting Complaints in Adult Patients, for Medical Students and Junior Doctors

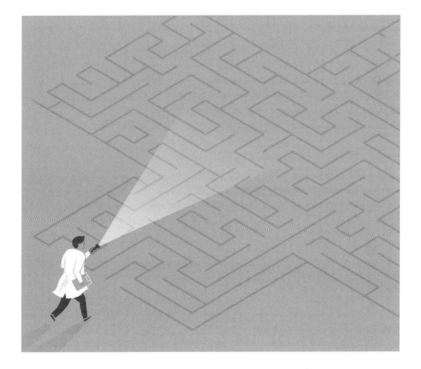

Dr. Nigel Fong

Singapore General Hospital, Singapore

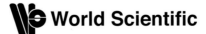 **World Scientific**

NEW JERSEY · LONDON · SINGAPORE · BEIJING · SHANGHAI · HONG KONG · TAIPEI · CHENNAI · TOKYO

Published by

World Scientific Publishing Co. Pte. Ltd.

5 Toh Tuck Link, Singapore 596224

USA office: 27 Warren Street, Suite 401-402, Hackensack, NJ 07601

UK office: 57 Shelton Street, Covent Garden, London WC2H 9HE

Library of Congress Cataloging-in-Publication Data
Names: Fong, Nigel (Nigel Jie Ming), author.
Title: Algorithms in differential diagnosis : how to approach common presenting complaints in
adult patients, for medical students and junior doctors / Dr. Nigel Fong.
Description: New Jersey : World Scientific, 2019. | Includes index.
Identifiers: LCCN 2018046261| ISBN 9789813232921 (hardcover : alk. paper) |
ISBN 9813232927 (hardcover : alk. paper) | ISBN 9789811200557 (pbk. : alk. paper) |
ISBN 9811200556 (pbk. : alk. paper)
Subjects: | MESH: Diagnosis, Differential | Algorithms | Adult | Case Reports
Classification: LCC RC71 | NLM WB 141.5 | DDC 616.07/5--dc23
LC record available at https://lccn.loc.gov/2018046261

British Library Cataloguing-in-Publication Data
A catalogue record for this book is available from the British Library.

Cover design by Jonathan Yong-Ern Lim

Disclaimer
This book is intended only for a professional audience, and should be used in conjunction with other reference texts and clinical experience. Accurate diagnosis and safe clinical practice is the physician's responsibility. Readers are urged to keep up to date with changes in medical knowledge and best practice. Additionally, junior physicians are advised to consult senior staff if unsure how to manage a patient. While the Author and Publisher have made every effort to ensure that the content of this book is accurate and up to date, neither the Author nor Publisher assumes liability for any error, omission, or harm resulting from the material in this book.

For any available supplementary material, please visit
https://www.worldscientific.com/worldscibooks/10.1142/10787#t=suppl

Printed in Singapore by Mainland Press Ptd Ltd.

Preface

This is a book for medical students and first-year doctors who wish to learn how to approach a patient's symptoms, and sharpen their skills of clinical reasoning and diagnosis.

Clinical medicine begins with the patient. Many of us learn one disease condition at a time, yet, patients present with symptoms and not a known disease. Many students know the correct evidence-based treatment of heart failure, yet are stumped when given a breathless patient on the ward, and told to 'figure out what is wrong'. Many can list the differentials for a symptom, but struggle to separate important diagnostic features from the irrelevant details that many patients throw at us. It is tempting to rely ever more heavily on our growing armamentarium of diagnostic tools. But testing without thinking not only confounds and misleads, it also costs our patients dear.

Having been a student myself not too long ago, I have experienced first-hand the struggles that a budding clinician faces in synthesising vast amounts of new information and applying it to real patients. In this book, I try to offer a toolkit to tackle this challenge.

Each chapter tackles one presenting complaint, identifying key differentials, providing a strategy to distinguish each differential from the other and setting out the thought process behind history, examination and initial investigations. Each approach cuts across different specialties, integrating approaches and conditions from various medical and surgical fields.

This book uses *algorithms* to aid diagnosis. This is a method of clinical reasoning that uses critical pieces of information as branch points to distinguish between groups of diagnoses. It complements (not replaces) clinical skills and knowledge of individual disease conditions. Junior diagnosticians particularly benefit from learning algorithms, because they not only provide a systematic and functional way to approach patients, but also serve as a scaffold to organise knowledge and learn the skills of clinical reasoning. I have written these algorithms to be usable for those who are just starting out, rather than theoretically complete but too complex to use.

Finally, always remember that if one hopes to develop clinical acumen, there is no substitute to seeing patients—they are our best teachers, inspiration and sources of creative inquiry.

Nigel Fong
2018

Subspecialty Reviewers

CARDIOLOGY	**Dr Wang Yue** *Senior Resident, Cardiology* *National Heart Centre, Singapore*
DERMATOLOGY	**Dr Oh Choon Chiat** *Associate Consultant, Dermatology* *Singapore General Hospital*
ENDOCRINOLOGY	**Dr Tan Zhen-Wei, Matthew** *Dr Matthew Tan Diabetes & Endocrine Care* *Farrer Park Medical Centre, Singapore*
GASTROENTEROLOGY	**Dr Ong Ming Liang, Andrew** *Associate Consultant, Gastroenterology & Hepatology* *Singapore General Hospital*
GERIATRIC MEDICINE	**Dr Lim Kim Hwa Jim** *Senior Consultant, Geriatric Medicine* *Changi General Hospital, Singapore*
GYNAECOLOGY	**A/Prof Tan Lay Kok** *Senior Consultant, Obstetrics & Gynaecology* *Singapore General Hospital*
HAEMATOLOGY	**Dr Dixon Grant** *Associate Consultant, Haematology* *Singapore General Hospital*
INFECTIOUS DISEASE	**Dr Benjamin Cherng Pei Zhi** *Consultant, Infectious Diseases* *Singapore General Hospital*
NEPHROLOGY	**Dr Jason Choo Chon Jun** *Senior Consultant & Program Director, Renal Medicine* *Singapore General Hospital*
NEUROLOGY	**Dr Wee Chee Keong** *Consultant, Neurology, National Neuroscience Institute* *Singapore* **Dr Gosavi Tushar Divakar** *Consultant, Neurology, National Neuroscience Institute* *Singapore*

OPHTHALMOLOGY

Dr Loo Jing Liang
Senior Consultant
Singapore National Eye Centre

ORTHOPAEDIC SURGERY

Dr Jerry Delphi Chen Yongqiang
Senior Resident, Orthopaedic Surgery
Singapore Health Services

OTOLARYNGOLOGY

Dr Toh Song Tar
Senior Consultant, Otolaryngology
Singapore General Hospital

PSYCHIATRY

A/Prof Ng Beng Yeong
Ng Beng Yeong Psych Med Clinic
Mount Elizabeth Medical Centre, Singapore

RESPIRATORY MEDICINE

Dr Ong Thun How
Senior Consultant & Program Director
Respiratory & Critical Care Medicine
Singapore General Hospital

A/Prof Koh Siyue, Mariko
Senior Consultant, Respiratory & Critical Care Medicine
Singapore General Hospital

RHEUMATOLOGY

Dr Fong Weng Seng, Warren
Consultant, Rheumatology and Immunology
Singapore General Hospital

SURGERY

Dr Lee Lip Seng
Consultant, General Surgery
Changi General Hospital, Singapore

EDUCATION ADVISORS

A/Prof Tan Choon Kiat, Nigel
Senior Consultant, Neurology
National Neuroscience Institute, Singapore

Deputy Group Director, Education (Undergrad)
Singapore Health Services

A/Prof Tay Sook Muay
Senior Consultant, Anaesthesia
Singapore General Hospital

Associate Dean, Yong Loo Lin School of Medicine
National University of Singapore

Acknowledgements

I praise God for his work in my life, which I scarcely deserve. He has blessed me greatly, and His grace sustains me each day. Each day in the wards, I marvel at how each of us are the work of His fingers, yet am reminded that to Him we will one day return. To Him be all glory.

I thank Marianne, my wife and closest companion, for being a wonderful blessing and support. I am also very grateful to my parents; to whom I owe so much.

I am indebted to the many senior clinicians from the SingHealth family (listed on page vii) who have taken personal time to review my writing. They have provided invaluable subspecialty input, refined the algorithms and corrected numerous errors and omissions. I am particularly thankful for Dr Ong Thun How and A/Prof Tay Sook Muay, both of whom first encouraged me to write this book, and who have mentored me in many ways.

Many peers and juniors have also contributed to this book (and its previous versions) as reviewers:

Dr Amanda Chin
Dr A. Sayampanathan
Dr Benjamin Nah
Dr Calida Chua
Dr Chang Zi Yun
Dr Chaung Jia Quan
Dr Chng Wei Qiang
Dr Chua Si Min
Dr Daniel Lim
Dr Darius Pan
Dr David Zhao
Dr Davin Ryanputra
Dr Dorothy Huang
Dr Edwin Chow
Dr Eugene Gan
Dr Gabriel Tan
Dr Goh Jiaying
Dr Graham Goh

Dr Hester Lau
Dr How Guo Yuan
Dr Huang Wenjie
Dr Jerold Loh
Dr Jiang Bochao
Dr Joel Goh
Dr Kara-Anne Tan
Dr Ke Yuhe
Dr Kevin Kwek
Dr Khoo Bo Yan
Dr Krystal Koh
Dr Lee Bing Howe
Dr Leong Jia Li
Dr Leong Yun Hao
Dr Liang Sai
Dr Marianne Tsang
Dr Michael Chee
Dr Michelle Sim

Dr Mohd Alimi
Dr Nicholas Ngiam
Dr Ng Qin Xiang
Dr Peng Siyu
Dr R. Chockalingam Jr
Dr Ryan Lee
Dr Samuel Ee
Dr Sharon Goh
Dr Stephen Sumarli
Dr Tan Pei Zheng
Dr Tang Wanchu
Dr Tony Li
Dr Tryphena Ng
Dr Wang Hankun
Dr Yii Zheng Wei
Dr Zhao Yang

I must thank my teachers. Over the years, I have had the benefit of many excellent clinical tutors, who have not only imparted medical knowledge, but more importantly, taught me how to think, and how to care for patients. I am also greatly indebted to my alma mater, the Yong Loo Lin School of Medicine, National University of Singapore.

Most of all, I thank my patients, who time and again have proven to be my best tutors, and who have given medicine its meaning.

Finally, I thank the publishing team at World Scientific for putting this book together. My editor, Lim Sook Cheng, has been particularly approachable and helpful. I also thank Jonathan Lim, a long-time friend and artist, who provided the cover illustration.

Contents

Introduction

Chapter

1 Learning How to Diagnose

Clinical Case

A final-year medical student has difficulty making clinical diagnoses. Although she is able to regurgitate a great deal about many conditions (having read the textbooks cover-to-cover), she has great difficulty pinpointing the correct diagnosis whenever she sees a patient on the ward. She says that she 'does not know where to begin', and 'just can't think of the right diagnosis'. What would you advise her?

Welcome! We must begin by learning how to diagnose. These skills are central to a physician's healing art—making an accurate and timely diagnosis allows the physician to administer appropriate treatment, which gets the patient better. Conversely, diagnostic errors harm patients.

This chapter opens with an exposition of how clinicians make diagnoses, and discusses the process of diagnostic reasoning, along with some other issues. Next, I offer some advice on how to use this book, and suggestions on how to learn the science and art of clinical diagnosis. We will use the clinical scenario (Box 1.1) as a starting point for discussion.

Box 1.1. Diagnostic Reasoning During Ward Rounds

Third-year student: Our next patient is a 70-year-old gentleman who complains of jaundice. It started 1 month ago, and has been getting worse. He does not have fever, abdominal pain, nausea or vomiting. He has been feeling lethargic and has also lost 10 kg in the last 3 months. His bowel movements are normal. He is a non-smoker, and has no travel or contact history. A sexual history is unremarkable. He has no past medical history. On examination, his abdomen is soft and there is no palpable liver. Liver function tests show elevated bilirubin, AST, ALT and ALP.

Consultant: What do you think it could be?

Third-year student: Hmm… does he have cirrhosis? He has jaundice and abnormal liver enzymes. Hepatitis? Haemolysis? Gallstones?

Final-year student: I've clerked him too. He has no stigmata of chronic liver disease, so cirrhosis is unlikely. I don't think he has haemolysis either, as his haemoglobin was normal. He has no abdominal pain, history of eating raw shellfish, unprotected sexual intercourse or hepatotoxic drug ingestion, so it's probably not hepatitis. His liver function test is actually

(Cont'd)

showing higher ALP than AST and ALT, suggesting biliary obstruction, maybe by gallstones or a mass.

Resident: Yes, this is a gentleman with obstructive jaundice. The causes of obstructive jaundice can be divided into painful and painless. He is painless, which makes gallstones less likely, and extrinsic compression of the bile ducts more likely. I would order an ultrasound next, looking for dilated bile ducts. If ducts are dilated, then we need to find out if there is biliary tree compression by an extrinsic mass, or if he has a stricture. If ducts are not dilated, then we should send off antimitochondrial antibody for primary biliary cholangitis.

Consultant: Alright. This is an elderly gentleman with painless progressive obstructive jaundice. You are right that in the absence of pain, bile duct compression is more likely than gallstones. Strictures and primary biliary cholangitis are possible, but in this patient with clinically significant weight loss, I am most worried about a pancreatic tumour with bile duct compression. Let's skip ultrasound and go straight to CT. That will tell us whether there is any pancreatic mass.

How Do Clinicians Diagnose?

Observe how each person in the ward round (Box 1.1) employed a different method of clinical problem solving. The third-year student was guessing, and had little chance of arriving at the correct diagnosis, except by fluke. The final-year student was testing one hypothesis at a time until he could find one to match the available information (*hypothetical-deductive* reasoning). The resident was using an *algorithm*, which divided the causes of jaundice based on key predictors (e.g., pre-hepatic, hepatic and obstructive jaundice; painful and painless). The expert clinician effortlessly *recognised this pattern of symptoms*, and synthesised his intuition with analytical decision rules (painful vs. painless). Understanding the diagnostic thought process is fruitful for all who wish to learn clinical diagnosis.

Hypothetical-Deductive Reasoning

Hypothetical-deductive reasoning is about generating and evaluating differential diagnoses. Every medical consult is an iterative process of information gathering, data interpretation, hypothesis generation and testing. Hypotheses so generated prompt a search for additional information (further history, examination or investigation); in turn, addition information may confirm or refute existing hypotheses, or trigger the generation of new hypotheses.

(a) **Hypothesis generation**: Do not simply take a history and examine the patient. Think! Think of: (i) what are the most likely diagnoses, and (ii) what are the most dangerous/important diagnoses that must not be missed (even if they are less likely).

(b) **Evaluating differentials**: Critically examine the differentials generated (Table 1.1). For every hypothesis, ask: (i) what information fits? (ii) what does not fit? (iii) what did I expect but could not find? Then rank the diagnoses in order of likelihood. Next, ask: (iv) what additional information do I need to confirm or refute this

Table 1.1. Hypothetical-Deductive Reasoning in a 60-year-old Presenting with Shortness of Breath and Wheeze

Hypothesis	What information fits the hypothesis?	What does not fit?	What did I expect but not find?	What additional information do I need?
Asthma	Acute-onset wheeze	Unusual to have new-onset asthma at 60 years old	There is no precipitating trigger	Is there an atopic history?
COPD	Smoker	Should be chronic, not acute		Is the chest X-ray hyperinflated?
Heart failure	Pedal oedema can cause wheeze		He has no known heart disease	Are there q-waves on his ECG?

hypothesis? This prompts a search for additional information (whether further history, examination or investigation), which would further allow one to distinguish between the possible differentials.

How to use: The ability to critically examine a list of differentials, rank them according to likelihood, and pick up 'what does not fit' is very important. *Drawing this table for every patient seen is a useful exercise in clinical reasoning.* Additionally, having a list of differentials guides physical examination (you can only find what you look for) and investigations.

Caveats: Generating differentials based simply on 'what I can think of' is a potential source of error, as the correct diagnosis may never be considered. Conversely, going through every possible differential for a certain symptom is inefficient and impractical. Therefore, while the hypothetical-deductive model is a helpful tool to evaluate differentials and identify 'what does not fit', it is best to augment this approach with a method to consistently generate the most important differentials.

Algorithms

Algorithms employ differentiating pieces of information (history, physical signs or investigations) as key branch points to distinguish between groups of diagnoses. The clinical consult begins by identifying the appropriate algorithm to use. Thereafter, information gathering is guided by the algorithm (Figure 1.1), with particular emphasis on deciding between diagnostic groups as made explicit by the branch points. After several branching points, only a small number of possible differentials are left, and hypothetical-deductive reasoning may be used to rank the remaining options.

How to use: Algorithms systematically and rapidly identify likely differentials, helping to reduce cognitive load and the chance of not considering the correct diagnosis. They reflect an organised knowledge structure. This book is about helping you develop algorithms and organise your knowledge, so that you may be able to use algorithms in your diagnostic process.

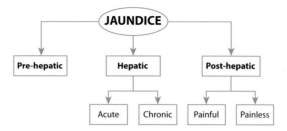

Figure 1.1. A simple algorithm for jaundice.
See Chapter 10 for complete algorithm.

Caveats: Algorithms are best used in conjunction with the critical lens of hypothetical-deductive reasoning. Algorithms identify the *most likely* diagnoses; the most dangerous diagnoses (that have to be excluded) may need to be considered separately via a hypothetical-deductive approach, even if deemed less likely by the algorithm.

Pattern Recognition

All of us can instantaneously recognise people we know, without conscious or effortful thought. In the same way, clinicians may instantly recognise a patient's diagnosis,[1] with little deliberate thought. This is an intuitive process involving matching the new patient's problem against similar ones solved previously. The ability to do so requires accumulation of 'illness scripts' (previous patients seen and mental prototypes) through clinical experience, as well as a well-organised knowledge structure so that correct matches can be retrieved rapidly based on salient cues.

How to use: To use pattern recognition, you must have accumulated a database of illness scripts through clinical experience, and organised your knowledge structure via deliberate reflection on patients seen. Furthermore, illness scripts are condition-specific (having seen thousands of fractures does not make one better able to diagnose chest pain) and context-specific (having seen 10 sick pneumonia inpatients does not help one diagnose and manage community-acquired pneumonia in a general practice setting). The accuracy of pattern recognition depends on the clinician's breadth and volume of condition-specific illness scripts; simply 'seeing many cases' is insufficient—these cases must encompass the variety of conditions encountered, and accurately represent the range of ways in which each condition presents. This is why developing pattern recognition takes time, and it is not something that can be taught in a book.

Caveats: Errors occur when the clinician is inexperienced, over-confident, distracted or fatigued. Patients who present atypically may be misdiagnosed, for example, acute coronary syndromes are more likely to be missed when the patient lacks chest pain.

---

[1] Referred to as 'pattern recognition', 'system one thinking' or 'non-analytical approach' in literature.

Combining Methods

There is good evidence that combining intuitive pattern-recognition with analytical strategies (algorithms and hypothetical-deductive reasoning) improves diagnostic outcomes. Most clinicians with some experience employ pattern recognition as a default, as it is faster and less effortful. But when faced with an atypical patient, or a novel clinical scenario, one is unfamiliar with, it is wise to abandon pattern recognition approaches in favour of conscious analytical thinking. Even when pattern recognition is used, safe diagnosis requires constant vigilance for information which 'does not fit', in which case analytical reasoning must take over.

The Process of Diagnostic Reasoning

Having understood the mental frameworks clinicians employ in making a diagnosis, this section delves further into the key elements of the diagnostic reasoning process: (i) information gathering, (ii) interpretation of the information to formulate a problem representation, (iii) making a diagnosis, (iv) searching for aetiologies and complications and (v) dealing with patients who have multiple issues.

(a) Information Gathering

Some students find that after an initial phase of allowing the patient to talk freely, they are not sure what questions to ask, or default to a memorised list of questions for each symptom. It is helpful to form an early impression of the patient's presenting complaint, and have some possible diagnoses in mind. Search for further information (history taking, examination and investigations) that would discriminate between the differentials. This is where an algorithm guides information gathering by specifying clinically important pieces of information that differentiate between diagnostic groups (i.e., the branch points). It is a useful maxim that *'the eye does not see what the mind does not think'*—clinically significant details often have to be explicitly solicited, or may be missed.

Information is interpreted as it is gathered; this is an iterative process culminating in the promotion of one differential as the 'most likely' and the relegation of others (Table 1.1).

(b) Problem Representation

Another early cognitive step is the creation of a one-sentence summary defining the case in specific terms. This may be explicitly articulated, or subconscious. Going back to our clinical scenario (Box 1.1), observes the consultant's problem representation—*an elderly gentleman with painless progressive obstructive jaundice and clinically significant weight loss.*

Notice how the third-year student's description of *'jaundice ... getting worse ... no abdominal pain'* has become *'painless progressive jaundice'*, and the final-year student's comment *'higher ALP than AST and ALT'* is now *'obstructive jaundice'*. These are abstract **semantic qualifiers**—painless, as opposed to painful; progressive, not time-limited. The consultant has interpreted the information gathered and recognised diagnostically significant details.

A sound problem representation using semantic qualifiers is associated with strong clinical reasoning. Conversely, failure to generate an accurate problem representation (whether explicit or subconscious) can lead to guessing possible diagnoses (as in the third-year student) based on isolated findings.

(c) Making a Diagnosis

The mechanics of making a diagnosis has been discussed in the previous section. Ideally, a combination of pattern-recognition and analytical methods should be used; for the novice clinician to whom pattern recognition is unavailable, analytical methods remain useful.

(d) Aetiologies and Complications

Don't stop at making a diagnosis. Many diseases have underlying aetiologies (although some are 'idiopathic'); keep asking *why, why,* and *why*—until no further *why* can be asked. Similarly, every diseases causes complications—search for them (Table 1.2).

Table 1.2. Asking 'Why' and 'So What' in Various Diseases

Scenario	'Why'—search for aetiology	'So what'—search for complications
40-year-old with acute cerebral infarct	*Why* does he have a stroke (e.g., cardioembolic, atherosclerosis) *Why* is getting a stroke this young?	Is there mass effect? Is he able to swallow?
21-year-old with an asthma exacerbation	*Why* did he get an exacerbation? (e.g., infection, allergen exposure)	Is he in respiratory failure?
70-year-old with iron deficiency anaemia	*Why* is there iron deficiency? (e.g., occult gastrointestinal bleeding)	Is he symptomatic?

(e) Patients with Multiple Issues

Patients can be complex. One disease leads to another, and multiple organ systems can be affected by ongoing disease processes. Add to that the potential for drug–disease and drug–drug interactions and things can get really confusing. Try to tease out cause–effect relationships and formulate a problem list to make sense of the madness.

For example, consider the scenario (Box 1.2).

Box 1.2. A Patient with Multiple Issues

A 75-year-old man suffers a fall while getting up from bed. He has been having diarrhoea and vomiting after eating some leftovers, and was given antibiotics by a general practitioner 2 days ago. When he got out of bed, he felt giddy and passed out momentarily. He recalls waking up on the floor, alert and in pain. Examination is normal except for marked postural hypotension and decreased skin turgor. ECG is normal. Initial blood tests show a creatinine level above his baseline, and an international normalised ratio (INR) of 5. A small subdural haemorrhage is seen on CT brain. He has a past medical history of diabetes, atrial fibrillation and heart failure, and is on metformin, bisoprolol, furosemide and warfarin.

A problem list might look as follows:

1. Subdural haemorrhage secondary to fall and over-anticoagulation.

2. Syncope secondary to postural hypotension.

3. Hypovolaemia due to gastroenteritis and diuretics, complicated by postural hypotension and acute kidney injury.

4. Over-anticoagulation? due to drug interaction (warfarin and antibiotic).

Formulating a problem list clarifies the issues on hand, and facilitates the creation of a management plan, which addresses all the problems.

Further Issues

Some other issues in diagnostic reasoning deserve brief mention—the use of diagnostic tests, diagnostic uncertainty and diagnostic error.

Using Diagnostic Tests

A few words about using diagnostic tests is in order. Unfortunately, the scenario in Box 1.3 is not uncommon. This young man has a very low clinical probability of prostate cancer, and prostate specific antigen (PSA) testing was inappropriate. The test is likely to be a false positive. Even with a positive test, he remains unlikely to have prostate cancer, but most clinicians (and patients) would consider themselves obliged to investigate further 'to rule out' cancer. On the other hand, in an 80-year-old gentleman with a hard nodular prostate, bony pain and weight loss, a raised PSA would only increase the clinician's confidence in a diagnosis of prostate cancer.

Box 1.3. The Fallacy of Prostate Specific Antigen Testing

A 25-year-old man seeks a consult for a mildly elevated prostate specific antigen (PSA). He is asymptomatic. It turns out that his company offers 'free' yearly health screening, and PSA was included in the standard package. He is anxious about the raised PSA level and upset because his application for a new health insurance policy had been denied on the basis of elevated PSA.

Diagnostic tests help refine a list of differential diagnoses (Table 1.1) by providing additional information to increase the probability of certain diagnoses while decreasing others. For example, amylase/lipase levels are useful in a patient complaining of epigastric pain radiating to the back; a positive test makes pancreatitis likely, but a negative test would prompt a search for alternative diagnoses. Diagnostic tests may also help to guide management (e.g., deciding if a transfusion is necessary), and identify aetiologies (e.g., if pancreatitis, are there gallstones?) and complications of disease. As a rule of thumb, *before ordering a diagnostic test, know what you are looking for*—be sure you know how to interpret the test, how it will help you with diagnosis, and how it will change your management of the patient.

Every diagnostic test performs differently; each has a certain false negative and false positive rate. For example, a negative CT scan does not rule out subarachnoid haemorrhage in a patient with high pre-test probability (false negative rate), and a moderately high troponin does not always imply myocardial infarction in a patient on chronic dialysis (false positive rate). As illustrated, interpretation of test results depends on the pre-test probability, and one should be familiar with the test characteristic before ordering it. Generally, a sensitive test (low false negative rate) helps to 'rule out' disease, while a specific test (low false positive rate) helps to 'rule in' disease. Some awareness of the issues in diagnostic testing is important, but a detailed discussion of probabilistic reasoning is beyond the scope of this text (but see 'GO FURTHER' at the end of this chapter).

Dealing with Diagnostic Uncertainty

Diagnostic uncertainty is a reality in clinical medicine. Information is limited and conflicting. Treatment decisions often have to be made before the results of clarifying investigations return. This unnerves many but every clinician must learn to be comfortable with diagnostic uncertainty. Some tools:

- Admit the uncertainty. Do not commit to one diagnosis and shut out all others, when this is not borne out by evidence. Rather, keep the differentials in mind.

- Look for a test that will increase the probability of one diagnosis and/or decrease the probability of another.

- When stakes are high and treatment has a favourable benefit/risk ratio, consider empirical treatment even if the diagnosis is uncertain. For example, patients with minor wounds often receive anti-tetanus toxoid even though the risk of tetanus is low, simply because the risk of treatment is smaller than the remote but catastrophic possibility of tetanus. Similarly, in acutely unwell patients with multiple competing differentials, consider treating both diagnoses in parallel if benefit/risk ratios are favourable. For example, in a patient presenting with fever, melena and hypotension; it will be prudent to treat for both septic shock and gastrointestinal bleeding.

- Reverse what is easily reversible. For example, if it is unclear whether a patient's weakness is due to hypoglycaemia or stroke, administer dextrose and re-examine in 10 min; if weakness persists then it is no longer due to hypoglycaemia. Similarly, if it is unclear whether a patient's breathlessness is due to pneumonia or progression of lung cancer, it is reasonable to treat pneumonia (even if the diagnosis is not 'definite'), as the latter would be difficult to treat.

- Remember that diagnosis is a dynamic process. The patient's response to ongoing treatment is usually very informative. Reassessment over an appropriate time period allows us to use time as a diagnostic tool; be prepared to re-consider the initial diagnosis if the patient fails to respond to treatment for the assumed diagnosis.

- Finally, realise that in some situations, it is not necessary to know the exact diagnosis. These situations include when the treatment for both differentials is identical, when the risk of diagnostic testing outweighs the benefit of information gained (e.g., subjecting patients with multiple comorbids to invasive investigations), or when there is no intention to initiate treatment even if a diagnosis is made (e.g., due to quality of life).

Diagnostic Error

Every clinician commits diagnostic errors. Wise clinicians learn from their errors, and learn the pitfalls so that errors are minimised. There are three sources of diagnostic error: (i) knowledge deficits, (ii) attitude problems such as overconfidence and (iii) cognitive bias. Apart from a good dose of humility and diligent work to improve knowledge, being aware of cognitive biases (Table 1.3) helps one to avoid them.

How to Use This Book

This book suggests sample diagnostic algorithms for several common presentations of disease. I hope that learning from these algorithms will help you to become a better diagnostician, and ultimately help patients. For maximal benefit, some advice is in order.

Five Things This Book Is NOT

1. This is NOT a guide to history taking and clinical examination. Basic history taking and examination skills are prerequisites before higher-order thought processes can be learnt.

2. This is NOT a replacement for standard clinical textbooks. The focus is on differential diagnosis, not on the presentation, diagnosis and management of individual disease entities. Familiarity with individual diseases will help greatly in differential diagnosis—an algorithm makes little sense if the diseases it leads to are completely alien to you.

3. This is NOT a protocol to rote-learn and follow rigidly, *in lieu* of the fullness of clinical reasoning. Algorithms are but one tool in the diagnostic toolbox, and must be used in conjunction with the other tools discussed in this chapter.

4. This is NOT a substitute for seeing real patients. That would be a tragedy. Students with extensive textbook knowledge but inadequate patient contact often find

Table 1.3. Common Cognitive Biases

Example		Cognitive bias	Mechanism of bias
1.	A patient is admitted from the emergency department for 'pneumonia'. Although he has no fever, the inpatient team continues to treat 'pneumonia'. Two days later, he is intubated for respiratory failure. A repeat chest X-ray shows worsening fluid overload.	Diagnostic momentum	Accepting a previous diagnosis without sufficient scepticism.
2.	A patient with diabetes and ischaemic heart disease presents with acute crushing chest pain. He is given loading doses of aspirin and Ticagrelor, while awaiting troponin results. One hour later, he collapses and a post-mortem finds aortic dissection.	Anchoring	Locking onto a diagnosis too early, based on initial information.
		Premature closure	Accepting the first diagnosis without considering whether there is a better answer.
		Under-adjustment	Failure to revise the diagnosis when new information becomes available.
3.	A young lady presents with symmetrical small joint polyarthritis and morning stiffness lasting 2 hr. Her general practitioner declines to refer her to a rheumatologist because her rheumatoid factor was normal.	Blind obedience	Undue deference to a false-negative diagnostic test (or other authority).
4.	After missing a pulmonary embolism, a physician orders CT pulmonary angiography for the next five patients with breathlessness.	Availability bias	Diagnosis influenced by ease of recollection of possible diagnoses.
5.	A 'frequent flyer' with borderline personality disorder, who is known to waste emergency department resources, presents with hip pain and difficulty walking. She is sent home with analgesia, with no X-ray done. She is later found to have a hip fracture.	Framing effect	Decision making unduly biased by the way it is presented.
		Affective bias	Personal emotions affecting judgement.

themselves unable to apply their knowledge to a clinical situation. Rather, seeing patients goes hand-in-hand with learning knowledge and knowledge structure—remember, patients are a clinician's best teachers.

5. This is NOT comprehensive or absolute. My goal is simply to help beginner diagnosticians develop a functional diagnostic framework. Therefore, I focus on common presentations of common conditions, downplaying rare diseases and uncommon exceptions to general rules. This book's *algorithms are generally written for adult patients*, and will lead to error if applied in paediatric contexts without modification.

Five Learning Aids to Help You

Apart from an algorithm to every symptom, and a discussion of the content of the algorithm, this book includes several elements to aid learning:

1. **Clinical case and case discussion**: Every chapter opens with a clinical vignette, and closes by applying the content of the chapter onto the clinical case. You are encouraged to pen down how you would approach the clinical vignette before reading the discussion.

2. **End-chapter summaries** of key learning points.

3. **Common pitfalls** highlighted at the end of each chapter.

4. **Illustrative ECGs and radiographs** are included in some chapters. For the sake of brevity, only a limited number of images can be included—looking up more examples can be helpful.

5. **Discussion questions** in several flavours are found at the end of each chapter.

    (a) REFLECT! questions encourage reflection on clinical cases previously encountered, so as to reinforce 'illness scripts' and encourage reflective practice.

    (b) EXPLORE! questions prompt reading up on topics related to the chapter, or prompt reinforcement and application of concepts discussed.

    (c) DISCUSS! questions should be discussed in small groups. They include differing opinions up for debate, as well as mini-exercises to synthesise and apply content learnt in the chapter.

    (d) GO FURTHER! questions suggest slightly more advanced concepts interested learners might wish to explore.

Five Ways to Use This Book

1. **As a primer**. Before beginning a new clinical rotation, flip quickly through relevant chapters. Use the approach discussed as a roadmap to read up on what you are unfamiliar with. Try to hit the ground running and learn as much as possible from the first patient you see.

2. **As a just-in-time aid**. Bring this book to the bedside. If you ever get 'stuck' while clerking a patient, whip out the relevant chapter and see if it can give you some ideas.

3. **Self-practice**. Read the clinical case at the beginning of each chapter. Jot down how you will approach the patient. Then read the chapter; as you read, continually edit your draft approach.

4. **Deliberate practice with patients**. Clerk patients (without referring to this book or the case notes); list and rank the top differentials. Next, refer to the relevant book chapter, and see if there is anything else it might prompt you to consider (other differentials to consider, important differentiating questions you did not ask, etc.). Go back to the patient and refine your differential list. Finally, open the case notes and investigations, and check if your diagnosis is similar to that of the expert clinician's (if it differs, ask why—the expert is not always right). *Repeated deliberate practice is essential in learning clinical diagnosis*.

5. **Critical reflection**. Examine the algorithms critically. Identify the key differentiators used (usually at branch points), and ask:

   (i) What is the pathophysiologic basis of these key differentiators? Understanding the pathophysiologic mechanisms for the presentation of diseases aids understanding.

   (ii) To what extent are they reliable? It is helpful to understand what are 'hard signs' with high specificity (e.g., upgoing plantars makes an upper motor neuron lesion *very* likely) and what are 'soft signs' with low specificity (e.g., a positive antinuclear antibody does not always mean that a patient has autoimmune disease).

 Using what you have learnt, **pen down your approach** to the Clinical Case at the start of the chapter **BEFORE reading the discussion** below.

Case Discussion

This student is not alone in having good content knowledge but struggling with clinical reasoning and the diagnostic process. Very often the root of the problem lies in (i) poor study habits—rote learning without processing to improve knowledge structure, and (ii) inadequate patient contact. She should immediately:

1. Put down the textbook and hit the wards. Try to clerk as many typical patients as possible, and for every patient, list three top differentials and complete Table 1.1.

2. Use algorithms to jump-start her journey in clinical reasoning. This book can help but it is not another textbook to be learnt by rote; rather, it is a teach-book to be used alongside seeing patients (page 13).

Key Lessons	1. Diagnosis requires content knowledge and knowledge structure. Combining analytical reasoning (via hypothetical-deductive methods and algorithms) with intuitive pattern-recognition increases the chance of diagnostic success.
	2. An appropriate search for underlying aetiologies, appropriate use of diagnostic tests, and problem list formulation can assist in diagnostic reasoning.
	3. Hard work, humility and an awareness of cognitive biases are helpful in minimising diagnostic error.
Common Pitfalls	1. Trying to memorise this book is not going to work.
	2. Trying to learn medicine without seeing patients is doomed to failure.
Questions	1. **REFLECT!** Recall one diagnostic error that you have made (or witnessed someone make). What were the factors that led to the error? What could have been done differently to prevent the error from being made?
	2. **EXPLORE!** What is the difference between surface learning and deep learning? When might one favour either approach?

3. **DISCUSS!** The explosion of medical knowledge in the past 10–20 years has made it difficult for any clinician (must less a beginner) to keep up. What are some strategies to cope with this volume of information and pace of progress?

4. **GO FURTHER!** Read up on Bayesian conditional probability. How does the pre-test probability influence interpretation of a given diagnostic test?

Heart and Lungs

Chapter

2

An Approach to Hypotension

Clinical Case

You are called to review a 64-year-old gentleman on the Renal ward for a blood pressure of 75/43. He has a history of end-stage renal failure on haemodialysis, diabetes, hypertension, ischaemic heart disease, atrial fibrillation and peripheral vascular disease with a left below-knee amputation. He was admitted 4 days ago for a thrombosed arteriovenous fistula. As thrombectomy of the fistula was unsuccessful, a tunnelled temporary dialysis catheter ('Permcath') was inserted in his right internal jugular vein 3 days ago. He is due for discharge tomorrow. How will you approach his hypotension?

Hypotension is a medical emergency. It indicates that the patient is severely ill, with a disease process causing physiologic compromise exceeding the body's compensatory mechanisms. Pathophysiologically, hypotension reflects a failure in preload (cannot fill left ventricle due to volume loss, inflow obstruction or excessive heart rate), contractility (heart muscle dysfunction or outflow obstruction) or afterload (decrease in systemic vascular resistance due to peripheral vasodilation).

In addition to hypotension, look out for tachycardia, oliguria, abnormal mental status and clammy peripheries, which are likewise indicators of shock—a state of tissue hypoperfusion that leads to organ dysfunction. High lactate indicates anaerobic metabolism due to insufficient tissue perfusion; in sepsis, levels above 4 mmol/L, even with normal blood pressure, has been shown to have a mortality rate comparable to overt septic shock.

The causes of hypotension can be classified as hypovolaemic, cardiogenic, obstructive and distributive (Table 2.1).

Initial Approach

Obtain a rapid clinical impression from history, examination and bedside investigations (including ECG and arterial blood gases). Focus initially on common causes of shock, and any cause that the patient may be particularly predisposed to. The temperature of the peripheries is a helpful differentiator—Warm peripheries indicate vasodilation, as mediated by bacterial endotoxin (septic shock), histamine (anaphylaxis) or loss of sympathetic tone (neurogenic shock and Addisonian crisis). Conversely, clammy peripheries indicate vasoconstriction, which is an appropriate response to hypovolaemic, cardiogenic and obstructive shock. Figure 2.1 provides an initial approach.

Table 2.1. Causes of Shock

	Hypovolaemic	Cardiogenic	Obstructive	Distributive
Aetiology	Haemorrhage—obvious or occult Dehydration Polyuria or over-diuresis	Acute myocardial infarct Arrhythmias Mechanical dysfunction e.g., acute valve rupture	Massive PE Tension pneumothorax Cardiac tamponade	Septic shock (common) Anaphylaxis Addisonian crisis Neurogenic shock Myxoedema crisis
Clinical history	Bleeding Abdominal pain Diarrhoea, vomiting	Chest pain Diaphoresis Dyspnoea Palpitations	Respiratory distress, pleuritic chest pain Unilateral swollen leg	Fever Angioedema, wheeze, new medication taken
Peripheries	Cold	Cold	Cold	Warm
Fluid status	Under-filled	Over-filled (usually) Under-filled (very acute)	Over-filled (tamponade) Euvolaemic (PE, pneumothorax)	Under-filled or euvolaemic
Other exam findings	Pallor Per-rectal bleeding Abdominal tenderness in occult bleeding	Arrhythmia Displaced apex beat Murmur	Calf swelling (PE) Hyper-resonant lung (pneumothorax) Beck's triad (tamponade)	Localising source of sepsis Angioedema, stridor (anaphylaxis)
Investigations	Haemoglobin + GXM Urine pregnancy test Consider abdominal imaging	ECG, cardiac enzymes Chest X-ray Consider echo	ECG Bedside echo CT pulmonary angiogram	Septic workup, lactate

GXM, group and cross-match; PE, pulmonary embolism.

Institute emergent management based on the bedside clinical impression; do not wait for blood tests to return. Return to review the patient, reviewing if the patient has responded to initial therapy, and if blood results support the initial diagnosis. Failure to respond to initial treatment should prompt reconsideration of the initial diagnosis, and escalation of initial treatment (e.g., more fluids and starting inotropes). Adjuncts to bedside clinical diagnosis, in particular bedside ultrasound scanning, can be helpful. Bear in mind that there may be multiple concurrent causes of shock, for example, sepsis precipitating an acute myocardial infarction.

The subsequent sections discuss individual classes of shock in greater detail.

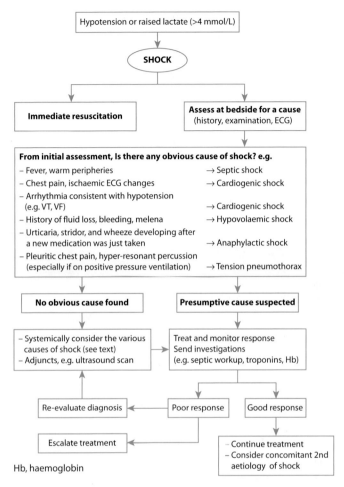

Figure 2.1. Initial clinical approach to hypotension.

Hypovolaemic Shock

In hypovolaemic states, examination reveals under-filled peripheries (decreased skin turgor, dry mucous membranes, flat jugular venous pressure (JVP) and clear lungs). Hypovolaemia can arise from:

Workup

- **Fluid loss**: There may be a clinical history of gastrointestinal losses (diarrhoea and vomiting), renal losses (polyuria e.g., in recovery phase of acute tubular necrosis, or hyperglycaemic emergencies). Victims of heat stroke and burns are also hypovolaemic.

- **Haemorrhagic shock**: This is easily suspected in the trauma victim, and if there is an obvious gastrointestinal bleed (e.g., haematemesis and melena).

  - Full blood count (FBC): A drop in haemoglobin is suggestive, but it may remain normal in acute blood loss

- **Occult haemorrhage**: This requires a high index of suspicion. Be alert to any complaint of abdominal pain in a hypotensive patient which may suggest a ruptured aortic aneurysm (examine for pulsatile mass and a rigid abdomen), a ruptured ectopic pregnancy (look for vaginal bleeding, examine for cervical motion tenderness), or a ruptured hepatocellular carcinoma. Do a digital rectal examination for melena.

  - Bedside ultrasound
  - CT abdomen/pelvis (if stable enough to be transported)
  - Urine pregnancy test

Cardiogenic Shock

The ECG is a critical bedside diagnostic tool.

Workup

- **Acute coronary syndromes**: This diagnosis is easy in the classic presentation of chest pain, dyspnoea and diaphoresis. However, many patients, especially those with diabetic neuropathy, present atypically. ECG reveals acute S-T changes (see Chapter 3).

  - Cardiac enzymes
  - Echocardiography

- **Unstable arrhythmias**: Certain tachycardias (ventricular tachycardia and fast atrial fibrillation) and bradycardias (high-grade atrioventricular blocks, i.e., type 2 second degree and third degree blocks) can cause hypotension (Chapter 5). Hypotension is less common with other arrhythmias (e.g., ectopic beats and low-grade atrioventricular blocks) and another cause should be sought.

  - Cardiac enzymes
  - Electrolytes

- **Poor cardiac contractility**: In decompensated heart failure and in severe metabolic disturbances (e.g., hyperkalaemia, acidosis and hypothermia).

  - Electrolytes
  - Echocardiogram

- **Structural catastrophe**: Acute valve rupture, ventricular septum or free wall rupture post myocardial infarction.

  - Echocardiogram

Distributive Shock

In distributive shock, cardiac output is normal but peripheral vasodilation and decreased systemic vascular resistance results in hypotension.

	Workup
• **Septic shock**: Immunocompetent patients may present with fever and localising symptoms. Immunocompromised hosts (e.g., neutropenia, immunosuppressed and HIV/AIDS), on the other hand, may not mount a febrile response. Sepsis should be considered in all immunocompromised patients regardless of fever. Look carefully for a source (see Chapter 35).	− Septic workup (inflammatory markers, blood cultures and look for a source, e.g., chest X-ray [CXR], urine formed element microscopy [UFEME] and urine cultures) − Lactate
• **Anaphylactic shock**: A clinical picture of rash, facial angioedema, flushing and stridor developing soon after a precipitant, such as a medication error or new drug.	− Mast cell tryptase (as a confirmatory test where diagnosis is unclear)
• **Neurogenic shock**: High spinal cord injury (usually above T6) compromises sympathetic outflow to the heart and peripheries. This should be apparent from the clinical history e.g., trauma.	− If suspected, treat with IV steroids. − Confirmatory testing (e.g., Synacthen test) inappropriate in hypotension.
• **Addisonian crisis**: Difficult to diagnose unless suspected. Consider especially in patients on chronic steroids (or traditional medicine with steroids) whose steroids are abruptly withdrawn, or who are suffering an intercurrent illness without receiving stress doses of steroids.	
• **Myxoedema coma**: Severe hypothyroidism may present with hypotension. Findings may include hypothermia, bradycardia (in spite of hypotension) and signs of chronic hypothyroid disease including coarse skin, facial oedema, eyelid oedema and thick tongue.	− Thyroid function tests

Obstructive Shock

	Workup
• **Massive pulmonary embolism**: This patient would be hypoxic and in respiratory distress. There may be evidence of deep vein thrombosis (DVT) (swollen and tender calf) and risk factors for DVT/PE (e.g., prolonged immobility, recent surgery and active malignancy). ECG may reveal an $S_1Q_3T_3$ pattern (most pathognomonic; Figure 3.2(f)), sinus tachycardia (most common) or T	− CT pulmonary angiogram (Figure 2.2)

inversions and signs of right heart strain (e.g., right bundle branch block).

- **Tension pneumothorax**: A patient with pleuritic chest pain, dyspnoea and hypoxia. Examination will reveal tracheal shift, unilateral absence of breath sounds and hyper-resonance to percussion. Mechanical ventilation of a tension pneumothorax rapidly worsens shock.

  − This should be a clinical diagnosis and not a CXR diagnosis

- **Cardiac tamponade**: Classically, Beck's triad describes a patient with distended jugular veins, muffled heart sounds and hypotension—but all three criteria are rarely fulfilled in practice. There may be a background of malignancy (lung or breast), myocarditis, recent myocardial infarction, autoimmune disease (e.g., lupus or rheumatoid arthritis) or uraemia. ECG may show small voltage complexes and electrical alternans.

  − Bedside echocardiogram

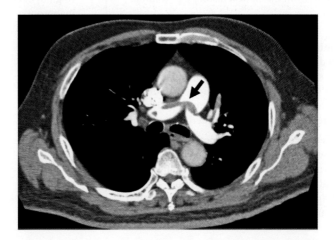

Figure 2.2. Pulmonary embolism—A premorbidly well 45-year-old gentleman presented with acute hypotension, chest pain and dyspnoea. There was no suggestion of infection or bleeding. ECG showed sinus tachycardia, CXR was normal and troponins were negative. A CT pulmonary angiogram revealed a large saddle embolus (arrow). He collapsed soon after this CT was taken and could not be resuscitated.

 Using what you have learnt, **pen down your approach** to the Clinical Case at the start of the chapter **BEFORE reading the discussion** below.

Case Discussion

This patient is at risk for multiple types of shock. With a central vascular catheter, he is predisposed to central-line associated sepsis. He is a vasculopath and at high risk of acute myocardial infarction. He may be hypovolaemic due to over-ultrafiltration during dialysis, and may have bled from procedural complications of dialysis catheter insertion.

First assess airway, breathing and circulation. Learn to recognise the toxic patient whose collapse is imminent—an obtunded patient with agonal breathing is clearly sicker than a conversant patient with the same blood pressure. Resuscitation proceeds simultaneously alongside diagnosis.

Review the vitals chart. History and examination should first target the most likely differentials. Ask for symptoms of myocardial ischaemia (e.g., chest pain), of sepsis (e.g., fever, dyspnoea and intradialytic rigours), bleeding and so on. Feel the peripheries (warm suggests sepsis), examine for sources of sepsis (e.g., pus coming from indwelling lines, lung crepitations, etc.), and look for bleeding from the procedural site. An ECG may reveal ischaemic changes or new arrhythmias (his known atrial fibrillation is unlikely to cause hypotension). Review if he has been given any new medication that could cause hypotension. Initial investigations, at a minimum, should include haemoglobin, inflammatory markers, blood cultures, cardiac enzymes, electrolytes and lactate (look for metabolic acidosis). Identify a likely diagnosis. If there are two competing diagnoses, it may be necessary to pursue both simultaneously (e.g., start antibiotics while awaiting troponin results).

Fluids are helpful in most types of shock but exercise caution with fluids in proven left ventricular infarction, aortic dissection (allow permissive hypotension), and where fluids would delay emergent treatment (i.e., giving adrenaline in anaphylaxis, decompressing a tension pneumothorax and cardioverting an unstable arrhythmia). Fluids should not be withheld from this patient just because he is on dialysis—hypotension kills before fluid overload does—and should be given unless he is already overtly fluid overloaded. Proceed with empiric treatment of the likely cause of shock, but re-evaluate the response to treatment frequently, and refine the working diagnosis as additional information becomes available.

Key Lessons	1. Faced with a hypotensive patient, think through the four main classes of shock: Hypovolaemic, cardiogenic, distributive and obstructive.
	2. Warm peripheries indicate vasodilation and hence distributive shock; cold peripheries suggest the other types of shock.
	3. Resuscitation proceeds alongside diagnosis. Begin empiric treatment with frequent review to assess for response.
Common Pitfalls	1. Occult bleeding is easy to miss. Be alert for any abdominal pain or tenderness in a hypotensive patient.
	2. Do not fixate on a working diagnosis—be ready to re-evaluate the diagnosis if the patient fails to respond to empiric treatment, and as new information becomes available.

3. There can be multiple causes of shock; all need to be treated simultaneously.

Questions

1. **REFLECT!** Obstructive shock can be difficult to recognise. Have you ever encountered a patient with obstructive shock? What was the initial impression, and what clues made you/your team suspect the diagnosis?

2. **DISCUSS!** 'The management of shock depends little on its aetiology'. To what extent do you agree?

3. **EXPLORE!** Look up the *Surviving Sepsis* guidelines (www.survivingsepsis.org). This provides a helpful overview of the approach to sepsis. Can you understand the rationale behind the recommendations given?

4. **GO FURTHER!** Bedside ultrasound can be extremely valuable in shock. How does ultrasound distinguish between the causes of shock, and assist in immediate management?

Chapter 3

An Approach to Chest Pain

Clinical Case

A 55-year-old Indian gentleman presents with sudden-onset chest pain and diaphoresis. His past medical history includes hypertension, obesity and heavy smoking. He has had intermittent episodes of chest tightness in the last few years, which was attributed to gastrointestinal reflux disease, but they had been getting worse of late.

On arrival at hospital 15 min later, his pain has improved markedly. His vital signs are: BP 170/94, HR 98, SpO2 98% on room air. ECG is as shown. How would you approach his chest pain?

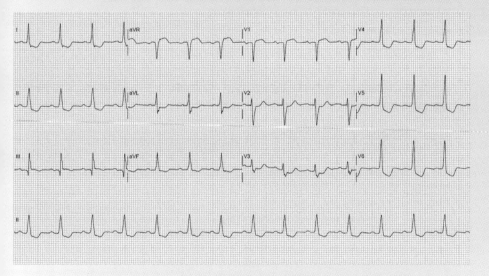

Patients with chest pain can be very sick. Learn to triage rapidly—the patient winced up in pain, panting in distress, and whose clothes are soaked with sweat is rather likely to have an acute myocardial infarction, and should be tended to immediately. At the same time, chest pain is a staple among the worried well—not all of whom require the customary two or three sets of cardiac enzymes. The causes of chest pain can be classified by organ system and presentation (Table 3.1).

Table 3.1. Major Causes of Chest Pain

Presentation		Cardiac	Respiratory	Gastrointestinal	Other
Acute	Potential emergencies	AMI, unstable angina Aortic dissection Cardiac tamponade	Pneumo-thorax PE	Oesophageal rupture	
	Require acute treatment	Myocarditis Pericarditis	Pneumonia	Cholecystitis Pancreatitis	Rib fracture Herpes zoster
Subacute or episodic	Serious	Angina AS HOCM			
	Other causes			GERD Oesophageal spasm Referred pain	Musculoskeletal Anxiety

AMI, acute myocardial infarction; AS, aortic stenosis; GERD, gastroesophageal reflux disease; HOCM, hypertrophic cardiomyopathy; PE, pulmonary embolism.

The approach to chest pain rests on a well-taken history and examination. The 'Socrates' questions (*s*ite, *o*nset, *c*haracter, *r*adiation, *a*ssociated symptoms, *t*ime course, *e*xacerbating and relieving factors, *s*everity) seem to have been written for chest pain—and work well here (Table 3.2).

Syndromes of Cardiac Ischaemia

The presentation and causes of cardiac ischaemia are worth further discussion. Ischaemic chest pain is classically a crushing, poorly localised retrosternal pain radiating to either arm or jaw, associated with diaphoresis and dyspnoea. Some patients (especially the elderly) may describe their symptoms as discomfort or tightness rather than pain, or may not have much chest pain at all. Not every ischaemic pain is equal—it may represent myocardial ischaemia or infarction, that is, cell death (Table 3.3).

Differentiating the Syndromes of Cardiac Ischaemia

History differentiates stable angina—of 'usual' quality and duration—from the acute coronary syndromes (i.e., unstable angina, non-ST-elevation myocardial infarction [NSTEMI] or ST-elevation myocardial infarction [STEMI]), which is anything new or more severe than before. ECG identifies a STEMI, and may show ischaemic changes in the other syndromes of cardiac ischaemia. Unstable angina vs. NSTEMI cannot be differentiated on history and ECG alone, and must wait for cardiac enzymes; troponins are elevated in NSTEMI, representing cell death.

Table 3.2. Differentiating the Causes of Chest Pain: The 'Socrates' Questions

	Ischaemic	Dissection	Respiratory	GERD	MSK
Onset and time course	Acute (AMI) Episodic (angina)	Acute, maximal pain at onset	Acute	Episodic	Variable
Character	Diffuse crushing	Tearing, migratory	Pleuritic	Burning	Localised
Radiation	Either arm, jaw	Interscapular	Lateral, back	Epigastrium	Nil
Associated symptoms	Diaphoresis Dyspnoea	Stroke, syncope Migratory pain	Dyspnoea	Reflux Heartburn	—
Exacerbating factors	Exertion		Inspiration	Meals, lying down	Coughing Palpation
Relieving factors	Nitrates	Time (pain max at onset)		Antacids	
Past medical history	Vascular risk factor	Hypertension Connective tissue disease	Young and thin COPD DVT risk factors	—	—

AMI, acute myocardial infarction; COPD, chronic obstructive pulmonary disease; DVT, deep vein thrombosis; GERD, gastrointestinal reflux disease; MSK, musculoskeletal.

Table 3.3. Syndromes of Ischaemic Chest Pain

	Pathophysiology	History	ECG	Troponins
Angina	Stable coronary occlusion	Episodic exertional chest pain, lasting 3–5 min, completely relieved by rest or nitrates		Normal
Unstable angina	Worsening coronary occlusion	New onset angina, worsening angina (increasing severity, frequency, duration of symptoms or triggered by less exertion) and angina at rest	ST depression or normal (if pain had resolved)	Normal
NSTEMI	Myocyte death			**Elevated**
STEMI	Myocyte death	Acute episode, more severe than usual angina, lasting > 30 min	**ST-elevation** with reciprocal changes	Elevated

NSTEMI, non ST-elevation myocardial infarction; STEMI, ST-elevation myocardial infarction.

Initial Approach

Resuscitate the patient—there may be hypotension (cardiogenic or obstructive shock), or hypoxia (pulmonary oedema from myocardial infarction, tension pneumothorax, massive pulmonary embolism). The immediate priority is to consider the life threatening causes of chest pain (Figure 3.1).

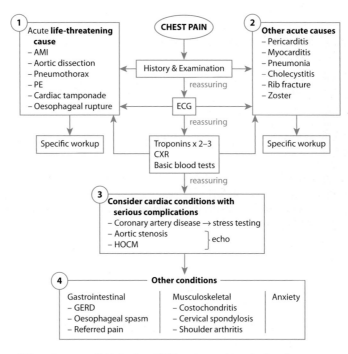

AMI, acute myocardial infarction; GERD, gastroesophageal reflux disease; HOCM, hypertrophic cardiomyopathy; PE, pulmonary embolism.

Figure 3.1. Approach to chest pain.

History and Examination

- **Acute coronary syndrome**: Crushing retrosternal pain radiating to arm or jaw, associated with diaphoresis and dyspnoea (syndromes of cardiac ischaemia, page 28). Cardiac and respiratory auscultation may be entirely normal.

- **Aortic dissection**: A sharp tearing pain radiating to the back between the scapulae. Onset is sudden, pain is maximal at onset and improves with time. If dissection involves the carotid artery origin, there may be neurological symptoms (stroke, transient ischaemic attack, syncope); if dissection involves the subclavian artery origin, there may be unequal blood pressure and pulses between the limbs (manifesting as radial–radial and radial–femoral delay on clinical examination). Retrograde spread of dissection causes aortic regurgitation (an early diastolic murmur) or myocardial infarction, and forward spread causes pain to migrate from chest to abdomen to legs.

- **Pneumothorax**: Acute-onset pleuritic (worse on breathing in/out) chest pain ± dyspnoea ± desaturation, with decreased chest expansion, hyper-resonance and decreased air entry on the affected side. A one-way valve may result in intra-thoracic pressure building up, obstructing venous return and causing hypotension— this is a tension pneumothorax, which manifests with hypotension, mediastinal shift and tracheal deviation, in addition to the signs of a simple pneumothorax. Pneumothorax may be primary (e.g., in tall young men), or secondary (e.g., in patients with chronic obstructive pulmonary disease, on positive pressure ventilation, or post-thoracic procedures).

- **Pulmonary embolism**: Classically pleuritic chest pain, dyspnoea and hypoxia with a normal lung examination; if massive, there may be hypotension. Presentations are often subtle with unexplained hypoxia, tachycardia and tachypnoea; absence of hypoxia makes pulmonary embolism less likely. Look for unilateral leg swelling (deep vein thrombosis) and risk factors (e.g., immobility, malignancy, pregnancy— see Chapter 47).

- **Cardiac tamponade**: Chest pain and dyspnoea, associated with hypotension, elevated jugular venous pressure, pulsus paradoxus (large fall in systolic blood pressure [> 10 mmHg] on inspiration) and muffled heart sounds. There may be a history of cancer, uraemia, autoimmune disease (e.g., lupus) or trauma.

- **Oesophageal rupture**: Chest pain following violent vomiting or oesophageal instrumentation.

Bedside ECG

This is immediately available and should be performed stat. It is always helpful to have old ECGs for comparison. Look for

- **ST-elevation**: ST-elevation with reciprocal depressions defines a STEMI (Figures 3.2a–b). Localise the infarct: ST-elevation in V1-3 in anterior STEMI (left anterior descending artery), V4-6 in lateral STEMI (left circumflex artery), II, III and aVF in inferior STEMI (right coronary artery). In inferior STEMI, do right-sided leads for right ventricular infarction (important to identify, as it carries implications for management).

- **ST-depression**: It implies coronary ischaemia, which may be angina, unstable angina or NSTEMI. Look out for widespread ST depressions with ST-elevation in aVR—this is a high-risk feature suggesting left main coronary artery or proximal left anterior descending artery disease, and is considered a STEMI-equivalent (see the ECG in Section 'Clinical Case').

- **T-wave changes**: T-wave inversions (Figure 3.2d) may be a sign of cardiac ischaemia, but are less specific than ST-elevations or depressions; they can also be seen in normal individuals, left ventricular hypertrophy, pulmonary embolism and other conditions. Repeat the ECG and compare against old ones—T-wave changes that are *new* (not present on old ECGs) or *dynamic* (changes with repeat ECGs) are more worrisome. Certain T-wave features are particularly high-risk: deeply inverted or biphasic T-waves in V2-3 (Wellens' syndrome), T-wave inversion in aVL (may precede development of ST-elevations in inferior leads) and hyperacute T-waves (very straight ST upslope rather than a curve).

- **Left bundle branch block**: Widened QRS (> 120ms) with dominant S in V1 and 'M' shaped QRS complex in V6[1] (Figure 3.2e). Chest pain plus left bundle branch block (LBBB; especially if new) is suspicious of myocardial infarction (MI). Look for old ECGs—in an old LBBB, interpreting ST changes can be tricky.[2]

- **Pulmonary embolism**: An $S_1Q_3T_3$ pattern (Figure 3.2f) is pathognomonic but rare; more commonly, the ECG shows sinus tachycardia, T inversion or evidence of right heart strain (e.g., right bundle branch block, P pulmonale).

- **Cardiac tamponade**: Low voltage QRS complexes.

- A normal ECG does not rule out myocardial infarction. Repeat ECGs for dynamic changes.

Figure 3.2. The ECG in chest pain.

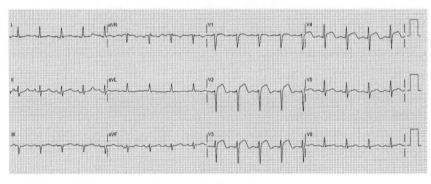

(a) **Anterior STEMI**: A 60-year-old gentleman presents with crushing chest pain and diaphoresis. ECG shows ST-elevations in V2-4. These ST-elevations are concave downwards ('sad face'), as compared to the concave upwards ('smiley face') ST-elevations in normal early re-polarisation. Coronary angiography revealed 99% stenosis in the left anterior descending artery.

(Cont'd)

---

[1] A helpful mnemonic: Wi**LL**iaM (in left bundle branch block, there is 'W' in V1 and 'M' in V6) vs. Ma**RR**oW (in right bundle branch block, there is 'M' in V1 and 'W' in V6).

[2] Consider the Sgarbossa criteria (beyond the scope of this text).

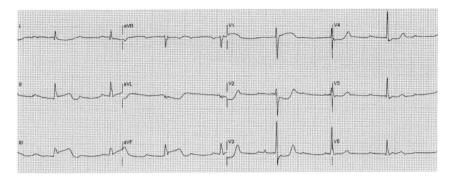

(b) **Inferior STEMI**: A 48-year-old gentleman presents with chest pain and dyspnoea. ECG shows ST-elevations in lead II, III and aVF, with reciprocal ST depressions in I and aVL. Deep ST depressions in V1-3 suggest concomitant posterior infarction. This patient should receive a right-sided ECG (for right ventricular infarction) and close monitoring for arrhythmias (an inferior STEMI may involve the sinoatrial and atrioventricular nodes). Coronary angiography revealed 100% stenosis in the right coronary artery.

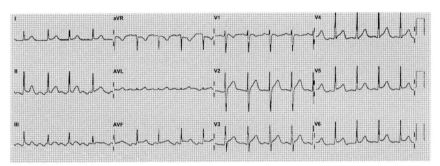

(c) **Pericarditis**: A 21-year-old infantry trooper presents with chest pain. His ECG shows widespread ST-elevations (lead II > III) and PR depression (best seen in inferior leads). Contrast this with the STEMI ECGs in (a) and (b). He recovered well with anti-inflammatory medication.

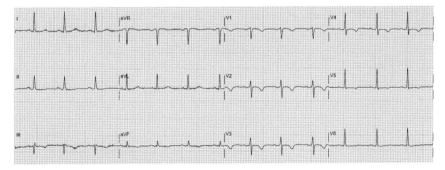

(d) **T-inversions**: A 70-year-old lady with a past medical history of diabetes presents with a 12-hr history of vague chest 'tightness'. ECG reveals T-inversions in V2-4 (the T-wave in V1 can normally be inverted) and q-waves in lead III. These changes were not present on old ECGs. Her troponin returned grossly elevated and coronary angiogram revealed 95% occlusion of the left anterior descending artery.

(Cont'd)

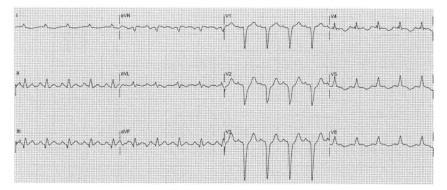

(e) **Left bundle branch block (LBBB)**: A 60-year-old gentleman presents with sudden-onset diaphoresis, but no chest pain. He is known to have diabetes, and had defaulted all medications. ECG shows a new LBBB (widened QRS, 'M-shape' notched QRS in V5-6, and 'W-shape' slurring in V1-2). Soon after this ECG was taken, he developed ventricular fibrillation and could not be resuscitated. Troponin subsequently came back grossly elevated. Because of diabetic neuropathy, he was pain-free despite having a myocardial infarction.

(f) **Pulmonary embolism**: A young lady with a history of multiple miscarriages presents with chest pain and dyspnoea after a long flight. ECG reveals $S_1Q_3T_3$ and a right bundle branch block. CT pulmonary angiogram confirmed pulmonary embolism. She was later found to have anti-phospholipid syndrome and received lifelong anticoagulation.

(g) **Underlying ischaemic heart disease**: This 50-year-old lady gave a history of stable angina. Serial ECGs showed no dynamic changes, and troponins were normal. However, her ECG shows q-waves in lead III, indicating an old inferior myocardial infarction, as well as small lateral R-waves in lateral leads (V4-6) with poor R-wave progression (these R-waves should be positive, rather than negative), suggesting loss of myocardium in the lateral wall of the left ventricle. She was eventually found to have triple vessel disease.

1. Acute life threatening causes: Subsequent investigations

Subsequent workup in the acute setting involves

- **Cardiac enzymes**: Do two sets of troponin, 3–6 hr apart. A negative first set does not exclude myocardial infarction, as values may take 3 hr to rise. Today's high-sensitivity troponins are good for picking up myocardial infarction (and ruling out if negative), at a cost of reduced specificity; they may be positive in renal failure, myocarditis, arrhythmias and pulmonary embolism.

- **Chest X-ray (CXR)**: For pulmonary oedema, pneumothorax (Figure 4.2f), widened mediastinum (dissection), pneumomediastinum (oesophageal rupture).

Other tests based on clinical suspicion:

- **For PE**: Bedside ultrasound is helpful to visualise right heart strain. CT pulmonary angiogram confirms pulmonary embolism. D-dimers are only useful to rule out PE if pre-test probability is low (i.e., do not order if PE is clinically suspected) (Chapter 4).

- **For aortic dissection**: Bedside ultrasound for a widened aortic root > 3 cm, and CT angiogram if stable.

- **CT thorax**: For oesophageal rupture.

- **Echocardiography**: For cardiac tamponade.

2. Other acute causes requiring treatment

The above evaluation will also identify these causes of acute chest pain which, while usually not as immediately life threatening as the prior ones, do require treatment.

- **Pneumonia with pleurisy**: Pleuritic chest pain with fever, cough ± sputum production and dullness and/or crackles on respiratory examination. CXR reveals consolidation. Continue with a septic workup including inflammatory markers (full blood count [FBC] and C-reactive protein [CRP]), sputum and blood cultures.

- **Pericarditis**: Chest pain is pleuritic in nature, and there may be a pericardial friction rub. The diagnosis is usually made when the ECG finds widespread ST-elevation (lead II > lead III), with reciprocal ST depression in aVR and V1, and PR depression (Figure 3.2c). Look for an underlying aetiology—infective, neoplastic, uremic, post-infarction and autoimmune.

- **Myocarditis**: Presentations vary and can be vague; a typical scenario is a young, previously healthy patient, who comes in with a viral prodrome (e.g., fever, malaise, arthralgia) and subsequently develops chest pain. Myocardial inflammation results in elevated troponins, arrhythmias (bundle branch block, high-degree atrioventricular blocks, etc.) and acute heart failure. Myocarditis can be mild or rapidly fatal.

- **Rib fractures**: Unfortunately, these are usually undiagnosed until a CXR is done *and looked at carefully*!

- **Referred pain from cholecystitis**: Consider if history is suggestive (Table 3.1) (see Chapter 9).

- **Herpes zoster**: Pain may precede the dermatomal vesicular eruption, such that patients receive work up for cardiac disease, without positive findings. The diagnosis is revealed days later when vesicles appear.

In the absence of red-flag history and examination findings, and normal initial investigations (ECG, CXR and troponins), move on to consider other less serious causes.

Reassuring Initial Workup

Having excluded the serious acute causes of chest pain, consider (3) whether chest pain could be due to an underlying cardiac disease, and (4) other diagnoses.

3. Cardiac Conditions with Serious Complications

- **Ischaemic heart disease**: Some patients with anginal symptoms have underlying ischaemic heart disease, and may require further testing. First, decide on the pre-test probability of ischaemic heart disease, which increases with age, a history of 'classic angina' (i.e., typical quality and duration, provoked by exertion or stress and relieved by rest or nitrates), cardiovascular risk factors (e.g., diabetes, hyperlipidaemia, hypertension) and suspicious ECG changes (Figure 3.2g). Next, if pre-test probability is at least moderate, consider non-invasive stress testing to confirm the diagnosis and obtain prognostic information. Choose an appropriate modality of stress test—for example, (a) treadmill ECG in patients who can exercise and have a normal rest ECG, (b) exercise stress echocardiography in patients who can exercise but have a non-interpretable ECG (e.g., bundle branch block or pacing) and (c) pharmacologic stress imaging for patients who cannot exercise. The results of the stress test determine the therapeutic approach taken; patients with intermediate to high-risk criteria on non-invasive testing generally receive coronary catheterisation, which is both diagnostic and therapeutic (stenting). A final consideration—in patients with ongoing symptoms, unstable angina or high-risk ECG (e.g., suspected left main occlusion), stress testing is risky and it may be preferable to proceed directly to coronary catheterisation.
- **Aortic stenosis (AS) or hypertrophic cardiomyopathy (HOCM)**: Identification of left ventricular hypertrophy on ECG (e.g., Sokolov criteria: S-wave V1 + tallest R-wave in V5–V6 > 35 mm), an ejection systolic murmur or concomitant syncope, prompts concern for AS or HOCM. Chest pain can develop in these conditions, and is usually a bad sign (implying myocardial hypoperfusion caused by increased wall stress and myocardial oxygen demand). Echocardiography confirms the diagnosis.

4. Consider Other Diagnoses

Non-cardiac diagnoses often present with chest pain.

Gastrointestinal causes commonly mimic cardiac ischaemia.

- **Gastroesophageal reflux disease**: Heartburn and reflux are classic, but may also present as 'chest pain'. Symptoms are exacerbated by lying down, food, alcohol and aspirin, and relieved by antacids.

- **Oesophageal spasm**: Mimics cardiac ischaemia or aortic dissection—pain is retrosternal ± radiating to the back, and relieved by nitrates.

- **Referred pain from sub-diaphragmatic aetiologies**: For example, biliary colic and peptic ulcer disease.

Musculoskeletal causes:

- **Costochondritis**: Pain localised to a single point on the chest wall, exacerbated by palpation and chest wall movement.

- **Cervical spondylosis causing nerve root compression**: Usually a shooting pain radiating from neck to arms, worse on neck movements (Chapter 51).

- **Shoulder joint arthritis**: Pain exacerbated on shoulder movements, may be localised on shoulder joint palpation (Chapter 49).

Psychiatric: Anxiety and related disorders (panic disorder, depression with anxious features, somatisation disorder) are relatively common causes of chest pain, but are diagnoses of exclusion.

Caveat: Due diligence must always be done to exclude serious causes of chest pain. The presence of known anxiety or gastroesophageal reflux does not exclude a serious cause of chest pain developing. Symptoms of myocardial infarction can be non-specific; vomiting can occur in acute myocardial infarction (AMI) and does not always point to a gastrointestinal aetiology.

 Using what you have learnt, **pen down your approach** to the Clinical Case at the start of the chapter **BEFORE reading the discussion** below.

Case Discussion

This is a middle-aged gentleman with multiple cardiac risk factors (hypertension, obesity, smoking, ethnicity). His pain is most likely due to cardiac ischaemia—it has a typical character, is relieved by rest and associated with diaphoresis. The history of intermittent chest tightness, which has been getting worse, may well be unstable angina instead of gastroesophageal reflux disease (GERD).

ECG is significant for diffuse ST-depression with ST-elevation in aVR; this is a high-risk ECG suggestive of left main coronary artery occlusion, proximal left anterior descending artery occlusion or severe triple vessel disease. He either has unstable angina or NSTEMI; troponin levels distinguish the two (normal in unstable angina, elevated in NSTEMI). While awaiting blood tests, he should receive emergent treatment (including antiplatelets). He will likely require an inpatient coronary angiogram and intervention (coronary stenting or coronary artery bypass grafting).

Key Lessons	1. Initial evaluation of chest pain focuses on the acute life threatening causes: acute coronary syndrome, aortic dissection, (tension) pneumothorax, pulmonary embolism, cardiac tamponade and oesophageal rupture.

2. Initial investigations in chest pain include an ECG, cardiac enzymes and CXR. Specific investigations (e.g., pulmonary angiogram and CT angiogram) may be considered if indicated by clinical suspicion. These may reveal the life threatening causes above, or other causes requiring treatment.

3. Consider cardiac stress testing in patients with symptoms of angina, and risk factors.

Common Pitfalls

1. Patients with acute myocardial infarction can have 'normal' ECG and troponin, when done very early. If there is a high clinical suspicion but a normal ECG, repeat serial ECGs (e.g., 15 min later), looking for dynamic changes.

2. Not every patient with an elevated troponin has myocardial infarction. There are other causes, especially renal failure, heart failure and arrhythmias.

Questions

1. **REFLECT!** Have you ever seen a STEMI patient wheeled through the Emergency Room door? How did the patient look? Would you have suspected the diagnosis even before an ECG?

2. **DISCUSS!** Two to three sets of cardiac enzymes (troponin and CK-MB) are routinely ordered. Do all patients with chest pain require cardiac enzymes, and is it necessary to order both troponin and CK-MB?

3. **EXPLORE!** A patient complains of episodic musculoskeletal-sounding chest pain. However, he has multiple cardiovascular risk factors. In this scenario, how do you differentiate cardiac chest pain requiring treatment, from musculoskeletal pain, for which he can be safely reassured?

4. **GO FURTHER!** Why do we distinguish between primary and secondary pneumothorax? What is the significance of this distinction?

Chapter

4

An Approach to Dyspnoea and Hypoxaemia

Clinical Case

A 56-year-old gentleman with a history of diabetes, ischaemic heart disease and chronic obstructive pulmonary disease (COPD), is admitted for breathlessness and cough. The cough had started 2 days ago; it was productive of thick sputum. Breathlessness started suddenly 5 hr ago. There is no chest pain or fever. On examination, his vitals are BP 154/92, HR 137, RR 27, SpO2 85% on room air. He appears uncomfortable; each breath is effortful and he is barely able to speak. Examination is remarkable for bilateral basal crepitations and scattered rhonchi. How would you approach his breathlessness?

Dyspnoea is a sensation of shortness of breath or difficulty breathing. 'Desaturation' refers to low peripheral oxygen saturation, as picked up by a pulse oximeter and reflects hypoxaemia, that is, low blood oxygen concentrations. Patients may have signs of respiratory distress (e.g., tachypnoea and use of accessory muscles of respiration).

The causes of dyspnoea may be divided by organ system and time course (Table 4.1).

Table 4.1. Causes of Dyspnoea by Organ System and Time Course

	Acute (min)	Subacute (hr)	Chronic
Respiratory	Upper airway obstruction Asthma Pneumothorax Pulmonary embolism	Pneumonia Asthma Exacerbation of COPD Pleural effusion	COPD Interstitial lung disease Tumour
Cardiac	Acute pulmonary oedema, including AMI	Decompensated heart failure	Heart failure
Others	Anaphylaxis Anxiety	Renal failure Decompensated cirrhosis Metabolic acidosis Neuromuscular weakness Anxiety	Anaemia Neuromuscular weakness

AMI, acute myocardial infarction; COPD, chronic obstructive pulmonary disease.

Initial Approach

Patients with dyspnoea can be unstable. Assess airway, breathing and circulation; look for features of respiratory distress and whether the patient is toxic. Decide if the patient requires immediate airway support (i.e., intubation in most cases), if there is time for an arterial blood gas (ABG) and quick evaluation before taking further decisions, or if one can afford a full history and examination. Providing supplemental oxygen is important, but remember that it will not address the underlying cause.

Clinical Pictures

Begin with a directed history, focused chest examination (Table 4.2), bedside investigations (ECG and blood gas) and a chest X-ray (CXR). Identify the likely clinical picture (Table 4.3). Bear in mind that patients may have multiple causes of dyspnoea, for example, myocardial infarction on top of chronic obstructive pulmonary disease (COPD).

Arterial Blood Gas

Consider performing an ABG if the patient looks unwell, or if peripheral oxygen saturations are low. It is rapid and provides a lot of information.

- **pO_2 and PaO_2/FiO_2 ratio ('P/F ratio')**: Low PaO_2 (< 60 mmHg) confirms hypoxaemia. This is only meaningful when read together with the inspired oxygen concentration (FiO_2)—for instance, a PaO_2 of 75 mmHg would be normal if the patient were on room air, but poor if he/she were on 50% oxygen. Use the ratio of PaO_2 to FiO_2 (i.e., PaO_2/FiO_2) to correct for varying FiO_2 concentrations (FiO_2 can be calculated: nasal prongs, 21% + 4% per 1L O_2; venturi mask, as set; face mask, ~50%; non-rebreather mask, 70–100%). Any P/F < 300 is worrying.

- **PCO_2**: If hypoxaemia is established, PCO_2 distinguishes type 1 (PCO_2 < 45 mmHg) vs. type 2 (PCO_2 > 45 mmHg) respiratory failure. Type 2 respiratory failure reflects hypoventilation and cannot simply be overcome by increasing FiO_2 (i.e., by providing supplemental oxygen).

- **pH**: For acidosis (pH < 7.35). Distinguish respiratory ($\uparrow PCO_2$) from metabolic ($\downarrow HCO_3$, compensatory $\downarrow PCO_2$) acidosis, both of which can present with dyspnoea (see Chapter 16).

- **Alveolar–arterial (A–a) gradient**: This can be calculated and helps to distinguish causes of hypoxaemia.
  - Reduced A–a gradient: Lung disease (ventilation/perfusion mismatch, diffusion abnormality) or shunts.
  - Normal A–a gradient: Hypoventilation, low inspired FiO_2. The implication of a normal A–a gradient is that the cause of hypoxaemia is not pulmonary.

Table 4.2. Chest Signs in Dyspnoea

	Collapse	Pneumothorax	Fibrosis	COPD	Bronchiectasis	Effusion	Consolidation
Trachea deviation	Towards affected side (if upper lobe)	Away from affected side (if tension)	Towards affected side (if upper lobe)	Nil. May have tracheal tug	Nil	Away from affected side (if massive)	Nil
Chest expansion	↓ On affected side	↓ On affected side	↓ On affected side	↓ Bilaterally Hyperinflated	—	↓ On affected side	↓ On affected side
Percussion	Dull	Hyperresonance	—	Hyperresonance	—	Stony dull	Dull
Added sounds	—	—	Fine crackles[a]	Expiratory wheeze ± coarse crackles	Coarse crackles, changes with cough[b]	Crackles if there is pulmonary oedema	Coarse late inspiratory crackles
Breath sounds	↓	↓	↓	↓ Or normal	Normal or bronchial[b]	↓	Bronchial
Vocal resonance	↓	↓	—	—	Normal or ↑[b]	↓	↑

[a] In severe pulmonary fibrosis, there may be traction bronchiectasis, leading to mixed fine and coarse crepitations.
[b] If there is superimposed consolidation, there may be bronchial breathing/increased vocal resonance.

Table 4.3. Clinical Pictures in Dyspnoea

Clinical Picture	History	Examination	Chest X-ray	Aetiologies
1. Chest pain + dyspnoea	**Chest pain** **Diaphoresis**	May be normal **ECG: S-T changes**	Normal Pneumothorax	Acute coronary syndrome Pneumothorax
2. Upper airway obstruction	Allergen or drug exposure Fever	**Stridor**	Not helpful	Anaphylaxis Epiglottitis Retropharyngeal abscess
3. Fluid overload	Orthopnoea Fluid indiscretion Known CCF/CKD/ cirrhosis	**Elevated JVP** **Basal** **crepitations** **Pedal oedema**	Fluid overload	Pulmonary oedema/CCF Renal failure Decompensated cirrhosis
4. Infection	**Fever** Cough	Consolidation	Consolidation	Pneumonia
5. Obstructive lung disease	Dyspnoea + **wheeze** Episodic dyspnoea (no wheeze)	Expiratory wheeze Hyperinflated lungs	Hyperinflation, normal or superimposed infection	COPD Asthma Heart failure
6. Other chest abnormality on physical exam	Variable	**Abnormal exam**, e.g., – Stony dullness – Hyperresonance – Fine crepitations	Specific findings, e.g., effusion, reticular opacities	Pleural effusion Pneumothorax Interstitial lung disease
7. Normal chest examination	Non-specific	Normal	Usually normal	Pulmonary embolism Metabolic acidosis Anaemia Hypoventilation Lung cancer Anxiety

CCF, congestive cardiac failure; CKD, chronic kidney disease; COPD, chronic obstructive pulmonary disease; JVP, jugular venous pressure.

1. Chest Pain Picture

This is discussed in Chapter 3. It is useful to always consider cardiac ischaemia as some patients (particularly diabetics with autonomic neuropathy) may actually be pain-free.

2. Upper Airway Obstruction Picture

Acute-onset inspiratory stridor, dyspnoea and/or wheeze, with respiratory distress is concerning for upper airway obstruction. This is a potential emergency with airway compromise.

Aetiologies to Consider

- **Anaphylaxis**: Stridor plus soft tissue swelling (facial swelling and angioedema), bronchoconstriction (wheeze), vasodilation (hypotension and syncope), developing acutely after allergen exposure (e.g., new drugs, pollen, food).
- **Epiglottitis**: Young children classically present with fever, stridor, drooling and anxiety. Symptoms are less typical in adults—fever, sore throat with odynophagia and difficulty swallowing saliva, and a muffled (hot potato) voice; stridor and dyspnoea are usually less marked than in children.
- **Retropharyngeal abscess**: Often a diabetic with infective symptoms (e.g., fever), together with neck pain and difficulty turning the neck. There may also be difficulty swallowing saliva and voice changes.
- **Retropharyngeal haematoma**: For example, after neck surgery or trauma.
- **Other causes**: Foreign body inhalation, smoke inhalation after escape from a fire.

Assessment and Workup

Investigate further only if the patient is stable. Intubate early if there is airway compromise (expect a difficult airway), and administer adrenaline immediately in anaphylaxis.

- **Lateral neck X-ray**: For thumb sign in epiglottitis (Figure 4.1) or soft tissue swelling anterior to vertebral body (retropharyngeal abscess). Foreign bodies may be radio-opaque or radiolucent.

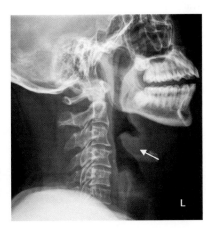

Figure 4.1. Epiglottitis. A 33-year-old man presented with sore throat, difficulty breathing and inability to swallow saliva. Lateral neck X-ray demonstrates a 'thumb sign' (the enlarged epiglottis itself), and loss of cervical lordosis (paravertebral muscle spasm). Nasoendoscopy by the otolaryngologist on-call confirmed a swollen epiglottis. He was admitted to High Dependency and a difficult airway set (including cricothyroidotomy sets) kept at his bedside, but he recovered rapidly with IV dexamethasone and antibiotics, and did not require intubation.

- **Nasoendoscopy**: May visualise uvula deviation and retropharyngeal anatomical distortion.

- **CT neck**: Allows better delineation of retropharyngeal abscess or haematoma. Ensure that the airway is patent before attempting a CT scan—it is not known as the 'donut for death' for no good reason!

- **Infective workup**: For example, inflammatory markers, blood cultures for infective aetiologies.

3. Fluid Overload Picture

Clinical findings of fluid overload include elevated jugular venous pressure, bibasal lung crepitations and pedal oedema. CXRs may show pulmonary oedema (perihilar opacities, costophrenic angle blunting, upper lobe diversion, Kerley B lines and cardiomegaly) and bilateral pleural effusions (Figure 4.2a).

Fluid overload may be due to cardiac, renal or hepatic aetiologies. It may occur *de novo*, in a patient without existing cardiac or renal disease, or due to the superimposition of an acute precipitant on underlying chronic disease.

Acute Event or Precipitant

Identify the acute event or precipitant that led to fluid overload. There may be multiple precipitants.

Workup

- **Acute myocardial infarction**: Typically with chest pain and diaphoresis, but this may be absent or vague (see Chapter 3).
  - − ECG
  - − Troponins

- **Acute kidney injury**: Due to hypovolaemia, nephrotoxic drugs, sepsis and so forth (see Chapter 18).
  - − Serum creatinine, compare with baseline

- **Arrhythmia**: Development of a new arrhythmia (e.g., atrial fibrillation) can worsen ejection fraction and lead to a decompensated fluid status.
  - − ECG

- **Acute valve dysfunction**: For example, acute mitral regurgitation due to papillary muscle rupture, for example, after a myocardial infarction. Auscultate for a murmur.
  - − Echocardiography

- **Non-compliance** to fluid restriction or medications.

- **Intercurrent illness**: Other medical illness (even an upper respiratory infection) can cause decompensation of heart failure or kidney disease.

Underlying Chronic Disease States

Workup

- **Congestive heart failure**: Patients have exertional dyspnoea, orthopnoea, paroxysmal nocturnal dyspnoea (patients often describe waking at night feeling that the room is 'stuffy', rather than breathlessness per se). Examination may reveal a displaced apex beat and third heart sound. Look for the cause—most commonly ischaemic heart disease with prior myocardial infarctions leading to reduced ejection fraction, but also hypertensive heart disease, cardiomyopathies, cor pulmonale, and so on.

  – pro-BNP: released in atrial stretch, high in cardiac failure
  – ECG for old infarcts (Q waves), hypertrophy
  – Echocardiogram: shows systolic and diastolic function, wall motion abnormalities, hypertrophy or dilation and valve abnormalities
  – Workup for risk factors and cause

- **Chronic kidney disease (CKD)**: Patients with late stage 4 or stage 5 chronic kidney disease usually have some degree of fluid overload. Patients already on dialysis may have fluid overloaded if dry weight is set too high, if they have missed dialysis or have been non-compliant to fluid restriction (see Chapter 18).

  – Serum creatinine

- **Decompensated cirrhosis**: Hypoalbuminaemia leads to accumulation of extravascular fluid, ascites and pulmonary congestion. There may be jaundice, splenomegaly and other stigmata of chronic liver disease (see Chapter 10).

4. Infective Picture

Pneumonia has a fairly obvious clinical picture. Dyspnoea develops over 1–2 days, accompanied with fever, rigours, cough and sometimes pleuritic chest pain. Examination reveals decreased breath sounds, dullness and crepitations. CXR may show lobar consolidation, patchy infiltrates or blurring of heart or diaphragmatic borders (Figure 4.2b). However, radiological findings may lag behind clinical findings, and findings may be atypical or subtle in immunosuppressed patients. Inflammatory markers (total whites, CRP, procalcitonin) are elevated.

Assessment and Workup

- **Severity**: Assess general clinical state especially adequacy of oxygenation. Lactate may be helpful to look for cryptic shock (see Chapter 2). The CURB-65 score (*c*onfusion, *u*rea > 7 mmol/L, *r*espiratory rate > 30, *B*P < 90 mmHg and age > *65*) predicts mortality in community acquired pneumonia; admission is suggested in CURB-65 scores of 2 or more.

- **Microbiological diagnosis**:
  - Bacterial: Features favouring bacterial infection include consolidation on CXR and elevated procalcitonin. Consider blood cultures (uncommonly positive but still done) and sputum gram stain and culture. Pneumococcal and legionella urinary antigen can be done but may not change management.
  - Viral: Upper respiratory tract infection (rhinorrhoea, sore throat, myalgia) is common; dyspnoea is not a typical feature in the absence of underlying chronic lung disease. Dyspnoea or opacities on CXR suggest a viral pneumonia or super-imposed bacterial infection.
  - Consider tuberculosis especially if there are upper lobe changes and a more chronic history. Send sputum for TB PCR, acid fast bacilli (AFB) smear and cultures.
  - Consider pneumocystis pneumonia in immunocompromised and HIV patients. It presents as fever, cough and dyspnoea, which may be fulminant (especially in non-HIV patients) or chronic (1–2 weeks). Hypoxia is prominent; patients desaturate when walking. The classic radiological picture is diffuse, bilateral, interstitial infiltrates; but imaging is often atypical or normal. Diagnosis is made via sputum or bronchoscopic recovery of organisms for staining or PCR.
- **For bacterial infections, consider risk factors for resistant organisms**: Stratify as community-acquired or hospital-acquired pneumonia (> 48 hr after admission). This is significant in terms of antibiotic choice. Patients from nursing homes, with dialysis unit contact, or recent hospitalisation (within 3 months) were previously classified as 'healthcare-associated pneumonia (HCAP)' but it was found that many of these patients are not truly at increased risk of resistant organisms.
- **Look for complications**: For example, parapneumonic effusion (Figure 4.2d)—diagnostic tap should be performed under ultrasound guidance if the effusion is large (> 25 mm on lateral decubitus film or CT), loculated, or associated with thickened parietal pleura (worrisome for empyema). Tap should be sent for biochemistry (pH, glucose, and lactate dehydrogenase [LDH]), cell microscopy, gram stain and culture.
- **Assess and treat underlying chronic lung disease**: Patients with chronic lung diseases (e.g., COPD, interstitial lung disease [ILD] or bronchiectasis) commonly suffer infective exacerbations; both the infection and underlying lung disease will need managing.

5. Obstructive Lung Disease Picture

Dyspnoea with expiratory rhonchi forms a distinctive clinical picture suggestive of obstructive lung disease. Unfortunately, an asthmatic will not have wheeze between episodes or during severe exacerbations ('silent chest')—in such cases, the diagnosis has to be made on history and bronchoprovocation testing. To complicate matters further, the distinction between asthma and COPD is not always straightforward; there is an overlap syndrome, and several mimics.

When patients present with acute exacerbations, two questions must be answered—(1) what precipitated the acute exacerbation—other differentials (including myocardial infarction, fluid overload and so forth) must be considered, and (2) what is the underlying disease and how has it been controlled?

Aetiologies

Workup

- **COPD**: A disease of longstanding smokers. Dyspnoea and decreased effort tolerance begins insidiously and progress slowly but relentlessly. On examination, there may be lung hyperinflation, wheeze and a tracheal tug. Patients are symptomatic at baseline, suffer intermittent infective exacerbations and are predisposed to secondary pneumothorax as well as lung cancer (which can present as rapid worsening of chronic dyspnoea).
  - See the following discussion
  - CXR may show hyperinflated lung fields (Figure 4.2c)

- **Asthma**: Classically, younger non-smokers with episodic dyspnoea and wheeze, precipitated by infection, allergen exposure, medication non-compliance or exercise. Patients are asymptomatic between attacks. Apart from wheeze, patients may also have cough or exertional dyspnoea. This sort of exertional dyspnoea has a delayed onset (15 min after starting exercise, vs. 5 min in other causes of exertional dyspnoea) and delayed resolution (30–60 min of rest). Patients may have a positive family history as well as other atopic disease (e.g., eczema and allergic rhinitis).
  - See the following discussion

- **Cardiac wheeze**: Heart failure may present with dyspnoea, wheeze and exertional dyspnoea, in addition to other findings of the fluid overload picture (e.g., elevated jugular venous pressure and pedal oedema). There is often a known history of heart disease.
  - Echocardiogram
  - NT-proBNP

- **Anaphylaxis**: A very acute presentation (page 43).

- **Asthma-plus syndromes and mimics**: These conditions mimic asthma and should be suspected in poorly controlled asthma or when there are atypical features
  - **Eosinophilic granulomatosis with polyangiitis** (EGPA, Churg–Strauss syndrome): A systemic vasculitis usually suspected in poorly controlled asthma, or when there is significant eosinophilia. There may be other clinical features including otolaryngological disease
    - Renal and liver chemistries to assess for organ involvement
    - Antineutrophil cytoplasmic antibodies (ANCA): positive

(otitis media, sinusitis, rhinitis), tender subcutaneous granulomas or rashes, mononeuritis multiplex, renal insufficiency or proteinuria and so forth.

– **Allergic bronchopulmonary aspergillosis (ABPA)**: Airway colonisation with Aspergillus fungi may result in a hypersensitivity reaction, presenting as recurrent exacerbations of asthma. Patients may also expectorate brownish mucus plugs.	– FBC: eosinophilia – Elevated serum IgE – Antibodies to aspergillus (aspergillus precipitins) – Imaging (CXR or High-resolution computed tomography [HRCT]) showing central bronchiectasis
– **Vocal cord dysfunction (paradoxical vocal cord motion)**: Inappropriate vocal cord movement resulting in functional airway obstruction and wheeze.	– Laryngoscopy
– **Intrathoracic airway obstruction**: A tracheal or endobronchial tumour may present with wheeze and dyspnoea. Be alert to red flag features including haemoptysis, loss of weight or chronic cough.	– CT thorax – Bronchoscopy

Assessment of Suspected Asthma/COPD

Acute Setting

- **Assess for life-threatening features**: For example, silent chest, altered mental state (drowsy, confused, agitated), severe respiratory distress, hypoxia requiring supplemental oxygen > 50%.

- **ABG**: Hypoxia may be present in both asthma and COPD, but there is an important difference in interpretation of pCO_2.

  - Asthma: Hypoxia drives hyperventilation, so pCO_2 is expected to be low during acute asthma attacks. A patient who is tiring out begins to hypoventilate—pCO_2 becomes normal, then high (> 40 mmHg). Therefore, normal or high pCO_2 during an asthma attack is a sign of impending respiratory collapse.

  - COPD: Patients have chronic hypercapnia and compensated respiratory acidosis. Review baseline ABG. Acidosis (pH < 7.25) or pCO_2 significantly elevated from baseline indicates decompensation and acute respiratory failure.

- **Assess for differentials, precipitant, complications**: Look for differentials (e.g., myocardial infarction), precipitant (e.g., infection and poor compliance) or complication (e.g., pneumothorax in COPD). This often entails blood work for infective markers, troponins and a CXR.

- Stabilise patient and assess as for outpatients. In poorly controlled disease, consider (ABCDE).

- Re-evaluate diagnosis: Is this really Asthma/COPD.
- Bronchial triggers and precipitants, for example, smoking in COPD, allergic rhinitis in asthma. Asthma better on weekends suggests an occupational component.
- Compliance to medication: Especially inhaled corticosteroids in asthma.
- Device technique: Patients may use their inhalers but not receive the drugs.
- Environment factors: For example, continued exposure to allergens, irritants, infective precipitants.

Stable Patient/Outpatient Setting

- **Consider differentials**: As earlier. Be particularly attentive if there are atypical features (e.g., first presentation of asthma in a middle-aged gentleman) or risk factors for other conditions (e.g., vasculopath with known ischaemic heart disease).
- **Assess severity**: Both asthma and COPD are assessed along two axes: (1) risk assessment, for example, previous intubation, multiple admissions, and (2) symptoms (see the GINA and GOLD guidelines).
- **Spirometry ± bronchoprovocation testing**:
  - Asthma: If spirometry shows an obstructive picture ($FEV_1/FVC < 70\%$), bronchodilator reversibility (increase in $FEV_1 > 12\%$ and > 200mL) supports asthma. Spirometry between attacks can be normal, in which case do bronchoprovocation testing e.g. methacholine challenge; fall in $FEV_1 > 20\%$ with a methacholine dose of 8 mg/mL supports asthma. A negative methacholine challenge test in a patient off inhalers makes asthma unlikely (low false negative rate). On the other hand, the methacholine challenge test is positive not only in asthma, but also bronchitis, COPD, heart failure, and allergic rhinitis (high false-positive rate).
  - COPD: Bronchial obstruction ($FEV_1/FVC < 70\%$) is a requirement for diagnosis; degree of FEV_1 limitation is a marker of severity. There may be a small component of bronchodilator reversibility (post bronchodilator increase in $FEV_1 > 12\%$), but usually not more than 400 mL.
  - At times a clear distinction between asthma and COPD cannot be made; this entity is known as 'asthma–COPD overlap'.
- **Other tests**: For example, exhaled nitric oxide, tests for differentials.

6. Other Chest Abnormality on Physical Exam

A number of other conditions have distinct abnormalities on physical examination (see page 41) and/or CXR.

Pleural Effusion

On examination, an effusion has reduced chest expansion, reduced breath sounds and a stony dull percussion note. On CXR, there is an opacified lower hemithorax with a meniscus sign (Figure 4.2d). Small bilateral effusions, with other clinical and X-ray manifestations of fluid overload, are usually due to fluid overload itself. Most other effusions should undergo diagnostic pleural tap, unless the cause is obvious.

An effusion may be identified as exudate or transudate based on its protein and LDH (with paired serum protein and LDH). Light's criteria states that an effusion is exudative if any one of three criteria are positive: (1) pleural fluid protein/serum protein > 0.5, (2) pleural LDH/serum LDH > 0.6 or (3) pleural LDH exceeds 2/3 of upper limit of normal for serum. The commonest causes are

Exudates:	**Pleural fluid tests**
• **Parapneumonic effusion**: Usually with infective symptoms, that is, fever and cough. The distinction between a simple or complicated (i.e., requires therapeutic drain) parapneumonic effusion is made based on appearance on diagnostic tap, biochemistry and microbiology (beyond the scope of this text).	− Gram stain + cultures − pH, glucose
• **Malignant effusion**: Look for red flags, for example, chronic cough, cachexia, haemoptysis, history of malignancy or nodules on CXR.	− Cytology and cell block
• **Tuberculous effusion**: May have history of chronic cough, night sweats, weight loss, upper lobe changes on CXR.	− Adenosine deaminase − AFB smear and culture
• **Hemothorax**: Frank blood seen on pleural tap. This can be due to malignancy or trauma.	

Transudate:

• **Fluid overload**: Heart failure, renal failure (see page 44). Usually bilateral, small pleural effusions.

• **Hepatic hydrothorax**: Usually a right-sided pleural effusion in cirrhotics with ascites. Small diaphragmatic defects allow ascites to pass from the peritoneal cavity into the pleural cavity. Spontaneous bacterial empyema (analogous to spontaneous bacterial peritonitis) can develop.

Interstitial Lung Disease

Patients may present with progressive breathlessness with exertional dyspnoea, and/or a persistent non-productive cough. Examination may find fine inspiratory crepitations ± clubbing. CXRs often show reticular changes (Figure 4.2e) but may be normal. There are many causes of ILD including

• ILD associated with exposures: For example, asbestosis, silicosis, hypersensitivity pneumonitis, and so forth.

• ILD associated with drugs: For example, bleomycin, amiodarone, methotrexate, busulfan.

- ILD associated with rheumatologic disease: For example, scleroderma, polymyositis/dermatomyositis, rheumatoid arthritis and so forth.
- Primary diffuse parenchymal lung disease (DPLD), including idiopathic interstitial pneumonias (many subtypes), granulomatous disease (e.g., sarcoidosis) and others.

The diagnosis of a specific aetiology of ILD is made via the intersection of clinical features (including identification of secondary causes of ILD), imaging findings and lung biopsy (where indicated). **A general approach would be to**

- **Assess for secondary causes** of ILD (exposures, drugs, rheumatologic disease): History, examination and diagnostic workup as indicated for rheumatologic disease.
- **High-resolution CT thorax** to assess for the pattern and distribution of ILD changes. Specific findings are associated with individual ILDs.
- **Spirometry**: The majority of ILDs show a restrictive pattern, that is, reduced FVC, reduced total lung capacity, but $FEV_1/FVC > 70\%$. Diffusing capacity (DLCO) is reduced.
- **Consider differentials** especially heart failure.
- Further testing including lung biopsy, bronchoalveolar lavage may be required.

Other Abnormalities

The CXR may identify many other abnormalities. More common ones are listed

- **Pneumothorax** (Figure 4.2f): See Chapter 3.
- **Lobar collapse** (Figures 4.2g and h): Identification of a lobar collapse would prompt a search for an aetiology, for example, obstruction of a lobar bronchus by tumour or secretions. This will not be discussed in further detail in this brief text.
- **Acute respiratory distress syndrome (ARDS)**: This is a syndrome of diffuse alveolar damage, precipitated by various clinical insults including sepsis, pneumonia, severe trauma and blood transfusion (transfusion-associated acute lung injury). Patients develop type 1 respiratory failure (P/F ratio < 300) within a week of the insult. CXR shows bilateral pulmonary opacities resembling pulmonary oedema (Figure 4.2i, also see Figure 4.2j). ARDS is a diagnosis of exclusion; cardiogenic pulmonary oedema and other lung disease should be ruled out as (these have disease-specific treatment, whereas, ARDS is managed supportively).
- **Cancer (lung or metastatic)**: A mass seen on CXR (Figure 7.2e). Usually these have to be quite large to cause significant dyspnoea.

7. Normal Chest Examination

These conditions present with dyspnoea ± hypoxaemia, but no abnormality detected on lung auscultation, and a normal CXR. They can be divided based on the A–a gradient (calculated from the ABG)

- **Elevated A–a gradient**: Implies a lung disease causing hypoxaemia (ventilation/perfusion mismatch and/or diffusion abnormality), or shunts (i.e., right to left heart shunting).

Figure 4.2. The CXR in dyspnoea.

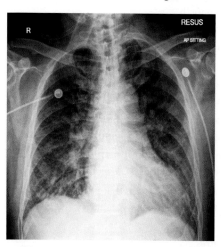

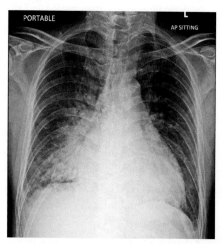

(a) **Fluid overload/Pulmonary oedema**: Bilateral perihilar opacities, upper lobe diversion, Kerley B lines and cardiomegaly. Bilateral pleural effusions may also be present (not visible in this X-ray).

(b) **Pneumonia, right middle lobe**: Right-sided consolidation with obliteration of the right heart border. The right diaphragmatic border is still visible, indicating right lower lobe sparing. Unlike lobar pneumonia, bronchopneumonia may appear as diffuse airspace opacities.

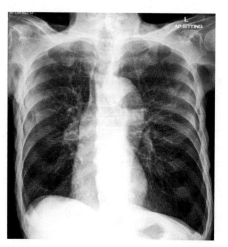

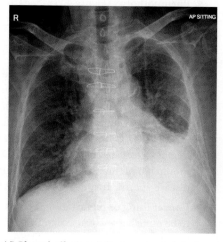

(c) **COPD**: Bilateral hyperinflated lung fields (> 6 anterior or > 10 posterior ribs in the midclavicular line), diaphragmatic flattening and mediastinal narrowing. This is consistent with chronic obstructive pulmonary disease.

(d) **Pleural effusion, left**: A moderate left pleural effusion with a concave-shaped top (meniscus sign), obliteration of the left diaphragmatic border and left heart border.

(Cont'd)

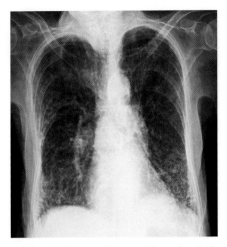

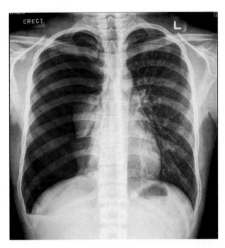

(e) **Interstitial lung disease**: Bilateral reticular opacities, predominantly in the lower zones, suggest an interstitial process. This was confirmed on high-resolution CT, which demonstrated the usual interstitial pneumonia pattern of idiopathic pulmonary fibrosis.

(f) **Pneumothorax, right**: Lung markings are absent in the right hemithorax. There is no tracheal or mediastinal shift (yet) to suggest tension.

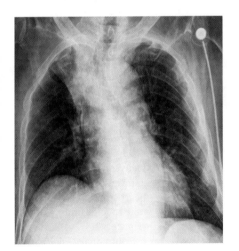

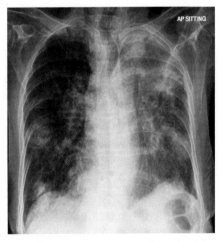

(g) **Collapse, right upper lobe**: Observe right upper zone density and right-sided volume loss. The trachea has been pulled to the right, and the right horizontal fissure has been pulled upwards.

(h) **Collapse, left upper lobe**: Unlike other lobes, the left upper lobe collapses anteriorly, causing a veil-like opacity over the entire left hemithorax ('veil sign'). Note tracheal deviation to the left. Incidentally, this X-ray also shows patchy opacities in the right middle and lower zones, suggestive of infection.

(Cont'd)

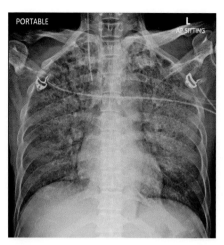

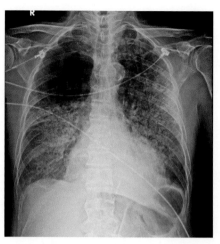

(i) **Acute respiratory distress syndrome (ARDS)**: Diffuse, bilateral pulmonary infiltrates. This patient had septic shock requiring vasopressors (hence the right internal jugular central line), and was intubated shortly after this X-ray was taken.

(j) **Pulmonary haemorrhage**: This patient had diffuse alveolar haemorrhage and massive haemoptysis. Note how the X-ray appearance resembles ARDS (and hence should be considered as a differential to ARDS), although in this case only certain lobes were affected.

- **Normal A–a gradient**: Implies that the cause of hypoxaemia is not pulmonary—for example, hypoventilation.

- **No hypoxaemia**—consider causes of normal A–a gradient.

Elevated A–a Gradient

	Workup
- **Pulmonary embolism** (PE): Classically pleuritic chest pain, dyspnoea ± haemoptysis. However, presentations are often subtle—for example, unexplained hypoxaemia and tachycardia. Examination is often normal; or there may be a swollen leg (deep vein thrombosis). *Severe acute dyspnoea with no clinical signs, normal CXR and non-specific ECG is very suspicious for PE.* This diagnosis is easily missed and a high index of suspicion if required especially in patients with risk factors (see Chapter 47). On the other hand, the absence of hypoxaemia makes PE less likely.	– ECG: $S_1Q_3T_3$, sinus tachycardia, T-inversions, right heart strain or non-specific findings (Figure 3.2f) – CT pulmonary angiogram
- **Consider right to left heart shunts**, for example, patent foramen ovale, ventricular septal defect and so forth. This is also a cause of a reduced A–a gradient, and may present with dyspnoea especially if complications develop. A murmur may be audible.	– Echocardiography

Normal A–a Gradient

	Workup
• **Metabolic acidosis**: Dyspnoea results from respiratory compensation for metabolic acidosis. The patient may hyperventilate—Kussmaul breathing. Look for diabetic ketoacidosis, uremic acidosis and other causes of metabolic acidosis (see Chapter 16).	
• **Hypoventilation**: This may be seen in a number of disease states	
– Neurologic disease: For example, myasthenic crisis, Guillain–Barre syndrome and motor neuron disease. There may also be other features of limb weakness and cranial nerve palsies (see Chapter 25)	– See Chapter 25
– Over sedation with opiates or sedatives	
– Traumatic brain or cervical spine injury	
– Mechanical causes: Obesity, kyphoscoliosis, diaphragmatic splinting from large ascites	
– Diaphragmatic palsy: Idiopathic, related to trauma (e.g., intra-thoracic surgery) or neurological disease. Diagnosis is usually suspected when the CXR shows a raised hemi-diaphragm	
• **Anaemia**: Dyspnoea may be a feature, in addition to pallor, and other symptoms of anaemia (see Chapter 32).	– Haemoglobin levels
• **Low inspired FiO$_2$**: For example, patients at high altitude.	
• **Anxiety and other psychiatric disorders**: A diagnosis of exclusion, but dyspnoea is a common complaint in patients with panic disorder.	

 Using what you have learnt, **pen down your approach** to the Clinical Case at the start of the chapter **BEFORE reading the discussion** below.

Case Discussion

This gentleman presents with acute dyspnoea on a background of COPD and ischaemic heart disease. Recognise that he is in respiratory distress. Provide supplemental oxygen and consider higher levels of ventilatory support if oxygen requirements are high, if respiratory status fails to improve, or if blood gas shows acidosis or hypercapnia (elevated from baseline).

The most obvious diagnosis would be an infective exacerbation of COPD, with dyspnoea, cough and increase in sputum volume or purulence (fever is not always present). However, other differentials should be considered. Examine carefully and scrutinise the CXR for a secondary pneumothorax (his emphysematous bullae can rupture), especially when he gives a history of 'sudden' breathlessness. Consider acute coronary syndrome and diabetic ketoacidosis as differentials. Initial investigations include a CXR, ECG, cardiac enzymes, blood glucose, inflammatory markers and sputum cultures.

Key Lessons	
	1. History, chest examination and CXR stratify the causes of dyspnoea into seven clinical pictures: dyspnoea with chest pain, upper airway obstruction, fluid overload, infection, obstructive lung disease, other respiratory abnormalities and dyspnoea with normal chest examination and CXR. This narrows down the aetiologies to consider.
	2. An ABG is valuable to establish severity of hypercapnia. Reduced A–a gradient suggests lung disease or cardiac shunts; normal A–a gradient implies an extra-pulmonary cause of hypoxia.
	3. Patients with an upper airway obstruction picture (i.e., stridor) may require early intubation; difficult intubation should be anticipated.
	4. Patients presenting with an exacerbation of asthma or COPD exacerbations should be assessed for: severity (clinical, ABG), differentials (cardiac wheeze, asthma plus syndromes, concomitant diseases), acute precipitants, compliance and inhaler technique issues.
Common Pitfalls	1. In a severe asthma exacerbation, a 'normal' pCO_2 is very abnormal and heralds impending respiratory collapse.
	2. Severe acute dyspnoea with a normal chest examination, normal CXR and non-specific ECG changes is very suspicions for pulmonary embolism.
	3. Metabolic acidosis is another cause of dyspnoea with normal chest examination, and can be easily missed without a high index of suspicion.
Questions	1. **REFLECT!** Have you ever encountered difficulty distinguishing between fluid overload and pulmonary infection? How did you decide which is the correct diagnosis?
	2. **DISCUSS!** 'When clerking the dyspnoeic patient, it is far easier to look at the CXR first before going to the bedside'. What are the merits and detriments of such an approach?
	3. **EXPLORE!** Intubating a patient with upper airway obstruction may be difficult. How do you assess for a difficult airway, and difficult bag-valve-mask ventilation? How would you manage a potentially difficult airway?
	4. **GO FURTHER!** Read up on how spirometry is performed. What are the findings in (a) restrictive lung disease, (b) asthma, (c) COPD, (d) intra-thoracic airway obstruction and (e) extra-thoracic airway obstruction?

Chapter 5

An Approach to Palpitations and Arrhythmias

Clinical Case

A 19-year-old female dance student walks into clinic complaining of intermittent palpitations. She has had four episodes in the last month, each lasting 5 min. Popping her ears (as one does in a landing aeroplane) apparently stops the palpitations. During episodes, she does not faint, feel giddy or have chest pain or diaphoresis. She feels perfectly normal between episodes, and has no other past medical history. Physical examination is normal. How would you approach her palpitations? She is currently asymptomatic.

Palpitations are an unpleasant awareness of the forceful, rapid and/or irregular beating of the heart. It may be due to both cardiac and non-cardiac disease. Most cases are benign, but there are a number of potentially life-threatening arrhythmias. A rational decision-making strategy is needed to quickly identify patients with life-threatening arrhythmias, then risk stratify and determine which patients require advanced investigations (Figure 5.1).

A. Unstable Tachyarrhythmias

Some arrhythmias can cause haemodynamic instability. First assess the patient for hypotension or serious signs or symptoms (e.g., drowsiness, shortness of breath, chest pain, syncope). An unstable tachyarrhythmia may require urgent intervention, usually cardioversion.

The next step is a 12-lead ECG.

Abnormal ECG

B. The Tachycardias

Two key differentiators are (1) is rhythm regular or irregular, and (2) is the QRS complex narrow or wide (normal = 80–120 ms = 2–3 small squares). The QRS width is the time taken for the complex to reach all ventricular myocardium. An impulse originating from or above the atrioventricular (AV) node, and going down the rapid conducting system, has a short conduction time and narrow QRS width; conversely, QRS is wide in a complex that originates in the ventricles and is not conducted through the rapid conducting system, or if there is a defect in the conducting system. (Note: patients with pacemakers are not discussed in this chapter).

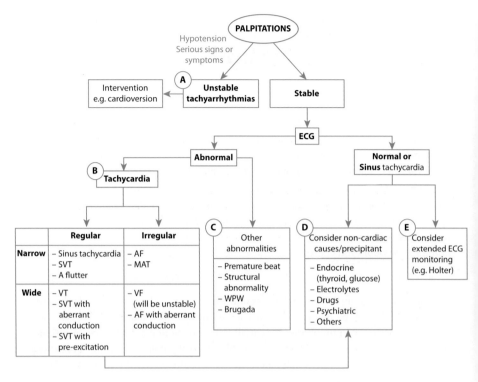

A. flutter, atrial flutter; AF, atrial fibrillation; MAT, multifocal atrial tachycardia; SVT, supraventricular tachycardia; VF, ventricular fibrillation; VT, ventricular tachycardia; WPW, Wolff–Parkinson–White.

Figure 5.1. Approach to palpitations.

(a) **Regular narrow-complex tachycardia**: Look at the timing and morphology of the P waves.[1]

- **Sinus tachycardia**: Sinus P waves present before each QRS, with 1 QRS complex for every P wave. This is usually a response to non-cardiac disease, for example, pain, infection, hypovolaemia, anaemia, hyperthyroidism, pulmonary embolism or anxiety (see page 62). Work up for these aetiologies.

- **Supraventricular tachycardia (SVT**; Figure 5.2a): P waves are absent or abnormal in morphology and/or timing. For instance, retrograde impulse conduction from the AV node to the atria results in inverted P waves (best seen in inferior leads) occurring soon after the QRS complex. There are different SVTs, including atrial tachycardia (AT), AV nodal re-entrant tachycardia (AVNRT) and orthodromic AV re-entrant tachycardia (AVRT); it is sometimes possible to determine the exact type of SVT from the 12-lead ECG, but this is not a diagnostic priority and usually does not change initial management.

---

[1] Is all lost when P waves cannot be found? → see 'GO FURTHER' question at the end of this chapter.

- **Atrial flutter** (Figure 5.2b): Rapid P waves (atrial rate: 250–300 beats/min) forming a saw-tooth baseline, most commonly with conduction of every second P wave (2:1 AV conduction), leading to a ventricular rate of 150 beats/min. Less commonly, there may be 3:1 or 4:1 AV conduction. The approach is as for atrial fibrillation (AF) (see the following).

(b) **Irregular narrow-complex tachycardia**

- **AF** (Figure 5.2c): Irregularly irregular R–R intervals with absent P waves. Search for a provoking cause, including non-cardiac (sepsis, electrolyte imbalance, hyperthyroidism) and cardiac (e.g., ischaemic heart disease and heart failure) aetiologies, as dictated by the clinical presentation.

- **Multifocal atrial tachycardia (MAT)**: An irregular tachycardia with ≥ 3 different P wave morphologies, and narrow QRS complexes following the P waves. This tends to occur in patients with lung disease (e.g., COPD and pneumonia) or heart disease with pulmonary hypertension.

(c) **Regular wide-complex tachycardia**

- **Ventricular tachycardia (VT**; Figure 5.2d): VT is the most common cause of regular wide-complex tachycardia, especially in patients with underlying ischaemic heart disease. Check vital signs—patients with VT may be unstable.

- **SVT with aberrant conduction**: SVT mimics VT in the presence of conduction delay, which prolongs the QRS complex. Consider SVT with aberrancy in young patients with structurally normal hearts,[2] especially if the QRS complex has a bundle branch block morphology. Conversely, features favouring VT over SVT include known ischaemic heart disease, very wide QRS complex (> 160 ms), northwest ECG axis, fusion or capture beats, AV dissociation (P waves seen with no relationship to QRS) or concordance (all precordial leads positive, or all negative). If in doubt, diagnose VT rather than SVT with aberrancy; managing VT as for SVT can cause haemodynamic instability.

- **SVT with pre-excitation**: Consider antidromic AVRT in patients with Wolff–Parkinson–White (WPW) syndrome; this is important as AV nodal blocking drugs should be avoided in WPW. Unfortunately, if there is no prior diagnosis of WPW, it is difficult to distinguish from VT.

(d) **Irregular wide-complex tachycardia**

- **Ventricular fibrillation**: Patient would have collapsed.

- **AF with aberrant conduction** (Figure 5.2e): Irregularly irregular rhythm.

Further workup: This would depend on the specific tachycardia. The majority of these aetiologies, except for sinus tachycardia and SVT, would require evaluation for cardiac function, and possible underlying ischaemic or valvular heart disease. This would include an echocardiogram ± stress testing, and at times electrophysiologic studies.

---

[2] Young patients with structurally normal hearts may also develop specific, uncommon types of VT. These include right ventricular outflow tract tachycardia, catecholaminergic polymorphic VT and so forth.

Figure 5.2. The ECG in tachycardia.

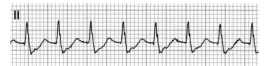

(a) **Supraventricular tachycardia**: Regular, with narrow QRS complexes. P waves are not well seen in this ECG.

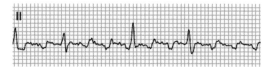

(b) **Atrial flutter**: Note narrow QRS complexes, saw-toothed P waves with 3:1 conduction.

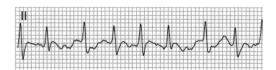

(c) **Atrial fibrillation**: Irregularly irregular, narrow QRS tachycardia.

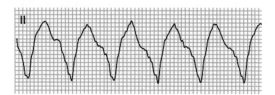

(d) **Ventricular tachycardia**: QRS complexes are very broad.

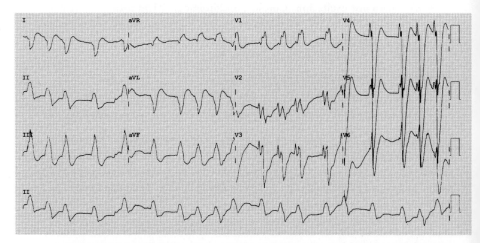

(e) **Atrial fibrillation with aberrant conduction**: The rhythm is irregularly irregular. QRS complexes are broad with suggestion of a right bundle branch block pattern.

C. Other ECG Abnormalities

Premature beats: May present with palpitations. These tend to occur suddenly and last for no more than an instant.

- **Premature ventricular contraction (PVC)**: A wide QRS complex, not preceded by P wave, followed by a T wave in the opposite direction, and then a compensatory pause. Isolated PVCs are common and do not require further workup. If frequent, consider ambulatory monitoring to determine the frequency and morphology of PVCs, and evaluation for an underlying aetiology—cardiac (hypertensive heart disease, myocardial infarction, heart failure) and non-cardiac disease (caffeine, COPD, hyperthyroidism, etc.).

- **Premature atrial contraction (PAC)**: A premature P wave triggering a normal or aberrant QRS complex. Isolated PACs are common and do not require further workup. If frequent, consider workup to rule out underlying structural heart disease.

Arrhythmia not captured: Many arrhythmias are intermittent and may not be captured on a single ECG. However, abnormalities in the rest ECG may suggest a diagnosis.

- **Structural cardiac abnormalities**: Q waves (old infarction), left ventricular hypertrophy (structural heart disease and hypertrophic obstructive cardiomyopathy) suggest that an arrhythmia may be the cause of palpitations. Attempts to capture the arrhythmia should be pursued (see page 62).

- **Wolff–Parkinson–White (WPW) syndrome**: Delta waves with a short PR interval may be seen (Figure 5.3). This is associated with a number of supraventricular and ventricular arrhythmias, and sudden cardiac death.

- **Brugada pattern**: Coved ST segment elevation > 2 mm, followed by a negative T wave, in more than 1 anterior lead (V1–V3). If symptomatic, this is associated with VT, AF and sudden cardiac death.

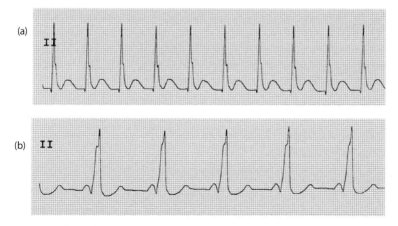

Figure 5.3. Wolff–Parkinson–White syndrome. A 17-year-old boy presents with palpitations. Initial ECG (a) shows a regular narrow-complex tachycardia for which IV adenosine is administered. Repeat ECG (b) uncovers underlying delta-waves, indicating an underlying WPW syndrome.

Normal ECG or Sinus Tachycardia

D. Consider Non-cardiac Causes

All patients with a normal initial ECG, and those with sinus tachycardia, should be evaluated for non-cardiac causes of palpitations. This includes

Workup

- **Endocrine disorders**:
  - **Hyperthyroidism**: Clinical features include heat intolerance, weight loss, diarrhoea, tremor (Chapter 36).
    - − Thyroid function tests
  - **Hypoglycaemia**: Usually a diabetic on insulin or oral hypoglycaemic agents who has missed meals or had recent dose adjustments.
    - − Blood glucose
  - **Phaeochromocytoma**: Episodes of palpitations, hypertension, headache and diaphoresis.
    - − Urine metanephrine screening

- **Drugs**: Beta-agonists or sudden cessation of beta-blockers, vasodilators, anticholinergics, recreational drugs (e.g., cocaine) and caffeine.

- **Hypovolaemia**

- **Anaemia**
  - − Full blood count

- **Psychiatric**: Panic attacks, anxiety disorders and somatisation. This is a diagnosis of exclusion.

E. Consider Extended ECG Monitoring

Many arrhythmias are intermittent, and may not be captured on a single 10-second ECG. The ECG is more likely diagnostic if captured when the patient has ongoing palpitations (e.g., in an emergency department setting). If an initial ECG is normal, the next decision is whether to pursue extended ECG monitoring. This would depend on the clinical suspicion of an arrhythmia (especially a malignant one).

Suggest extended monitoring in patients with:

- Severe symptoms (syncope, chest pain, diaphoresis) during episodes of arrhythmia.
- Known structural heart disease including ischaemic heart disease, valvular heart disease, cardiomyopathies.
- Family history of sudden cardiac death.
- Abnormal physical examination, including murmurs, heart failure, displaced apex beat.
- Abnormal rest ECG.
- Recurrent bothersome symptoms.

Extended ECG monitoring can be accomplished via Holter devices (24 or 48 hr), trans-telephonic monitoring (2 weeks) or implantable loop recorders (even longer duration, but invasive).

 Using what you have learnt, **pen down your approach** to the Clinical Case at the start of the chapter **BEFORE reading the discussion** below.

Case Discussion

This young lady gives a history of episodic tachycardia, which she has learnt to terminate using a Valsalva manoeuvre. This history, together with her demographic, makes SVT the most likely diagnosis. An ECG now (while asymptomatic) is unlikely to capture the SVT, however, look for rest abnormalities especially any delta wave, Brigade pattern or hypertrophic obstructive cardiomyopathy. Ensure that she has no family history of sudden cardiac death. Obtain thyroid, glucose and haemoglobin levels, and rule out any recreational drug use. Transtelephonic ECG monitoring can be offered to capture the arrhythmia, if she is bothered or wants a diagnosis.

Key Lessons	1. The tachycardias can be divided as (1) regular vs. irregular, (2) narrow vs. wide QRS complex. The most common types are: sinus tachycardia (regular narrow QRS), SVT (regular narrow QRS), VT (regular wide QRS) and AF (irregular narrow QRS).
	2. A single rest ECG may not capture the arrhythmia responsible for palpitations. If there is high clinical suspicion of an arrhythmia, consider extended ECG monitoring.
	3. Consider non-cardiac causes of palpitations, including hyperthyroidism, hypoglycaemia, phaeochromocytoma, drugs, hypovolaemia and anaemia.
Common Pitfalls	1. Sinus tachycardia is usually a response to non-cardiac disease. It is more important to identify this precipitant, than attempt serial troponins or cardiac testing.
Questions	1. **EXPLORE!** With this book closed, attempt to draw out the ECG tracing for each type of tachycardia. Then check your answers. (This tests if you understand the key features of each tachycardia; if you can draw it, you probably can recognise it when you see one!)
	2. **GO FURTHER!** The regular narrow-complex tachycardias can be difficult to tell apart, because P waves are hard to find when the rate is rapid. In this situation, IV adenosine is helpful—apart from its therapeutic utility in terminating supraventricular tachycardias—it can be used diagnostically to slow the ventricular rate and uncover the underlying rhythm.

Exercise: In the following rhythms, is IV adenosine diagnostic (uncovers the rhythm) or therapeutic (i.e., terminates the rhythm)? Please circle (one, both, or none)

(a) Sinus tachycardia	Diagnostic vs. Therapeutic
(b) Supraventricular tachycardia	Diagnostic vs. Therapeutic
(c) Atrial flutter	Diagnostic vs. Therapeutic
(d) Atrial fibrillation	Diagnostic vs. Therapeutic

Chapter **An Approach to**

6 **Hypertension**

Clinical Case

A 23-year-old university student consults the general practitioner for a viral upper respiratory tract infection. Her blood pressure is opportunistically measured, and it is 160/93 mmHg. A repeat blood pressure on a separate day is 158/90 mmHg. She is asymptomatic and has no past medical history. Her body mass index is 19.5. How would you approach her hypertension?

Hypertension is a common and treatable cardiovascular risk factor. All patients who consult a physician for other ailments should have their blood pressure opportunistically screened. The majority have essential hypertension, with only a minority having a secondary cause of hypertension.

Diagnosis of Hypertension

The diagnosis of hypertension is made on blood pressure readings above systolic 130 mmHg, or diastolic 80 mmHg, at two or more visits. Many patients are anxious when visiting the doctor, leading to spuriously elevated clinic blood pressures ('white coat' hypertension). Home blood pressure monitoring or formal ambulatory blood pressure monitoring can be valuable to remove the 'white coat' effect.

Severe Hypertension

At blood pressures of systolic ≥ 180 mmHg and/or diastolic ≥ 120 mmHg, a single reading is sufficient to diagnose hypertension. At these levels, patients may be symptomatic. Look out for

- **Hypertensive emergency**: Severe hypertension with end organ damage. This may be neurological (stroke and hypertensive encephalopathy), cardiac (aortic dissection and acute heart failure), renal (acute hypertensive nephrosclerosis) or pre-eclampsia. Symptoms would be apparent.

- **Hypertensive urgency**: Symptomatic hypertension (e.g., headache and giddiness) without overt end organ damage. Do not assume that these symptoms are due to hypertension alone; consider and exclude other differentials.

Secondary Hypertension

The majority of patients with hypertension have essential hypertension; it is neither necessary nor cost effective to screen every patient for secondary causes. However, the following features would prompt suspicion of secondary causes:

- **Young hypertension**: Especially if before 30 years old.
- **Resistant hypertension**: Blood pressure that remains above target with optimal doses of three antihypertensives from different classes, including a diuretic.
- **Abnormal renal panel**: Elevated creatinine, rise in creatinine > 30% after starting angiotensin-converting enzyme inhibitors, or hypernatraemia with hypokalaemia.
- Clinical features of the diseases below—many are identifiable on clinical history.

The secondary causes of hypertension include renal, endocrine and other causes. Begin with a renal panel and clinical examination for recognisable endocrine syndromes (Figure 6.1):

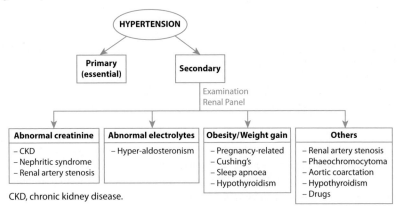

Figure 6.1. Approach to hypertension.

Abnormal Creatinine

	Workup
- **Chronic kidney disease**: Hypertension is common due to impaired autoregulation and hypervolaemia; hypertension itself accelerates progression of kidney disease.	- See Chapter 18
- **Renal artery stenosis**: One clinical hallmark is a deterioration of renal function (rise in creatinine > 30%) after starting ACE inhibitors or angiotensin receptor blockers. There may be an abdominal bruit. Renal artery stenosis may develop in both older patients (due to atherosclerotic disease), as well as young patients (fibromuscular dysplasia).	- Doppler ultrasound renal artery: shows decreased flow - Ultrasound kidney: unilateral shrunken kidney

- **Nephritic syndrome**: Hypertension accompanies raised creatinine, haematuria, proteinuria and oliguria (see Chapter 20).

  – UFEME for haematuria
  – Other workup (see Chapter 20)

Abnormal Electrolytes

- **Primary hyperaldosteronism (Conn's syndrome)**: Overproduction of aldosterone increases sodium reabsorption (hypernatraemia), in exchange for increased potassium excretion (hypokalaemia and metabolic alkalosis). Renin is suppressed. This can occur due to an adrenal tumour or adrenal hyperplasia. Hypokalaemia is an inconsistent feature and many patients have 'normal' potassium.

  – Screening: plasma aldosterone (elevated) and renin (suppressed)
  – Confirmatory: salt loading or saline suppression test
  – CT adrenal gland: look for adrenal tumour

Obesity or Weight Gain

- **Pregnancy**: The spectrum of pregnancy-related hypertensive disease ranges from pregnancy induced hypertension, to pre-eclampsia (new-onset hypertension and proteinuria after 20 weeks' gestation), to eclampsia (pre-eclampsia and seizures).

  – Urine pregnancy test
  – Urine for protein
  – Liver function test (LFT) (for HELLP syndrome)

- **Cushing's syndrome**: A clinically recognisable syndrome—central obesity with dorsocervical and supraclavicular fat pads, thin skin, proximal muscle weakness. It may be due to exogenous steroid ingestion, or endogenous steroid production (see Chapter 38).

  – Low-dose dexamethasone suppression test
  – See other testing (see Chapter 38)

- **Obstructive sleep apnoea**: (Usually) overweight patients with night-time snoring, witnessed apnoea, day-time somnolence and morning headaches. Sleep apnoea is not an innocent disease, but is associated with hypertension, arrhythmias and adverse cardiovascular outcomes.

  – Sleep study

- **Hypothyroidism**: Look for weight gain, lethargy and cold intolerance.

  – Thyroid panel

Clinically not Overt

The following aetiologies tend not to be clinically obvious at first glance, and have a normal renal panel.

- **Renal artery stenosis**: Creatinine can be normal, especially if ACE-inhibition has not been given (see earlier).

  – See earlier

- **Phaeochromocytoma**: Paroxysmal episodes of hypertension, headache, tachycardia and diaphoresis.

    – Urinary or plasma fractionated metanephrines

- **Aortic coarctation**: Upper limb hypertension with low limb normotension. Examine for radial–femoral pulse delay, and interscapular systolic murmur. There may be features of other congenital heart disease.

    – Echocardiography

- **Hypothyroidism**: Worthwhile to screen as its features are non-specific.

    – Thyroid panel

- **Drugs**: Oral contraceptive pills, stimulants, non-steroidal anti-inflammatory drugs (NSAIDs) and some other drugs are associated with hypertension.

No Obvious Cause of Secondary Hypertension

Further testing should be based on the clinical suspicion of underlying causes of secondary hypertension. Additionally, it is reasonable to do renal panel, plasma renin and aldosterone and renal Doppler ultrasound for most patients. The more atypical the patient profile (e.g., very young and very severe hypertension), the more extensively a diagnosis of secondary hypertension should be pursued. If clinical examination and all investigations are normal, then essential hypertension remains the diagnosis.

The workup for all forms of hypertension should be completed with an evaluation of other cardiac risk factors (diabetes, lipids, smoking), all of which should be addressed at the same time.

 Using what you have learnt, **pen down your approach** to the Clinical Case at the start of the chapter **BEFORE reading the discussion** below.

Case Discussion

This lady has young hypertension. She should be encouraged to monitor her home BP, which would remove the effect of white coat hypertension, and subsequently aid monitoring of response to antihypertensive medications. Secondary causes of hypertension must be considered. In particular, perform four-limb blood pressure (coarctation), ask about episodes of headache, tachycardia and diaphoresis (phaeochromocytoma), drug use (e.g., contraceptive pills) and rule out pregnancy. Examine for an abdominal bruit. Obtain a renal panel, looking for elevations in serum creatinine (whether at baseline or after starting ACE-inhibition), and plasma renin/aldosterone ratio. Obstructive sleep apnoea and Cushing's syndrome are less likely given her low BMI. Further tests depend on the findings of initial examination.

Key Lessons	1. Essential hypertension is the commonest cause of hypertension. Secondary hypertension should be considered in young patients, resistant hypertension and if there are suggestive clinical features or an abnormal renal panel.
	2. The commonest causes of secondary hypertension are chronic kidney disease, renal artery stenosis, primary hyperaldosteronism and obstructive sleep apnoea.
Common Pitfalls	1. Failure to consider secondary causes in the presence of suggestive clinical features. Older patients do not *always* have essential hypertension.
Questions	1. **REFLECT!** Have you ever met a patient with resistant hypertension? How was the aetiology of hypertension uncovered?
	2. **DISCUSS!** How does the identification of an aetiology of secondary hypertension change management?
	3. **EXPLORE!** A mild rise in creatinine (up to 30%) is expected after starting ACE-inhibitors or angiotensin receptor blockers. Why is this so?

Chapter

7

An Approach to Cough

Clinical Case

A 57-year-old gentleman presents with a 2-month history of cough, productive of small amounts of non-bloody sputum. This cough started after a particularly bad flu, and never went away. It occurs throughout the day, but seems to be worse when he lies down. He has no fever, dyspnoea, weight loss or other symptoms, and maintains good effort tolerance. He saw a general practitioner 1 week ago, and was given a week of antibiotics, with little response. He is a lifelong smoker of 80 pack years, with a past medical history of hypertension, hyperlipidaemia and gout. His drugs include amlodipine, enalapril, simvastatin and as-needed colchicine; there are no recent dose or drug changes. How would you approach his cough?

Cough originates as a protective respiratory tract reflex. It is a common symptom, often due to self-limiting causes, but may also be due to insidious causes like tuberculosis (TB) and malignancy. Diagnostically, divide the causes of cough by time course (Figure 7.1).

Acute Cough

Acute cough is common and mostly due to time-limited causes:

- **Infective**: This may be an upper respiratory tract infection (URTI) or pneumonia. Rhinorrhoea, nasal congestion and a sore throat suggest a viral upper respiratory infection, while dyspnoea, hypoxia, respiratory distress or consolidation on examination suggests pneumonia.

- **Allergen exposure**: For example, pets or pollen in susceptible people. Cough may be accompanied by wheezing and shortness of breath.

- **Irritant exposure**: Exposure to smoke, haze and so forth. The diagnosis is usually fairly obvious.

- **Asthma exacerbation**: Cough is a possible manifestation (see page 75).

- **Foreign body aspiration**, including secretions.

Trial of therapy for the above causes is appropriate. Reassess the patient; if cough fails to resolve, then the causes of chronic cough need to be considered.

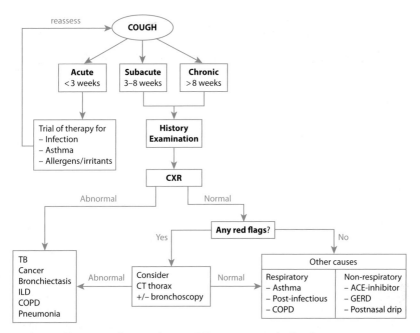

COPD, chronic obstructive pulmonary disease; GERD, gastrointestinal reflux disease; ILD, interstitial lung disease; TB, tuberculosis.

Figure 7.1. Approach to cough.

Subacute and Chronic Cough

Chronic cough is not in keeping with the natural history of a simple infection. It may represent other respiratory pathology (e.g., asthma, cancer, bronchiectasis) or non-respiratory pathology (e.g., gastrointestinal reflux). A clinical approach would be to

1. **Begin with a detailed history** focusing on the cough (onset, timing, exacerbating and relieving factors), associated symptoms, past medical history, exposures (smoking, occupation, hobbies, contact history for TB) and personal and family history (of TB or cancers). In particular, pay attention to the following features:

   - **Weight loss, night sweats or persistent fever** are red flags for TB and cancer (but their absence does not rule out these causes).

   - **Haemoptysis** is a red flag; causes include cancer, bronchiectasis and TB (see Chapter 8).

   - **Sputum production**: Bronchiectasis (especially if copious), TB, pneumonia.

   - **Dyspnoea** suggests lung pathologies such as obstructive airway disease, interstitial lung disease, malignancy and so forth.

   - **Timing of cough**: For example, immediately after lying down (gastrointestinal reflux), early dawn (asthma), after beginning an angiotensin-converting enzyme inhibitor.

- **Past medical history**: For example, known airway disease, rheumatologic disease (interstitial lung disease), systemic malignancy (pulmonary metastases).

- **Occupational and recreational exposure** for causes of interstitial lung disease and precipitants of asthma.

- **Response to prior treatment**: Whether previous courses of antibiotics or inhalers ameliorated cough.

2. **Physical examination**: May identify bronchiectasis (coarse crepitations which change on coughing), interstitial lung disease (fine crepitations), lobar collapse or pleural effusion (malignancy or TB). See Table 4.2 in Chapter 4.

3. **Obtain chest X-ray (CXR)** in all patients with chronic cough. The causes of chronic cough may then be stratified into those with normal vs. abnormal CXR.

CXR Abnormal

An abnormal CXR allows identification of

Workup

- **Pulmonary TB**: Some patients have florid constitutional symptoms (fever, night sweats, weight loss), others present only with chronic cough. Examination may reveal upper lobe fibrosis or collapse, but this is not sensitive. CXR is the key to show upper lobe infiltrates, scarring or consolidation (Figure 7.2a). TB may also present as lobar pneumonia in immunocompromised or HIV patients.

  - Sputum for TB PCR, acid fast bacilli (AFB) smear and culture (×2 sets); induce sputum if necessary
  - If TB positive, test for HIV and diabetes

- **Cancers**: Patients may have chronic cough, haemoptysis and constitutional symptoms. Dyspnoea is a late feature. Unfortunately, lung cancer is often asymptomatic until late. CXR may reveal a nodule (Figure 7.2e), lung collapse (Figure 4.2g and h), or pleural effusion (Figure 4.2d). If there are multiple pulmonary nodules (Figure 7.2f), consider metastatic disease rather than a primary lung cancer.

  - CT thorax
  - If concerned about metastatic cancer, look for a primary
  - Consider biopsy

- **Bronchiectasis**: The classic presentation is a long-standing history of daily cough and copious sputum production. Examination may reveal clubbing and coarse crepitations. CXR shows dilated thickened airways (tram track lines and ring shadows) (Figure 7.2c and d). Aetiology includes:

  - CT thorax

  - **Generalised**: Abnormal secretion clearance (e.g., cystic fibrosis and Kartagener's syndrome), immune deficiency, rheumatic disease (rheumatoid arthritis, Sjogren syndrome, Crohn's disease).

- **Focal**: Post-pneumonia (especially if repeated or severe) or TB, aspiration, bronchial obstruction (e.g., foreign body or cancer).

- **Interstitial lung disease**: Patients present with chronic non-productive cough and/or progressive exertional dyspnoea. Examination may find fine inspiratory crepitations, clubbing and pulmonary hypertension in late disease. CXR shows reticular shadowing (Figure 7.2b). Evaluate for secondary causes (see discussion on page 50).

- **COPD**: A longstanding smoker with cough, exertional dyspnoea, wheeze on examination and hyperinflation on CXR (see discussion on page 48).

- **Pneumonia**: This can cause chronic cough in the presence of underlying chronic infection, immunocompromised state or recurrent aspiration.

Figure 7.2. The CXR in chronic cough.

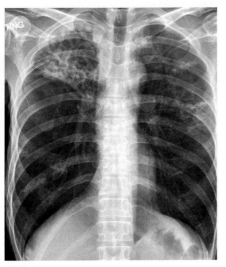
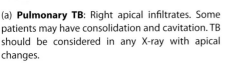
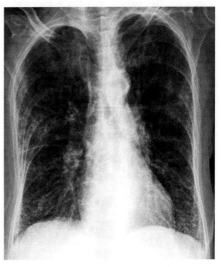

(a) **Pulmonary TB**: Right apical infiltrates. Some patients may have consolidation and cavitation. TB should be considered in any X-ray with apical changes.

(b) **Interstitial lung disease**: Bilateral, diffuse reticular changes. These are better visualised on a CT scan.

(Cont'd)

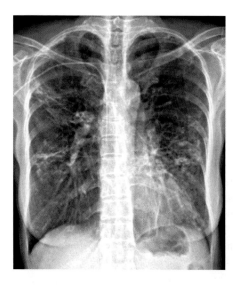

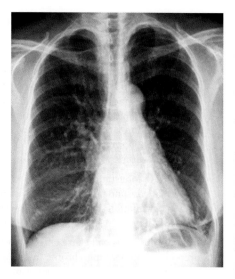

(c) **Bronchiectasis, generalised**: Tram-track opacities and several ring shadows (bronchioles seen end-on), seen throughout the lung fields. Incidentally, this patient also has a peripherally inserted central catheter for treatment of non-tuberculous mycobacterial infection.

(d) **Bronchiectasis, focal**: Similar tram-track changes and coarsened lung markings, but seen only in the left retrocardiac region. This patient's bronchiectasis was due to a previous pneumonia.

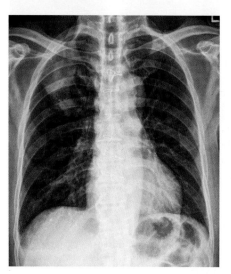

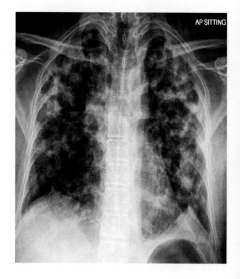

(e) **Lung mass**: The irregular right upper zone opacity proved to be a lung cancer. The appearance of a lung mass may resemble that of pneumonia; malignancy should be considered if 'pneumonia' does not resolve radiologically.

(f) **Lung metastases**: Multiple, bilateral lung nodules. These may be irregularly-shaped (as in this X-ray) or nodular ('cannonball'). This patient had metastatic breast cancer.

CXR Normal

1. **Are there any red flags?** In the presence of red flags (e.g., weight loss, haemoptysis, fever—see history earlier), consider further investigation with CT thorax ± bronchoscopy, as CXRs are insufficiently sensitive for small tumours, bronchiectasis and other abnormalities.

2. **No red flags**—Consider respiratory and non-respiratory causes

   (a) **Respiratory causes:**

   - **Cough-variant asthma:** Asthma can present without wheeze or dyspnoea, but instead with cough—typically a dry cough, worst in the early dawn (when bronchioles are most reactive). Look for other atopic symptoms, for example, eczema, allergic rhinitis, allergic conjunctivitis and for a positive family history. Consider spirometry with bronchodilator reversibility or provocation testing (see discussion on page 49).

   - **Chronic obstructive pulmonary disease** (COPD): The cardinal features are chronic cough, sputum production, and dyspnoea in a longlasting smoker; some patients may complain of cough before dyspnoea becomes noticeable. Consider spirometry (see page 49).

   - **Post-infectious cough:** Cough may persist for weeks after a URTI.

   (b) **Referred cough syndromes:**

   - **ACE-inhibitor:** Look at the drug history for any ACE-I (especially a newly started one). ACE-I cause cough in 5%–30% of patients due to inhibition of bradykinin metabolism; angiotensin receptor blockers do not inhibit bradykinin and do not cause cough. Stopping ACE-I should solve the cough—if not, look hard for another cause.

   - **Chronic rhinitis + post-nasal drip (upper airway cough syndrome):** Upper airway secretions may trigger the cough reflex. Cough is usually triggered immediately upon lying down. These patients may have symptoms of allergic rhinitis (morning 'stuffy nose', rhinorrhoea, frequent throat clearing and sneezing), and may even feel a sensation of liquid dripping into the back of the throat. Examination of the nose may reveal excess secretions, inflammation of nasal mucosae or nasal polyps.

   - **Gastroesophageal reflux disease (GERD):** Causes cough associated with food, burping and lying down (or early in the morning just after waking up). This may also be heartburn, a sour taste in the mouth, and relief of cough with antacids.

Using what you have learnt, **pen down your approach** to the Clinical Case at the start of the chapter **BEFORE reading the discussion** below.

Case Discussion

This is a smoker with chronic cough, who should have received a chest X-ray (CXR) rather than a course of antibiotics. A CXR may reveal upper lobe changes suggestive of pulmonary TB, which is common and may not always present with night sweats and weight loss. Any nodules on the CXR would be worrisome for cancer, especially with his florid smoking history. Chronic obstructive pulmonary disease (COPD) is less likely given the lack of dyspnoea and good effort tolerance. If his chest examination and CXR were normal, possible diagnoses include a post-infectious cough (since it started after a flu), post-nasal drip (cough worse when he lies down). He appears to have been on ACE-inhibitors for a while, so it is less likely the cause of cough.

Key Lessons	1. Acute cough (< 3 weeks) is common and most often due to viral upper respiratory infections or pneumonia.
	2. Chronic cough is not in keeping with a simple infection. Red flags include haemoptysis, weight loss, persistent fevers, night sweats and dyspnoea. All patients with chronic cough should receive a CXR. This may identify TB, cancers or other lung pathology.
	3. Cough may be due to non-pulmonary causes, for example, ACE-inhibitors, post-nasal drip and gastroesophageal reflux disease.
Common Pitfalls	1. Failure to obtain an early CXR in chronic cough can result in community transmission of TB and late diagnosis of cancers.
	2. Cough should not be attributed to smoking or ACE-I without consideration of other treatable causes.
Questions	1. **REFLECT!** Have you ever met a patient with post-nasal drip? How do they describe their cough? (usually quite different from someone with an infective cough)
	2. **DISCUSS!** A systematic approach to CXR interpretation is helpful to reduce the chance of missing any abnormality. What is your approach to interpreting a CXR?

Chapter

8

An Approach to Haemoptysis

Clinical Case

A 55-year-old gentleman presents with a 1-day history of coughing blood. He had been well with no symptoms of cough, weight loss, fever or dyspnoea prior to this episode. He is a chronic smoker of 30 pack years. How would you approach his haemoptysis?

Haemoptysis is the expectoration of blood from the lower respiratory tract. This can range from small amounts of blood-streaked sputum in the context of pneumonia, to massive haemoptysis requiring intubation. Major causes of haemoptysis include neoplasms, infections (bacterial, tuberculosis [TB] and fungal), bronchiectasis, auto-immune disorders and pulmonary vascular disorders (Figure 8.1).

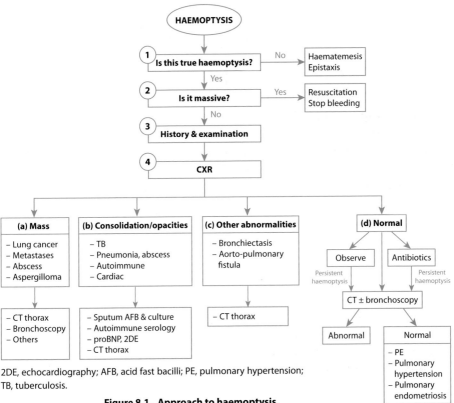

2DE, echocardiography; AFB, acid fast bacilli; PE, pulmonary hypertension; TB, tuberculosis.

Figure 8.1. Approach to haemoptysis.

Clinical Approach

1. Is This True Haemoptysis?

Haemoptysis is coughing out blood from the respiratory tract. This must be distinguished from haematemesis (blood vomited from the upper gastrointestinal tract) and epistaxis (nose bleed), which may mimic haemoptysis.

2. Is This Massive Haemoptysis?

Massive haemoptysis ($\geq$ 500 mL over 24 hr, or $\geq$ 100 mL/hr) is a medical emergency with high mortality. Patients die from airway obstruction, not exsanguination. The approach would be

- **Resuscitation**: Intubate to protect the airway.

- **Bleeding cessation**: Usually via bronchial artery angiography and embolisation (most massive bleeds are arterial rather than venous). Many clinicians perform bronchoscopy prior to embolisation; this helps to localise the bleeding site (hence making subsequent angiography easier) and allows an attempt at haemostasis.

- **Find the underlying cause**: See the following section.

3. Initial History and Examination

Obtain a history and examine the patient, focusing on broad groups: neoplastic, infective, bronchiectasis, autoimmune and vascular

- **Infective**: Fever, blood streaks mixed with purulent sputum.

- **Systemic symptoms**: Chronic cough, weight loss, night sweats (suggest TB or malignancy), chronic sputum production (bronchiectasis).

- **Autoimmune**: Other autoimmune manifestations including renal impairment, sinusitis, otitis media, rash, purpura, neuropathies and so forth.

- **Cardiac aetiologies**: Congestive fluid overload, murmurs on examination.

- **Injuries**: Chest trauma, foreign body inhalation, cocaine inhalation, iatrogenic injuries (e.g., pulmonary artery catheterisation and complication of tracheostomy) or related to leukaemia chemotherapy or bone marrow transplant.

4. Obtain Chest X-ray and Consider Aetiologies

Initial investigations include a full blood count, renal panel, liver panel, coagulation profile and chest X-ray (CXR). The causes of haemoptysis can be stratified based on the CXR picture: (a) mass, (b) consolidation or opacities, (c) other defined abnormalities or (d) a normal CXR. The commonest causes are marked *. In many cases further investigation with CT imaging ± bronchoscopy would be suggested.

(a) CXR: Mass or Nodule

	Workup
• **Lung cancer**[*]: A single new or enlarging nodule (Figure 7.2e), especially if large and irregular in a chronic smoker, is suggestive of a primary lung cancer. Also consider bronchial carcinoid in a young non-smoker, Kaposi's sarcoma in patients with AIDS and keep metastases as a differential.	− CT thorax − Bronchoscopy and biopsy, or image-guided transthoracic biopsy
• **Lung metastases**: If there are multiple nodules (Figure 7.2f), or a clinical history compatible with other cancers, consider metastatic disease.	− Look for a primary lesion
• **Infective**: These may mimic cancer. Pulmonary abscesses appear as cavities with air-fluid levels, patients may have fever and cough. Aspergillomas appear as a rounded mass in a pulmonary cavity, the air-crescent or halo sign are classic but better appreciated on CT imaging.	− CT thorax − Inflammatory markers, blood cultures, sputum gram stain and culture − Aspergillus IgG levels

(b) CXR: Consolidation or Opacities

Diffuse opacities on a CXR may be due to water, pus or blood. Certain appearances may suggest specific aetiologies. In general, consider

	Workup
• **Infective**:	
− **TB**[*]: A relatively common cause of haemoptysis, when granulomas erode into bronchial arterial vessels. There may be chronic cough, weight loss and night sweats. CXR classically shows upper lobe cavitation or fibrosis (Figure 7.2a).	− Sputum for acid-fast bacilli smear and cultures, TB polymerase chain reaction (PCR)
− **Bacterial**[*]: For example, bronchitis, necrotising pneumonia and lung abscess. There may be fever, cough, dyspnoea and putrid or sour-tasting sputum in lung abscesses. Many clinicians empirically cover patients with minor haemoptysis (and no other apparent cause) with a course of antibiotics.	− Sputum and blood cultures − Consider CT thorax − Bronchoscopy can be helpful
− **Other**: Fungi (e.g., aspergilloma and others) and parasites (e.g., paragonimiasis and leptospirosis).	− As per clinical suspicion − Consider bronchoscopy and bronchoalveolar lavage especially if there are cavitatory opacities

- **Autoimmune disease**: Can cause diffuse alveolar haemorrhage, which may be seen on CXR as lung infiltrates (Figure 4.2j). These include the anti-neutrophil cytoplasmic antibody (ANCA) vasculitides (e.g., granulomatosis with polyangiitis, i.e., Wegener's granulomatosis), Anti-GBM disease (Goodpasture's) and others (including lupus, scleroderma, etc.). These disorders tend to involve multiple organs; for example, glomerulonephritis in anti-GBM disease, or sinusitis, otitis media, rash, purpura and neuropathy in Wegener's granulomatosis.

  - UFEME for haematuria
  - Autoantibodies: antinuclear antibody (ANA), ANCA, anti-GBM, dsDNA
  - Screen for other organ involvement: renal panel, liver function studies, coagulation profile
  - Other testing as indicated: skin or kidney biopsy, bronchoscopy

- **Cardiac causes**: A pulmonary oedema CXR picture (Figure 4.2a) prompts consideration of cardiac aetiologies. Elevated pulmonary capillary pressures can cause alveolar capillary rupture and pink frothy haemoptysis. Causes include mitral valve disease especially mitral stenosis, and acute heart failure (haemoptysis is less likely in chronic heart failure, which allows for pulmonary vasculature adaptation). Examine for a murmur.

  - NT-proBNP
  - Echocardiography

(c) CXR: Other Abnormalities

The CXR may reveal other abnormalities

Workup

- **Bronchiectasis***: Chronic productive cough, coarse crepitations, clubbing and CXR showing dilated thickened airways (tram track lines, ring shadows; Figure 7.2c and d). In bronchiectasis, airway dilation brings bronchial arteries closer to mucosal surfaces; erosion of capillary plexus causes blood-streaked sputum, while bronchial artery rupture may give massive bright red haemoptysis.

  - High resolution CT thorax

- **Aortic aneurysm with aortopulmonary fistula**: Suspect if there is a widened mediastinum.

  - CT thorax or CT angiogram

(d) CXR: Normal

A normal CXR does not entirely exclude malignancy. A clinical decision ought to be made on whether to pursue further investigation with high-resolution CT and/or bronchoscopy. Consider the following scenarios

- A patient with first episode haemoptysis, and no risk factors for malignancy: Observation or investigation would both be reasonable; discuss with the patient.

- A patient with infective symptoms suggestive of bronchitis: It would be reasonable to treat infection, and hold off further investigation unless haemoptysis persists.
- Haemoptysis in a chronic smoker or with strong family history of lung cancer: Pursue high-resolution CT and/or bronchoscopy.
- Persistent haemoptysis: Proceed with high-resolution CT and/or bronchoscopy.

Persistent haemoptysis with normal CT: Aetiologies in this scenario include

- Pulmonary embolism: Haemoptysis is an uncommon presentation.
- Pulmonary hypertension.
- Pulmonary endometriosis: Monthly haemoptysis in a reproductive-aged lady.
- Systemic coagulopathy: Usually not sufficient to cause haemoptysis on its own.

 Using what you have learnt, **pen down your approach** to the Clinical Case at the start of the chapter **BEFORE reading the discussion** below.

Case Discussion

This is a smoker with a first episode of haemoptysis, and no other symptoms. First, confirm that he has haemoptysis, not haematemesis or epistaxis. Quantify the volume of haemoptysis—if massive, he may require intubation for airway protection, bronchoscopy and bronchial artery embolisation.

If non-massive, begin with history, examination and a CXR. If CXR shows upper lobe fibrosis suggestive of TB, isolate the patient and obtain sputum for acid-fast bacilli smears, cultures and TB PCR. If CXR shows a nodule, evaluate with CT thorax and consider bronchoscopic or transthoracic biopsy. Even if CXR is normal, he is at high risk of malignancy; consider offering CT thorax, with re-evaluation after a course of empiric antibiotics.

Key Lessons	1. Massive haemoptysis threatens the airway. Patients should be intubated, and undergo bronchial artery embolisation ± bronchoscopy.
	2. The commonest causes of haemoptysis are cancer, TB, bronchitis and bronchiectasis. A CXR is helpful in stratifying the possible causes of haemoptysis.
	3. Many cases of haemoptysis require further investigation with CT thorax or bronchoscopy.
Common Pitfalls	1. Mistaking haematemesis for haemoptysis.
	2. Failure to recognise that a normal CXR does not exclude malignancy.
Questions	1. **REFLECT!** Have you ever seen a patient with haemoptysis? How did you assess if his/her airway is under threat?

2. **EXPLORE!** What are the risks of bronchial artery embolisation? Why is it only performed for massive haemoptysis, whereas no haemostatic methods are not discussed in non-massive haemoptysis?

3. **GO FURTHER!** In a patient with haemoptysis, pulmonary nodules should generally be investigated. Do asymptomatic pulmonary nodules always require further investigation?

Gut and Abdomen

Chapter 9 An Approach to Abdominal Pain

Clinical Case

A 23-year-old female presents with a 1-day history of right iliac fossa (RIF) pain. Her pain has progressively worsened over the past 8 hr and she is now unable to walk. She also complains of nausea and vomiting, but does not have any diarrhoea, rectal bleeding or abdominal distension. She has no past medical history. On examination, her vitals are: BP 112/71, HR 121, T 38.1, RR 18. She appears diaphoretic and pale. Abdominal examination is significant for tenderness and guarding over the RIF. No masses are palpable. Bowel sounds are sluggish. What are your differentials, and how would you approach her abdominal pain?

Abdominal pain is not an easy symptom to approach. The abdomen consists of many structures, each of which may cause pain—some serious, others not. Danger lurks at every corner for it may well be an acute abdomen requiring emergent surgery, a gynaecological surprise, or a medical cause arising from anywhere but the abdomen. Helpful strategies include

- Identify unwell patients early, and evaluate for the most life-threatening causes first.

- **Pattern recognition of symptom complexes** helps to narrow down the differentials—for instance, pelvic pain with vaginal bleeding suggests a gynaecological cause, right upper quadrant pain with jaundice and fever is cholangitis until proven otherwise, generalised colic with abdominal distension, constipation and vomiting suggests intestinal obstruction.

- Have a **systematic approach** to avoid missing anything important—one technique is to consider differentials in organ systems (gastrointestinal [GI], urological, reproductive and others) and categories (e.g., structural vs. non-structural).

- Keep an open mind, and do not 'rule out' diagnoses too early. Be aware that certain findings (e.g., nausea, leucocytosis, dysuria) are 'soft' signs and often non-specific. Remember that a normal CT abdomen does not guarantee the absence of serious pathology—critical entities (diabetic ketoacidosis [DKA], testicular torsion, etc.) may elude the CT scanner!

Two methods are useful: (1) a systematic approach, and (2) pattern-recognition of symptom complex.

Method 1: The Systematic Approach

Clinical categories of abdominal pain: The causes of abdominal pain can be divided into

1. **Acute generalised peritonitis**: A sick patient who suddenly developed severe abdominal pain, exacerbated by movement or palpation. On examination, the abdomen is guarded with board-like rigidity, but signs can be subtle in the elderly or obtunded. A rigid abdomen is important to recognise; it indicates widespread peritoneal irritation by intraperitoneal blood or inflammatory fluid—often the result of a catastrophic event.

2. **Acute non-peritonitic abdominal pain**: Pain may be vaguely localised, or focal ± localised guarding. Crucially, the rest of the abdomen is soft.

3. **Episodic abdominal pain**: Episodic recurrences of abdominal pain with complete resolution in between.

4. **Chronic progressive abdominal pain**.

In each category, consider the causes of abdominal pain by system—whether upper GI, lower GI, urological, testicular (in men), gynaecological (in women) and other causes (Table 9.1).

Method 2: Pattern Recognition of Symptom Complexes

Using a symptom complex facilitates rapid pattern recognition and clinical decision-making. It is most useful in classical presentations of straightforward cases. Where history is vague, presentation is atypical, or available information contradicts, it may be necessary to fall back on a more systematic approach, pursuing multiple possible differentials in parallel. Always keep an open mind, and do not jump to conclusions if there is insufficient evidence.

A suggested algorithm is outlined (Figure 9.1 for acute abdominal pain, Figure 9.5 for episodic abdominal pain). In acute abdominal pain

- First distinguish peritonitic vs. non-peritonitic acute abdominal pain. Peritonitis suggests either a surgical emergency or infected peritoneal fluid, both of which require urgent intervention.

- Consider the 'cannot miss' diagnoses early, via deliberate examination and simple investigations. These 'cannot miss' diagnoses are easy to miss, often with serious consequences, but also easy to exclude if searched for.

- Then identify if abdominal pain is (a) focal or non-localised, (b) colicky (i.e., waxing and waning with pain-free intervals, which is characteristic of intermittent peristaltic contractions of hollow viscera) or constant and (c) if there are any localising symptoms (e.g., jaundice, vaginal discharge, dysuria).

1. Acute Generalised Peritonitis

These are catastrophic pathologies with widespread peritoneal irritation, causing sudden, severe abdominal pain and guarding.

Table 9.1. Causes of Abdominal Pain by Category and Organ System

	Character and time course of abdominal pain			
	1. Acute peritonitic	**2. Acute non-peritonitic**	**3. Episodic**	**4. Chronic progressive**
Gastrointestinal				
Hepatobiliary	Perforated viscus (ulcer, IO, tumour, appendix, diverticulitis)	Cholecystitis Cholangitis Hepatitis Hepatic abscess	Biliary colic	
Pancreatic		Pancreatitis		Pancreatic cancer Chronic pancreatitis
Gastric			Functional dyspepsia Peptic ulcer disease GERD	Gastric cancer
Intestinal		IO Strangulated hernia Appendicitis Diverticulitis Gastroenteritis Constipation colic Adhesion colic Mesenteric ischaemia	IBS IBD Mesenteric ischaemia	Other enlarging masses
Urological	SBP PD peritonitis	Urolithiasis Pyelonephritis Pyonephrosis Urinary retention		
Reproductive				
Male		Testicular torsion Epididymo-orchitis		
Female	Ruptured ectopic pregnancy	Ectopic pregnancy PID Ovarian torsion	Dysmenorrhoea	Ovarian cancer
Others		AMI DKA Dengue Zoster Hypercalcaemia		
	Ruptured AAA	Leaking AAA Adrenal crisis Porphyria	Porphyria	

AAA, abdominal aortic aneurysm; AMI, acute myocardial infarction; DKA, diabetic ketoacidosis; GERD, gastrointestinal reflux disease; IBD, inflammatory bowel disease; IBS, irritable bowel syndrome; IO, intestinal obstruction; PD, peritoneal dialysis; PID, pelvic inflammatory disease; SBP, spontaneous bacterial peritonitis.

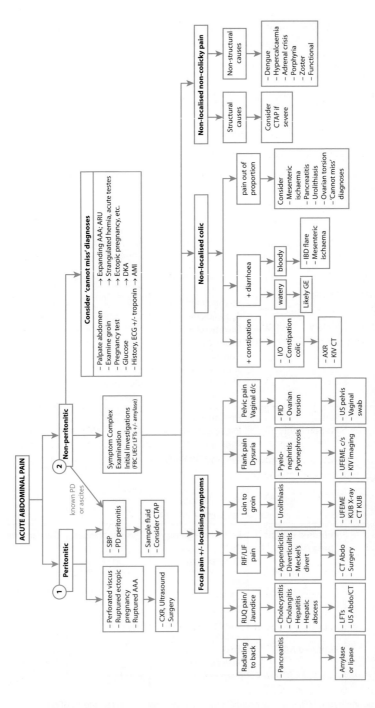

Figure 9.1. Approach to acute abdominal pain by symptom complex.

AAA, abdominal aortic aneurysm; AMI, acute myocardial infarction; ARU, acute retention of urine; DKA, diabetic ketoacidosis; GE, gastroenteritis; IBD, inflammatory bowel disease; I/O, intestinal obstruction; LIF, left iliac fossa; PID, pelvic inflammatory disease; RIF, right iliac fossa; RUQ, right upper quadrant.

Aetiologies

- **Perforated viscus**: Just about any GI organ can perforate, spilling digestive contents, bacteria or blood throughout the peritoneum. Culprits include

    − Perforated intestinal obstruction: Due to pressure build up, especially in a closed-loop obstruction.

    − Perforated peptic ulcer: Due to erosion of the ulcer through the stomach or duodenal wall.

    − Ruptured appendix or diverticulitis.

    − Ruptured hepatocellular carcinoma.

- **Ruptured abdominal aortic aneurysm (AAA)**: Presents with severe peritonitis and hypotension from blood loss. At times, however, the presentation is non-classical (especially with retroperitoneal rupture, in the elderly or obtunded). Many patients do not survive long enough to undergo treatment.

- **Ruptured ectopic pregnancy**: Classically vaginal bleeding plus abdominal pain, but vaginal bleeding is not always present. Pregnancy is frequently a surprise to the patient—but it should not catch a wary physician by surprise!

- **Spontaneous bacterial peritonitis (SBP) and peritoneal dialysis (PD) related peritonitis**: Patients on PD, or who have ascites (e.g., from liver cirrhosis) may develop bacterial infection of the intra-peritoneal fluid. This may present with generalised severe peritonitis, or with abdominal pain of lesser severity.

Approach

Bedside tests: After resuscitating the patient, consider

- **Pregnancy test** in a female of child-bearing age (do not accept a history of celibacy or faithful contraceptive use as a reason to omit a pregnancy test). Generalised peritonitis with a positive pregnancy test should be assumed to be a ruptured ectopic pregnancy, until proven otherwise.

- **Bedside ultrasound (US)** to identify intra-abdominal free fluid.

- **Erect chest X-ray**: May reveal air under the diaphragm (Figure 9.2), indicating intra-abdominal perforation. This is also seen in PD patients, or if there is recent abdominal surgery, and may not indicate perforation in these circumstances.

Suspected perforated viscus, AAA or ruptured ectopic pregnancy:

- If there is a high clinical suspicion—emergent laparotomy is the diagnostic and therapeutic modality of choice.

- If the clinical situation is more doubtful—consider contrasted abdominal CT, if it can be obtained urgently. This should not delay laparotomy where indicated. Note that impaired renal function may preclude contrasted CT; a non-contrast CT is frequently not helpful; very often, all that is seen is free air and fluid suggestive of a perforated viscus, which does not add very much to the clinical indication for laparotomy.

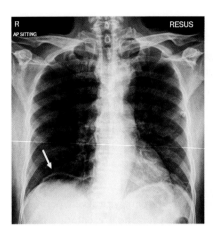

Figure 9.2. Air under diaphragm. A 40-year-old man presented with severe abdominal pain and guarding. He was too unwell to do an erect chest X-ray; a sitting film shows air under the right hemidiaphragm. Laparotomy eventually revealed a perforated peptic ulcer.

Suspected SBP or PD peritonitis:

- **Sample peritoneal fluid**: Peritoneal fluid may be obtained via a diagnostic para-centesis (in SBP), or through the Tenckhoff catheter (for PD peritonitis—drain existing PD fluid or dwell dialysate for 2 hr). Fluid should be sent for cell count and differential, biochemistry (albumin, protein, glucose), gram stain and culture.

  - SBP is diagnosed in a patient with ascites and a cloudy ascitic tap, ascitic fluid neutrophils > 250 cells/mm^3 or positive gram stain.

  - PD peritonitis is diagnosed in a patient on PD who has a cloudy effluent, PD cell count > 100 cells/mm^3 (0.1 cells/mL), neutrophils > 50% (even if cell count < 100 cells/mm^3) or positive gram stain. (Observe that these criteria are stricter than for SBP.)

- **Consider secondary bacterial peritonitis**: Patients on PD or with ascites may still develop 'surgical' peritonitis (e.g., perforated viscus, diverticulitis, etc.) with spillage of gut flora. Features worrisome for secondary bacterial peritonitis include (i) focal abdominal symptoms suggestive of surgical causes, (ii) sudden onset of symptoms, (iii) polymicrobial gram stain or culture result, (iv) very low glucose (< 2.8 mmol/L) or very high protein (> 1 g/dL in ascitic fluid). If there is concern for secondary bac-terial peritonitis, consider performing CT abdomen to look for a perforated viscus.

- Other causes of acute abdominal pain should also be considered, including diabetic ketoacidosis (DKA), myocardial infarction and so forth.

2. Acute Non-Peritonitic Abdominal Pain

Warning: The causes of acute peritonitic abdominal pain should always be considered before moving on to this section!

The Concept of 'Cannot Miss' Diagnoses

These serious conditions can be missed, because their symptoms are non-specific and may not lead one to suspect the diagnosis. On the other hand, they are easy to exclude on bedside examination or point-of-care tests. It is advantageous to look for these diagnoses early and deliberately. In any patient presenting with acute abdominal pain, remember to do the following.

(a) **Palpate the abdomen**: Deliberately look for

- **Peritonitis** (see page 89).

- **AAA**: Look for an expansile pulsatile midline mass, radio-femoral delay and 'trash feet' (embolic infarcts or hypoperfusion to the toes). AAAs are commonly asymptomatic and cause pain only if rapidly expanding or leaking; it should not always be assumed to be the cause of abdominal pain.

  Workup
  - Bedside ultrasound
  - CT aortogram

- **Acute urinary retention**: Examine for a palpable bladder. Somewhat embarrassing if only diagnosed on CT scan.

(b) **Examine the groin**:

- **Strangulated hernia**: Look for a hernia. Most hernias are asymptomatic, but if tender, erythematous and irreducible, strangulation must be suspected.

- **Acute testes**:

  o **Testicular torsion**: The testis is tender, high-riding and lies transversely, with loss of cremasteric reflex. This is more common in post-pubertal teenage boys, in whom an acute testes should be assumed to be torsion until proven otherwise.

    - Doppler US shows absence of blood flow
    - Surgical exploration

  o **Epididymo-orchitis**: Pain develops more gradually, and is associated with symptoms of a urinary tract infection (e.g., fever and dysuria). The testis is not high riding and does not lie transversely. More common in older men.

    - Urine: pyuria

  o **Torsion of appendix testes** (cyst of Morgagni): Tenderness localised to upper pole ± blue dot sign.

(c) **Bedside tests**

- **Pregnancy test (females)**: If positive, consider pregnancy-related diseases especially an ectopic pregnancy, which may rupture.

  − US pelvis for an extra-uterine gestation sac

- **Glucose for DKA**: Abdominal pain is a relatively common presentation.

  − Electrolytes with bicarbonate, glucose and ketones

- **ECG for myocardial infarction**: Pain may be referred to the epigastrium (see Chapter 3).

  − Troponins

The remaining causes of acute non-peritonitic abdominal pain are sorted by organ system. Both the systematic/categorical (Table 9.1) and pattern-recognition approaches (Figure 9.1) should be used in conjunction to arrive at a differential list.

Hepatobiliary Tree Causes

Right upper quadrant pain:

Workup

- **Cholecystitis**: Chemical *inflammation of the gallbladder* (due to irritation by gallstones) causing right upper quadrant pain lasting hours (may radiate to the right shoulder) ± low-grade fever. Murphy's sign is classic (but not sensitive). There may be mild transaminitis, but there should not be marked jaundice.

  − US: gallbladder wall thickening and oedema, calculi *in situ*
  − CTAP usually unnecessary

- **Acute cholangitis**: *Biliary tree infection* causing right hypochondrial pain, fever, jaundice (Charcot's triad) ± shock and altered mental state (Reynold's pentad). There is a cholestatic pattern of raised liver enzymes (alkaline phosphatase [ALP] and gamma-glutamyl transferase [GGT] > alanine aminotransferase [ALT] and aspartate aminotransferase [AST]) and patients are sicker than in cholecystitis. (See Explore! question, page 101.)

  − US or CT demonstrating dilated common bile duct
  − Septic workup, blood cultures
  − Endoscopic retrograde cholangiopancreatogram visualises stones and allows therapeutics

- **Acute hepatitis**: Fever, jaundice, tender small hepatomegaly and non-specific symptoms, for example, nausea/vomiting. Liver enzymes show a marked derangement in a hepatocellular pattern (ALT and AST > ALP). See Chapter 10.

  − Acute hepatitis serology (Hep A IgM, HBsAg, HBcAg, anti-HBs)

- **Hepatic abscess**: Fever, right hypochondrial pain, sometimes with jaundice or hepatomegaly.

  − US or CT rim-enhancing collection
  − Blood cultures

Central pain, radiating to back:

- **Acute pancreatitis**: Steady epigastric and peri-umbilical pain, classically radiating to the back, relieved on bending forward, accompanied by frequent vomiting and persistent nausea. Flank or umbilical bruising (Grey Turner's and Cullen's signs) are rare signs of retroperitoneal haemorrhage. Search for an aetiology—gallstones, alcohol, post-instrumentation and so forth.

  - Amylase (rises earlier, normalises in 3 days) or lipase (stays positive up to 7 days)
  - Severity scoring (e.g., Glasgow)
  - Imaging not required unless to consider differentials or complications

Intestinal Causes

Think of the gut as a tube that can be obstructed, ischaemic, inflamed or infected.

Focal right iliac fossa (RIF) or left iliac fossa (LIF) pain:

Workup

- **Appendicitis**: Classically a dull periumbilical pain (referred pain) that migrates to the RIF, with localised RIF guarding and rebound tenderness. Non-specific symptoms of fever and nausea may be present. The Alvarado score is helpful as a clinical decision tool (Table 9.2).

  - CT abdomen (Figure 9.3), especially if old patient
  - Or: proceed directly to appendectomy (see Discuss!, page 101)

- **Diverticulitis**: LIF or RIF pain, associated with nausea and anorexia. This can form an abscess or even perforate.

  - CT abdomen–pelvis

- **Meckel's diverticulum**: Indistinguishable from acute appendicitis.

Table 9.2. Alvarado Score for Appendicitis

M	Migration	1 pt
A	Anorexia	1 pt
N	Nausea and Vomiting	1 pt
T	Tenderness in R lower quadrant	2 pt
R	Rebound tenderness	1 pt
E	Elevated temperature > 38.0	1 pt
L	Leukocytosis (WBC > 10)	2 pt
S	Shift to left (neutrophil > 75%)	1 pt

Likelihood of Appendicitis:
5–6 possible | **7–8** probable | **9–10** v probable

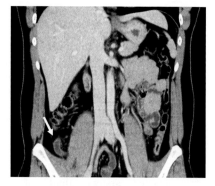

Figure 9.3. CT abdomen—acute appendicitis.

Generalised colic:

- **Intestinal obstruction (IO)**: The four cardinal features are abdominal colic (usually poorly localised), distension, nausea/vomiting and lack of passage of stool or flatus (incomplete IO may allow some output). The clinical tasks are to localise the IO, identify its aetiology and look for complications (see Chapter 12).

  – AXR demonstrates dilated bowel loops (Figure 12.2)

- **Constipation colic**: A diagnosis of exclusion, common in the elderly.

  – AXR shows faecal loading but no overt dilation of bowel loops

- **Adhesion colic**: Patients with prior abdominal surgery may develop adhesions between bowel loops. These may cause intermittent colicky pain, even in the absence of frank intestinal obstruction (i.e., no vomiting, able to pass stool and flatus). This is a diagnosis of exclusion.

Generalised non-specific pain:

- **Mesenteric ischaemia**: The classic scenario is a patient with atrial fibrillation (or other embolic risk factors) who develops severe abdominal pain with a normal abdominal examination (i.e., *pain out of proportion*). As bowel ischaemia progresses, bowel sounds become sluggish, the abdomen distends, peritoneal signs develop and the patient turns hypotensive. This is a difficult diagnosis. Lactate is raised due to tissue hypoperfusion; this is an important clue (tip: always send lactate in a sick patient with abdominal pain).

  – Serum lactate
  – CT mesenteric angiogram

Urological Causes

	Workup
• **Urolithiasis**: Loin to groin colic, often severe, causing patients to roll around in pain. Higher obstruction may result in flank pain rather than loin to groin colic. If there are signs of infection—consider pyonephrosis, a urological emergency.	– X-ray KUB (Figure 9.4a) – Non-contrast CT KUB (Figure 9.4b) – UFEME may show haematuria
• **Pyelonephritis**: Flank pain, fever and positive renal punch. Consider systemic bacteraemia (urosepsis) in a sick patient. If there is an obstructed system, think of pyonephrosis. Pyelonephritis may require further workup to look for anatomical abnormalities (see Chapter 21).	– UFEME – May require further imaging (see Chapter 21)

Figure 9.4. Urolithiasis.

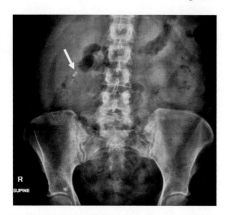
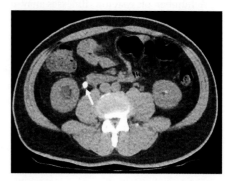

(a) **X-ray**: A 40-year-old lady presented with loin to groin colic. X-ray showed a radiopaque right renal stone (arrow). Not all stones are radio-opaque; radio-lucent (non-calcium) stones may be missed.

(b) **CT**: Non-contrast CT kidneys–ureter–bladder (KUB) was later performed on the same patient. This confirmed a right upper ureteric stone (arrow) with mild right hydronephrosis.

Gynaecological Causes (Female)

Gynaecological causes should be considered in reproductive-aged ladies. The first consideration is to exclude ectopic pregnancy (do a pregnancy test).

With negative pregnancy test: Consider

- **Pelvic inflammatory disease (PID)**: A young, sexually active lady with lower abdominal pain ± features of infection (fever, ↑white blood cell [WBC], ↑C-reactive protein [CRP]). Bimanual pelvic examination may find cervical excitation, adnexal tenderness or adnexal masses (suggests tubo-ovarian abscess), and a vaginal speculum may find vaginal discharge. PID can also present as right hypochondrial pain, should inflammation reach the hepatorenal pouch (Fitz-Hugh–Curtis syndrome).

- **Ovarian torsion and ruptured ovarian cyst**: These conditions both present with acute-onset unilateral pelvic pain ± an adnexal mass. Ovarian torsion is a gynaecological emergency as it can permanently impair ovarian function, but it is a difficult diagnosis.

Workup

- Vaginal discharge microscopy, gonorrhoea and chlamydia PCR
- US pelvis for tubo-ovarian abscesses
- HIV and syphilis screen

- US pelvis: engorged ovary with diminished blood flow (torsion) vs. adnexal mass with free fluid in pelvis (ruptured cyst)
- Surgery if suspected torsion

Other Causes

A number of systemic illnesses may present with non-specific abdominal pain

Workup

- **Dengue**: Abdominal pain is a warning sign, which may heralds the onset of dengue shock syndrome. Suspect dengue in an acute febrile illness with nausea/vomiting, arthralgia/myalgia and rash. If full blood count (FBC) is done, thrombocytopenia is characteristic.

  − Serological confirmation (i.e., dengue PCR and NS1 antigen)

- **Hypercalcaemia**: Abdominal pain is a cardinal feature, along with altered mental state, urolithiasis, bony pain and constipation.

  − Serum calcium
  − Further workup (see Chapter 17)

- **Adrenal crisis**: It can present with abdominal pain. Other clues include borderline hypotension, postural hypotension, hyponatraemia, hyperkalaemia and hypoglycaemia.

  − Take serum electrolytes, cortisol, Adrenocorticotropic hormone, renin, aldosterone (treat while awaiting results)
  − Search for a cause/ precipitant

- **Herpes zoster**: This is hard to diagnose until the characteristic dermatomal rash appears a couple of days later.

- **Pelvic bone injuries**: A pelvic or hip fracture may masquerade as lower abdominal pain.

  − X-ray pelvis

- **Porphyria and related disorders**: Acute intermittent porphyria arises from impaired heme metabolism due to an enzyme defect. It presents with acute-onset abdominal pain, red–brown urine and neurological symptoms (neuropathy, autonomic dysfunction, seizures, coma). Lead poisoning presents with similar symptoms.

  − Begin with urinary porphobilinogen (further testing to differentiate the porphyrias is out of the scope of this text)

When No Serious Organic Cause Is Found

This is a relatively common scenario. Many patients present acutely with mild, non-specific epigastric or peri-umbilical pain, a soft abdomen and normal blood tests (omitted in primary care, but usually done if the patient presents to Emergency); no specific clinical entity is suspected, and the patient responds to symptomatic treatment. The majority of these patients have either functional dyspepsia or a self-limiting viral illness, and can indeed be safely sent home. It would be unreasonable to investigate every one. What is important is—(1) to be sure to exclude the 'cannot miss' diagnoses especially ectopic pregnancy, DKA and myocardial infarction, (2) ensure that the abdomen is truly soft and (3) be prepared to re-assess if pain worsens or new symptoms develop (i.e., provide appropriate return advice to the patient).

3. Episodic Abdominal Pain

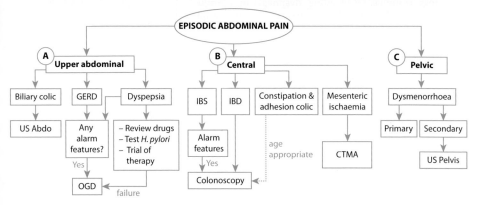

CTMA, CT mesenteric angiogram; GERD, gastroesophageal reflux disease; IBD, inflammatory bowel disease; IBS, irritable bowel syndrome; OGD, oesophagogastroduodenoscopy.

Figure 9.5. Approach to episodic abdominal pain.

(a) Episodic Upper Abdominal Pain

These aetiologies present in well patients with normal blood tests (liver enzymes, bilirubin and amylase). It can be classified into three main symptomologies: biliary colic, gastroesophageal reflux (GERD) and dyspepsia.

	Workup
• **Biliary colic**: This is episodic right hypochondrial or epigastric pain, often after fatty meals, peaking over an hour and then resolving. 'Colic' is a misnomer, the pain of biliary 'colic' is constant without pain-free intervals. There may be nausea and vomiting, but no jaundice, and liver enzymes are normal.	− US to demonstrate biliary stones
• **GERD**: Typical symptoms are post-prandial epigastric or retrosternal discomfort, exacerbated by lying flat, with regurgitation of acidic gastric contents into the oropharynx (leading to a sour taste). It may also present with cough or chest pain.	− Generally a clinical diagnosis − Oesophagogastroduodenoscopy (OGD) if concerned about oesophageal cancer (anaemia, weight loss, dysphagia, vomiting)
• **Dyspepsia**: This is a poorly characterised symptom of epigastric pain and/or post-prandial fullness, and/or early satiety. The majority of cases are functional (i.e., no structural GI disease), but dyspepsia may also arise from peptic ulcers,	− Stop contributory drugs (e.g., NSAIDS) − Test and treat for H pylori

gastric cancer and other sinister causes. *Alarm features* including age > 60 years, anaemia, weight loss, jaundice, GI bleeding, dysphagia or a family history of upper GI malignancy would prompt further investigation. In the absence of alarm features, a positive diagnosis of functional dyspepsia can be made without unnecessary endoscopy or scans.

— OGD if alarm symptoms present, or empiric therapy fails

(b) Episodic Central Abdominal Pain

Workup

- **Irritable bowel syndrome (IBS)**: Recurrent abdominal pain (1 or more days/week in last 3 months), classically relieved by defecation, with changes in stool frequency and consistency (either predominant constipation, predominant diarrhoea or alternating constipation and diarrhoea). It is a clinical diagnosis.

  — Nil if no alarm symptoms
  — Colonoscopy if there are alarm features, for example, age > 50 years, rectal bleeding, bloody diarrhoea, anaemia, weight loss

- **Inflammatory bowel disease**: Crohn's Disease and ulcerative colitis present with flares of abdominal colic and bloody diarrhoea (see Chapter 13).

  — Colonoscopy (see Chapter 13)

- **Mesenteric ischaemia**: Post-prandial abdominal pain and nausea, with weight loss and food aversion. Patients often have atherosclerotic risk factors.

  — Doppler US or CT mesenteric angiogram demonstrates arterial occlusion

- **Constipation colic**: Colicky pain associated with severe constipation, relieved by defecation. This is a diagnosis of exclusion, more common in the elderly.

  — Advocate for age-appropriate colonoscopic screening

- **Adhesion colic**: Intermittent colicky pain, without other signs of intestinal obstruction, in a patient with prior abdominal surgery. Another diagnosis of exclusion.

  — Advocate for age-appropriate colonoscopic screening

(c) Episodic Pelvic Pain

Workup

- **Dysmenorrhoea** may be a cause of cyclical pelvic pain in females. This may be primary, or secondary to endometriosis or leiomyoma (fibroids). These secondary causes may also feature heavy menstrual bleeding, and examination may find pouch of Douglas tenderness, adnexal masses or an enlarged uterus (see Chapter 52).

  — Transvaginal US if suspecting secondary causes

4. Chronic Progressive Abdominal Pain

This symptomology is worrisome for a relentlessly worsening disease process.

Malignant causes: Should these present as chronic abdominal pain, disease is usually advanced.

- **Gastric cancer:** Asymptomatic early, then vague constant epigastric pain, with no relationship to meals. Friable malignant tissue may bleed, causing anaemia, haematemesis and melena. Late symptoms include early satiety, vomiting of undigested food (in gastric outlet obstruction or linitis plastica), dysphagia (in tumours near the cardia), loss of appetite and weight or symptoms from metastatic disease.

- **Pancreatic cancer:** A cancer in the body or tail of pancreas presents late, with severe weight loss and constitutional symptoms, as well as chronic progressive epigastric pain radiating to the back (vs. head of pancreas tumour, which more likely presents with obstructive jaundice).

- **Ovarian cancer:** Patients present late with abdominal distension, palpable pelvic mass and mass-related symptoms (bloating, discomfort, constipation, urinary frequency) and constitutional symptoms (weight loss and anorexia).

- **Hepatocellular carcinoma:** Capsular stretch can cause abdominal pain. There may not be jaundice until very late. Patients with chronic hepatitis and cirrhosis are at elevated risk.

- **Other enlarging masses:** For example, atypical presentations of colon cancer (usually change in bowel habit or anaemia rather than abdominal pain).

Non-malignant causes:

- **Chronic pancreatitis:** Epigastric pain, steatorrhoea (pancreatic exocrine insufficiency) and new-onset or worsening diabetes (endocrine insufficiency). Patients may have significant weight loss, mimicking pancreatic cancer. Abdominal imaging reveals pancreatic calcification.

- **Gynaecological disease:** Endometriosis may be chronic instead of episodic (see page 98), and pelvic inflammatory disease (page 95) may not show features of acute infection.

Approach: Suspicion of these aetiologies would prompt abdominal CT as the diagnostic modality of choice.

Using what you have learnt, **pen down your approach** to the Clinical Case at the start of the chapter **BEFORE reading the discussion** below.

Case Discussion

This is a young, reproductive-aged female with acute right iliac fossa (RIF) pain and guarding. The critical differentials are appendicitis and ectopic pregnancy (which may have ruptured, considering her pallor and tachycardia). Other differentials include

- *GI—diverticulitis, Meckel's diverticulum, Crohn's disease (more likely to have had prior episodes).*
- *Gynaecological—ovarian torsion, pelvic inflammatory disease (PID) ± tubo-ovarian abscess.*
- *Renal colic and DKA are less likely to cause focal RIF signs.*

The next step is a pregnancy test to rule out ectopic pregnancy. Once this is ruled out, the most likely diagnosis becomes appendicitis (consider CT scan—see DISCUSS! below). If her pain worsens and she develops generalised abdominal guarding, consider ruptured appendicitis.

Key Lessons	1. Recognise a peritonitic abdomen. It suggests a surgical emergency (e.g., perforated viscus, ruptured aortic aneurysm or ruptured ectopic pregnancy), or infected peritoneal fluid (spontaneous bacterial peritonitis or PD-related peritonitis).
	2. In acute abdominal pain, consider differentials from every organ system (gastrointestinal, urological, reproductive, and others. Attention to the nature of pain (focal vs. generalised, colic vs. non-colicky) and localising symptoms is helpful in narrowing the differentials.
	3. Episodic abdominal pain in an otherwise well patient with normal blood tests is often functional, but pay attention to alarm symptoms which would prompt further investigation.
	4. Chronic progressive abdominal pain is worrisome for malignancy or other worsening disease processes.
Common Pitfalls	1. Every patient with *severe* acute abdominal pain must have his/her abdomen palpated (for AAA), groin examined (for hernia, testicular torsion) and sent for pregnancy testing, glucose and ECG. Missed diagnoses are common, especially in the elderly.
	2. A normal CT abdomen does not guarantee the absence of serious pathology. It may miss mesenteric ischaemia (send lactate), testicular torsion, early pancreatitis and non-structural causes (e.g., AMI and DKA).

Questions

1. **EXPLORE!** Gallstones present in many different ways. *Cholelithiasis* refers to the presence of gallstones in the gallbladder, which can cause pain (*biliary colic*) if impacted against the gallbladder outlet. This can result in chemical inflammation of the gallbladder—*cholecystitis*—which, left long enough, becomes infected. Stones leaving the gallbladder may lodge in the common bile duct—*choledocholithiasis*. If this is distal and blocks the pancreatic duct, *gallstone pancreatitis* ensues. Finally, stasis of bile flow predisposes to ascending infection of the biliary tree—*cholangitis*. Compare and contrast the features of these entities by completing the table.

	Location of gallstone	Nature of pain	Jaundice?	Fever?	Liver enzymes
Biliary colic		Episodic post-meal RHC pain			
Cholecystitis				None or mild	
Choledocho-lithiasis	Common bile duct—blocks biliary drainage				
Cholangitis			Yes		Elevated, cholestatic picture
Gallstone pancreatitis			No		

2. **EXPLORE!** What are the most important diagnoses to consider in a patient who presents with abdominal pain and hypotension? What will your approach be?

3. **DISCUSS!** Appendicitis was traditionally a clinical diagnosis, with high clinical suspicion prompting appendectomy and uncertain cases subjected to serial abdominal examination (with the expectation that in appendicitis, RIF tenderness declares itself with time). However, the current trend is that all patients receive a CT scan for confirmation of diagnosis. Discuss the advantages and downsides of CTAP prior to appendectomy in (a) a 70-year-old man with recent functional decline, and (b) an 18-year-old boy with no prior medical history.

4. **GO FURTHER!** Bedside US is emerging as a rapid diagnostic tool. In the approach to abdominal pain, how might a bedside US be helpful?

Chapter
10

An Approach to Jaundice and Abnormal Liver Function Tests

Clinical Case

A previously well 30-year-old gentleman presents with a 1-week history of jaundice, discoloured urine and malaise. Liver function tests (LFTs) reveal bilirubin 65 mmol/L (direct 50 mmol/L), albumin 38 g/L, aspartate aminotransferase (AST) 184 IU/L, alanine amino-transferase (ALT) 265 IU/L and alkaline phosphatase (ALP) 80 IU/L. How would you approach his complaint?

There are a hundred causes of jaundice and/or abnormal liver enzymes—surgical hepatobiliary disease, various causes of liver injury and haematological disease with haemolysis—but a few basic principles are sufficient for one to begin telling these causes apart (Figure 10.1).

Distinguishing Pre-Hepatic, Hepatic and Post-Hepatic Jaundice

The first step is to distinguish pre-hepatic, hepatic and post-hepatic jaundice (Table 10.1).

1. Pre-Hepatic Jaundice

Raised unconjugated bilirubin may be due to increased bilirubin production, or impaired hepatic uptake.

(a) **Is there haemolysis?** A classic example would be the patient with G6PD deficiency who develops jaundice after inadvertently taking trimethoprim–sulphamethoxazole (Bactrim), which causes haemolysis. Look for

- **Predisposition or known haemolytic disease**: G6PD deficiency, thalassemia, chronic lymphoid leukaemia, recent exposure to drugs causing haemolysis, recent blood transfusion and so forth.

- **Biochemical evidence of haemolysis**: Apart from raised unconjugated bili-rubin, this includes raised lactate dehydrogenase (LDH), low haptoglobin, raised reticulocyte count, peripheral blood film findings of haemolysis (e.g., schistocytes and bite cells) and a positive direct Coombs' test.

The causes of and approach to haemolytic anaemia are discussed in Chapter 32.

(b) **Look for causes of impaired hepatic uptake**. If there is no evidence of haemolysis, consider other causes of impaired hepatic uptake of bilirubin.

- **Medications**: For example, rifampicin and probenecid.

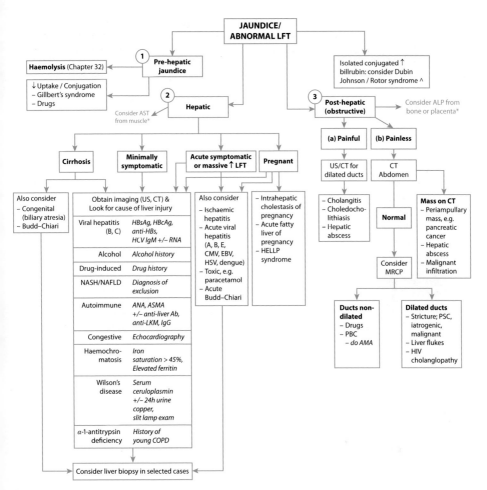

*Aspartate aminotransferase (AST) and alkaline phosphatase (ALP) are not liver-specific. Isolated raised AST or ALP, with the other liver function test (LFT) components normal, should prompt consideration of non-liver disease.

- **AST**: AST is found in muscle (cardiac and skeletal), blood, kidney and brain. In a patient with isolated raised AST (and normal alanine aminotransferase [ALT], bilirubin), consider rhabdomyolysis, myositis and myocardial infarction. ALT is a more specific marker of liver injury than AST.
- **ALP**: ALP is found in liver, bone and placenta. In isolated raised ALP, consider bone disease (e.g., osteomyelitis, fracture, hyperparathyroidism) and pregnancy. To distinguish liver from other sources of ALP, (i) perform gamma-glutamyl transferase (GGT)—elevated GGT suggests that ALP is of liver origin, or (ii) fractionate ALP into heat stable (liver) vs. heat labile (bone) fractions.

^Isolated conjugated hyperbilirubinaemia in a well patient, with normal AST, ALT and ALP, may be due to Dubin–Johnson syndrome or Rotor syndrome. These are rare genetic conditions, which do not require treatment. Other conditions, including cirrhosis, should first be excluded.

ALP, alkaline phosphatase; ALT, alanine aminotransferase; ANA, antinuclear antibody; ASMA, anti smooth muscle antibody; AST, aspartate aminotransferase; LDH, lactate dehydrogenase; LFTs, liver function tests; MRCP, magnetic resonance cholangiopancreatography; NAFLD, non-alcoholic fatty liver disease; NASH, non-alcoholic steatohepatitis; PBC, primary biliary cholangitis; PSC, primary sclerosing cholangitis.

Figure 10.1. Approach to jaundice and abnormal LFTs.

Table 10.1. Pre-Hepatic, Hepatic and Post-Hepatic Jaundice

	1. Pre-hepatic	2. Hepatic	3. Post-hepatic
Patho-physiology	Increased bilirubin production or impaired liver uptake	Hepatocyte damage and impaired function	Obstruction to biliary flow
Bilirubin type	Unconjugated (indirect) *Rate of bilirubin production exceeds that of hepatic conjugation*	Conjugated (direct) *As the rate limiting step is excretion, not conjugation, liver disease results in increased conjugated bilirubin*	
Pattern of deranged LFT	LFTs normal *The liver is normal*	Hepatocellular pattern: ↑↑AST and ALT > ↑ALP *AST and ALT are found in hepatocytes and are released when hepatocyte damage occurs*	Cholestatic pattern: ↑↑ALP >> ALT and AST *ALP is found on the hepatic canalicular membrane, and is released when there is bile stasis*
Urine and stool colour	Normal urine (dark in intravascular haemolysis with haemoglobinuria)	Tea-coloured urine *Only conjugated bilirubin is water-soluble and excreted in urine*	Dark urine Pale stools if obstruction is near-total
Other clinical features	May have haemolysis (anaemia, ↑LDH)	Ascites, coagulopathy, encephalopathy	Pruritus may be prominent

ALP, alkaline phosphatase; ALT, alanine aminotransferase; AST, aspartate aminotransferase; LDH, lactate dehydrogenase; LFTs, liver function tests.

- **Gilbert's syndrome**: This is a genetic defect of UDP-glucuronyltransferase, resulting in decreased hepatic conjugation of bilirubin, which can be more marked in times of stress. A presumptive diagnosis can be made in an asymptomatic patient with mildly elevated unconjugated bilirubin levels and otherwise normal LFTs, if haemolysis and medications causing raised bilirubin are excluded. It is a benign disorder with no untoward consequence. Additional evaluation is not routinely necessary.

2. Hepatic Jaundice/Hepatocellular Pattern of Raised LFT

Conjugated hyperbilirubinaemia with raised ALT and AST reflects hepatocellular injury. Note that the normal upper limit of ALT is 29 to 33 IU/L for males and 19 to 25 IU/L for females. Levels above this are associated with increased liver-related mortality and should be investigated.

Clinical Syndromes

Hepatic injury may be acute or chronic, fulminant or subclinical. Consider this range of clinical syndromes

- **Minimally symptomatic**: Many patients have minimal symptoms.

- **Cirrhosis**: Recurrent episodes of liver damage and regeneration results in gradual progression from chronic hepatitis to fibrosis and eventually cirrhosis. Look for evidence of cirrhosis (Table 10.2) especially splenomegaly, ascites, thrombocytopenia and features of chronic hyperoestrogenism. Abdominal imaging reveals liver nodularity. Severity of cirrhosis may be graded by the Child–Pugh and *M*odel of *E*nd-stage *L*iver *D*isease (MELD) scoring systems.

- **Acute symptomatic**: Some patients present with an acute onset of jaundice or fulminant liver failure (encephalopathy, coagulopathy, hypoglycaemia; Table 10.2). This can occur *de novo*, or from a new insult superimposed on chronic hepatitis/cirrhosis.

- **Massive transaminitis**: While 4- or 5-digit AST and ALT levels inspire fear, liver dysfunction (coagulopathy, hypoglycaemia, etc.) provides a far better reflection of disease severity than AST/ALT levels *per se*. Massive transaminitis tends to be seen in ischaemic, viral and toxic (especially paracetamol) causes.

- **Hepatic jaundice in pregnancy**: A number of additional differentials apply.

Table 10.2. Complications of Liver Dysfunction

Mechanism	Complication	Present in acute liver injury?	Present in cirrhosis?
Synthetic dysfunction	Hypoalbuminaemia	At times (albumin is a negative phase reactant)	Almost always
	Coagulopathy	Yes	Yes
	Hypoglycaemia	Yes (a late feature)	Yes (a late feature)
Catabolic dysfunction	Encephalopathy	Yes	Yes
	Hyperoestrogenism	No	Yes, e.g., gynaecomastia, spider naevi, testicular atrophy, loss of axillary hair
Portal hypertension	Splenomegaly	No	Yes
	Ascites	No	Yes
	Oesophageal varices	No	Yes
	Thrombocytopenia	Not directly due to liver injury	Yes (due to hypersplenism)

Aetiology

A workup for the aetiology of liver injury begins with a history for liver insults (alcohol, drugs, sexual history, IV drug use, family history), examination for features of cirrhosis and multi-organ disease, serological tests (Table 10.3) and abdominal imaging (ultrasound or CT). Liver biopsy may be considered to confirm a diagnosis, when diagnosis is unclear or multiple diagnoses are possible, or to stage a condition.

Table 10.3. Aetiologies of Hepatic Jaundice/Hepatocellular Pattern of Transaminitis

Aetiology	Time course	Comments	Workup
Viral	Chronic with acute flares	Hepatitis B and C. May be transmitted vertically (mother–child), sexually or blood-borne (e.g., IV drug use).	HBsAg, HBcAg, anti-HBs, HCV IgM ± RNA
	Acute	Hepatitis A, B and E CMV, EBV, HSV and dengue	HBsAg, HBcAg, anti-HBs Hepatitis A and E IgM CMV, EBV, HSV, dengue
Alcoholic	Chronic with acute flares	Longstanding heavy alcohol use (> 100 g/day). AST:ALT ratio typically > 2. There may be tender hepatomegaly and fever	—
Toxic/drug	Acute or chronic, mild or fulminant	Many drugs, including paracetamol, TB drugs (pyrazinamide, rifampicin, isoniazid), anti-epileptics and traditional medicine	Paracetamol levels (plot on Rumack–Matthew nomogram) Toxicology screen (blood and urine)
Ischaemic	1–3 days after insult	Precipitated by hypotensive episode (e.g., sepsis). Transaminitis can be massive but resolves over a week	—
Congestive	Chronic	Patients with severe right heart failure, tricuspid regurgitation	Echocardiogram
Non-alcoholic fatty liver disease/ steatohepatitis	Chronic, usually insidious, can progress to cirrhosis	Common and under-recognised. Patients often have metabolic risk factors. A diagnosis of exclusion—exclude viral, alcoholic and other causes	Screen hypertension, diabetes, hyperlipi-daemia, obesity

(Cont'd)

Aetiology	Time course	Comments	Workup
Autoimmune	Acute or chronic, mild or fulminant	Diagnosis made based on autoantibodies, elevated IgG, exclusion of viral hepatitis ± biopsy. There may be other auto-immune disease	ANA, ASMA, immuno-globulin levels ± anti-LKM, anti-liver Ab
Hemochromatosis	Chronic	Hereditary or secondary to chronic iron overload (e.g., recurrent transfusions in thalassemia). Apart from hepatitis/cirrhosis, there may be endocrine disease (diabetes, hypopituitarism, hypogonadism), cardiomyopathy, pseudogout/arthropathy and bronzing of skin	Screen: Iron saturation (> 45%), ferritin (> 200 ng/mL in men, > 150 ng/mL in women) Confirmatory: gene testing for hereditary hemochromatosis
Wilson's disease	Acute or chronic	Young patient with liver disease, neurologic features (dysarthria, cerebellar, extrapyramidal and psychiatric) and haemolytic anaemia. There may be a family history	Screen: serum ceruloplasmin, 24 hr urine copper, slit lamp exam for Kayser–Fleischer rings
α-1-Antitrypsin deficiency	Chronic	Consider in a patient with history of young COPD	Serum α-1-antitrypsin levels or genetic testing
Budd–Chiari syndrome	Acute, subacute or chronic	Hepatic vein obstruction, most commonly thrombotic. Acute Budd–Chiari syndrome presents with RHC pain, hepatomegaly and acute liver failure. Subacute or chronic Budd–Chiari syndrome presents with ascites and features of cirrhosis	Hepatic venous Doppler ultrasound Evaluate for aetiology: hypercoagulable state, hepatocellular carcinoma, extrinsic compression
Congenital	Chronic	e.g., biliary atresia	

ANA, antinuclear antibody; anti-LKM, anti-liver-kidney microsome-1 antibody; ASMA, anti-smooth muscle antibody; CMV, cytomegalovirus; EBV, Epstein–Barr virus; HSV, Herpes simplex virus; RHC, right hypochondrial.

Additional considerations in pregnancy: In addition to the earlier causes of liver injury, consider

- **Intrahepatic cholestasis of pregnancy**: Presents in second to third trimester with pruritus and raised bilirubin, but women are otherwise well.

- **Acute fatty liver of pregnancy**: Presents in third trimester with liver dysfunction (jaundice, elevated AST/ALT, coagulopathy), abdominal pain, nausea/vomiting and often renal impairment.

- **HELLP syndrome**: Presents in third trimester with *h*aemolysis, *e*levated *L*FTs and *l*ow *p*latelets. This is thought to be a severe form of pre-eclampsia, often with hypertension, proteinuria, abdominal pain and vomiting.

3. Post-Hepatic Jaundice/Obstructive Pattern of Raised LFT

Conjugated hyperbilirubinaemia with raised ALP and GGT reflects biliary tree obstruction. As this is often a disease amenable to surgical intervention, post-hepatic jaundice is also known as obstructive or surgical jaundice.

(a) Painful Obstructive Jaundice

Aetiology: Painful obstructive jaundice is almost always due to gallstone disease.

- **Cholangitis**: Infection of an obstructed biliary system presents with right hypochondrial pain, jaundice and fever (Charcot's triad). Obstruction is usually due to gallstones (which acts as a nidus for infection), and less commonly from tumour or other causes of biliary obstruction (page 109).

- **Choledocholithiasis**: Gallstones obstructing the common bile duct, without evidence of infection.[1]

- **Hepatic abscess**: May also present with right hypochondrial pain and jaundice.

Hepatobiliary imaging (ultrasound or CT) distinguishes between these aetiologies. Note that marked jaundice is inconsistent with biliary colic or simple cholecystitis (see Chapter 9), if present, cholangitis must be considered.

Approach to Suspected Cholangitis

- **Early treatment of sepsis**: Cholangitic patients deteriorate rapidly, so empiric treatment must be instituted without awaiting imaging confirmation. Obtain blood cultures (these are frequently positive) and begin antibiotics urgently.

- **Hepatobiliary imaging**: The next step is to do ultrasound or CT scan. In this setting, a dilated common bile duct confirms the clinical diagnosis of cholangitis;

---

[1] Some patients experience a transient episode of painful obstructive jaundice; symptoms are improving and serial LFTs down-trending by the time they are seen. This frequently represents spontaneous passage of a gallstone.

gallstones may be visible in the common bile duct as hyper-echoic lesions casting an acoustic shadow, or may be obscured (especially on ultrasound as gastric air obscures the distal common bile duct). Imaging may also identify a ring-enhancing hepatic lesion, diagnostic of hepatic abscess.

- **Biliary drainage**: After confirmation of dilated ducts, pursue endoscopic retrograde cholangiopancreatography (ERCP) or percutaneous transhepatic biliary drainage (PTBD). While useful to confirm biliary dilation and intra-ductal stones, these are invasive and not performed solely for diagnosis. Their main utility is therapeutic—achieving source control of infection. ERCP allows stenting or sphincterotomy with stone extraction, while in PTBD, an external drain is inserted into the dilated biliary tree (favourable in unstable patients in whom sedation is risky).

(b) Painless Obstructive Jaundice

Painless obstructive jaundice has a wider differential, including

(i) **Extrahepatic biliary obstruction**:

- **Periampullary mass**: Painless progressive jaundice is the classic presentation of a periampullary cancer, for example, of the head of pancreas, ampulla of vater, a distal cholangiocarcinoma or malignant periampullary lymph nodes (as in lymphoma). These patients often have constitutional symptoms and weight loss.

- **Strictures**: In primary sclerosing cholangitis (an autoimmune disease associated with inflammatory bowel disease), strictures complicating prior biliary intervention or cholangiocarcinoma presenting as a stricture.

- **Other causes**: Liver flukes, AIDS cholangiopathy (in advanced HIV with CD4 < 100).

(ii) **Intrahepatic cholestasis**:

- **Primary biliary cholangitis** (PBC): An autoimmune disease classically presenting in middle-aged females with cholestatic jaundice, pruritus, xanthelasma and hepatosplenomegaly. Anti-mitochondrial antibodies are sensitive (positive in almost all cases of PBC) and specific (rarely positive in other diseases).

- **Drugs**: A number of drugs cause intrahepatic cholestasis including antibiotics (beta-lactams, rifampicin, erythromycin), anti-thyroid drugs, immunosuppressants (azathioprine and cyclosporine), the oral contraceptive pill and others.

(iii) **Other causes**: Diffuse liver infiltration with metastatic cancer, hepatic abscess, and so forth.

Suggested Approach

- **Begin with CT abdomen**: To identify dilated biliary ducts (suggesting extrahepatic biliary obstruction) and any cause of extrahepatic compression (i.e., any periampullary mass) or other disease (e.g., hepatic abscess and liver infiltration).

- **If CT abdomen normal, consider magnetic resonance cholangiopancrea-tography (MRCP)**: This interrogates the bile ducts; strictures may not be visible on CT.

- **If strictures seen without mass**: Consider primary sclerosing cholangitis and sec-ondary causes of strictures (e.g., cholangiocarcinoma).

- **If there are no dilated extrahepatic bile ducts**: Consider drugs and PBC (send anti-mitochondrial antibody).

- If there is a mixed picture of transaminitis (elevated AST, ALT and ALP), consider pursuing investigations for hepatocellular jaundice as well.

 Using what you have learnt, **pen down your approach** to the Clinical Case at the start of the chapter **BEFORE reading the discussion** below.

Case Discussion

This is a young gentleman with a hepatocellular pattern of jaundice and transaminitis. He may have an acute hepatitis, or a flare of a chronic hepatitis. Begin by considering common aetiologies. Take a history for alcohol use, drugs including traditional supplements, recent travel, exposure to uncooked shellfish (hepatitis A), IV drug use and unprotected sexual intercourse or tattoos (hepatitis B and C). Examine for abdominal tenderness, hepatomegaly and features of cirrhosis. Send hepatitis serology (hepatitis A IgM, HBsAg, HBcAg, anti-HBs and HCV IgM), and investigations for complications of liver disease (PT/aPTT and platelets). Consider liver ultrasound to exclude obstruction and cirrhosis.

Findings that should prompt consideration of less common aetiologies include ataxia, chorea or psychiatric disease (Wilson's disease), bronzing of skin, hypogonadism, early onset diabetes or hypothyroidism (hemochromatosis) and other autoimmune disease (autoimmune hepatitis).

Key Lessons	
	1. Jaundice is classified as pre-hepatic, hepatic and post-hepatic (obstructive) based on whether bilirubin is conjugated or unconjugated, and the pattern of raised LFTs (hepatocellular vs. cholestatic).
	2. In pre-hepatic jaundice, look for haemolysis, and consider causes of reduced hepatic uptake/conjugation of bilirubin.
	3. Hepatocellular jaundice may present acutely, as chronic hepatitis, or as cirrhosis. Search for a cause of liver injury including viral hepatitis, alcohol, drugs, non-alcoholic fatty liver, autoimmune, ischaemic and other causes of liver injury.
	4. Painful obstructive jaundice is almost always due to gallstones, for example, cholangitis. Painless obstructive jaundice may be due to a compressive tumour, stricture or primary biliary cirrhosis; CT is the initial investigation of choice.

Common Pitfalls

1. Isolated raised AST and ALP may not be due to liver disease.

2. The normal upper limit of ALT is 29 to 33 IU/L for males and 19 to 25 IU/L for females. Levels above this are associated with increased liver-related mortality and should be investigated. Non-alcoholic fatty liver disease can progress to cirrhosis and is under-diagnosed, which leads to missed opportunities for treatment.

Questions

1. **REFLECT!** Compare and contrast the history, physical findings and investigation results in (a) cholangitis, and (b) pancreatic cancer presenting with obstructive jaundice.

2. **DISCUSS!** A patient presents with jaundice and confusion, and cannot give any history. How would you approach him/her?

3. **GO FURTHER!** Read up on hepatitis B and C. (a) What is their natural history, and at which stages are LFTs abnormal? (b) How do you interpret hepatitis B serological results? Complete the table:

	HBsAg	anti-HBs	HBcAg	HBeAg	anti-HBe	Interpretation
a	−	−	−	−	−	
b	−	+	−	−	−	
c	−	+	+	−	−	
d	+	−	+	+	−	
e	+	−	+	−	+	

Chapter
11

An Approach to Gastrointestinal Bleeding

Clinical Case

A 53-year-old odd-job worker presents with a 1-day history of giddiness, lethargy and black, foul-smelling stools (which he is unable to quantify). He has no past medical history, apart from longstanding back pain, for which he has been taking naproxen. He drinks, on average, eight bottles of beer plus some hard liquor each day.

On arrival in the Emergency Department, his vitals are: BP 102/54, HR 132, SpO2 98% on room air, Temp 37.5°C. On examination, he is alert and anxious. Conjunctival pallor, palmar erythema and mild abdominal distension with shifting dullness are noted. His abdomen was soft with no masses. Blood is drawn for full blood count (FBC), coagulation studies, electrolytes, liver function and group and cross-match. How would you approach his presenting complaint?

Acute gastrointestinal bleeding manifests overtly with **haematemesis** (vomiting of fresh blood or coffee-ground material), **melena** (black, sticky, foul-smelling stools) or fresh **per-rectal bleeding** (haematochezia). This can be massive, leading to hypotension and death. Do not be misled by *normal* haemoglobin levels here—haemoglobin takes time to fall.[1] Conversely, gastrointestinal bleeding may be occult, presenting with trace amounts of rectal bleeding and chronic anaemia, which may or may not be symptomatic (Figure 11.1).

Distinguishing Upper vs. Lower Gastrointestinal Bleeding

Following resuscitation, confirm that bleeding is from the gastrointestinal tract (haemoptysis and epistaxis may mimic gastrointestinal bleeding) and distinguish clinically between an upper and a lower gastrointestinal bleed (Table 11.1). Initial investigations should include a full blood count (FBC), coagulation profile, urea and electrolytes, liver enzymes and group cross-match.

---

[1] Acutely, both red cells and plasma are proportionally lost, so haemoglobin remains normal. Only after fluid resuscitation (by physicians or by the body's own fluid conservation mechanisms), when a fixed amount of red cells is diluted in an increased plasma volume, does the haemoglobin fall.

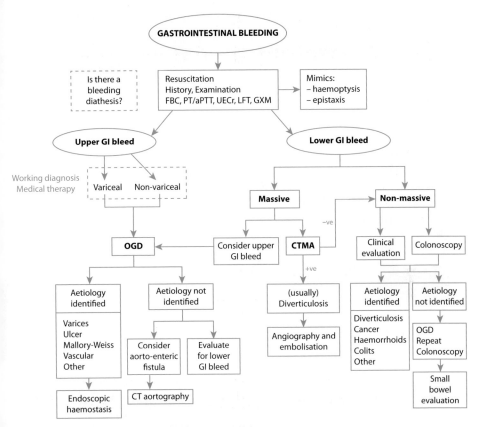

See text for details of clinical evaluation and/or identification of aetiologies.

CTMA, CT mesenteric angiography; FBC, full blood count; GXM, group and cross match;
LFT, liver function test; OGD, oesophagogastroduodenoscopy; UECr, urea, electrolytes and creatinine.

Figure 11.1. Approach to gastrointestinal bleeding.

Is There a Bleeding Diathesis?

Features that prompt consideration of a systemic bleeding diathesis include

- Bleeding from multiple sites—for example, mucocutaneous or intracranial bleeding in addition to gastrointestinal bleeding.
- Clinical context predisposing to bleeding—dengue infection, sepsis with disseminated intravascular coagulopathy.
- Laboratory findings—significant coagulopathy, severe thrombocytopenia.

In such situations, further evaluation for a cause of systemic bleeding may be necessary (see Chapter 33). On the other hand, gastrointestinal bleeding should not simply be blamed on a known bleeding diathesis or drugs (e.g., anticoagulation or antiplatelets) without consideration for gastrointestinal workup, as the presence of these contribu-

Table 11.1. Distinguishing Upper vs. Lower Gastrointestinal Bleeding

	Upper gastrointestinal bleed	Lower gastrointestinal bleed
Anatomic location	Oesophagus, Stomach, Duodenum (proximal to ligament of Treitz at duodenojejunal junction).	Jejunum, Ileum, Colon, Rectum (distal to ligament of Treitz at duodenojejunal junction).
Clinical symptoms	Haematemesis, melena. May also present with per-rectal bleed if rate of bleed is too quick for digestion of blood to occur.	Per-rectal bleed, slow or brisk. Blood clots in stool makes a lower gastrointestinal source more likely.
Laboratory clues	Urea elevated out of proportion to creatinine (due to gastric digestion of blood). Deranged liver enzymes or history of cirrhosis.	—
Notes	Massive bleeding or hypotension should be presumed as upper until proven otherwise.	

tory factors does not rule out an anatomical abnormality in the gastrointestinal tract that is responsible for bleeding.

Upper Gastrointestinal Bleeding

The approach to upper gastrointestinal bleeding, in most patients, centres around adequate resuscitation followed by early endoscopic haemostasis.

Initial Plan: Variceal vs. Non-Variceal Bleed

The aims of initial management are to (a) maintain haemodynamic stability, (b) risk stratify, (c) optimise the patient for endoscopy (including blood transfusion as necessary) and (d) institute pre-endoscopic medical therapy. As pre-endoscopic management differs between variceal and non-variceal bleeding, it is important to make an early working diagnosis of variceal or non-variceal bleeding.

- **Variceal bleeding**: Oesophageal varices are a consequence of portal hypertension. Suspect variceal bleeding if there is (a) a history of cirrhosis ± known varices, (b) signs of chronic liver disease, for example, jaundice, ascites or splenomegaly, (c) abnormal liver function tests or (d) coagulopathy or thrombocytopenia.

- **Non-variceal bleeding**: In the absence of the factors above, patients can be initially managed as a non-variceal bleed (pre-endoscopic medical therapy differs).

In either case, patients should proceed to oesophagogastroduodenoscopy (OGD), after considering risk and benefit.

OGD: Bleeding Lesion Found

OGD will, in many cases, identify the source of upper gastrointestinal bleed, including

- **Peptic ulcers**: Common and treatable. Hunt down *why* the patient has peptic ulcer disease—test for *Helicobacter pylori* (e.g., a rapid *CLO* test), look for drugs that cause peptic ulceration (e.g., Non-steroidal anti-inflammatory drugs [NSAIDs], antiplatelets, steroids), and a history of smoking. As gastric cancer can present as an ulcer with irregular margins, gastric ulcers are usually biopsied. A repeat OGD may be performed to document healing of a gastric ulcer (failure to heal prompts suspicion of cancer); biopsy or repeat OGD is not necessary for a duodenal ulcer.

- **Complications of portal hypertension**: Oesophageal varices and portal hypertensive gastropathy (diffuse oozing from friable vessels) occur in cirrhotics with portal hypertension.

- **Oesophagitis**: Oesophageal inflammation can present with bleeding. This may be due to gastroesophageal reflux, drugs (e.g., tetracyclines and bisphosphonates), or infection.

- **Mallory–Weiss tear**: A longitudinal oesophageal mucosal tear, classically after an episode of binge drinking leading to violent vomiting or retching.

- **Vascular lesions**: For example, angiodysplasia, Dieulafoy's lesion, gastric antral vascular ectasia (GAVE).

Note: 'Gastritis' is an endoscopic description of mild mucosal erythema suggesting inflammation. It is common and rarely leads to significant bleeding—gastrointestinal bleeding should usually not be ascribed to gastritis alone, without a search for other sources.

Apart from its diagnostic utility, OGD also allows for therapeutic manoeuvres to secure haemostasis (e.g., banding of varices, clipping of ulcers, etc.).

OGD: Bleeding Lesion Not Found

If the OGD is negative, consider

- **Colonoscopy**: Evaluate for lower gastrointestinal causes of bleeding. Blood from right-sided colonic lesions may appear altered, resembling melena.

- **CT scan for aorto-enteric fistula**: Patients who have received prior aortic surgery and grafting (e.g., for repair of dissection) may develop an aorto-enteric fistula, which is an anomalous connection between aorta and intestine that leads to gastrointestinal bleeding. If there is a history of aortic disease or surgery, consider CT aortography to look for an aorto-enteric fistula.

Lower Gastrointestinal Bleeding

Begin by triaging the severity of bleeding. Practically, a massive per-rectal bleed is one which causes haemodynamic instability (including tachycardia), an acute and significant fall in haemoglobin (e.g., > 2 g/dL over 24 hr), or is large volume and persistent.

Massive Lower Gastrointestinal Bleed

The usual cause of massive lower gastrointestinal bleeding is diverticular disease, as diverticula can form at the site of penetrating arteries and cause an arterial bleed. The other aetiologies of lower gastrointestinal bleed tend not to be as massive. The approach is to

1. **Exclude upper gastrointestinal bleeding**: Some large upper gastrointestinal bleeds present with per-rectal bleeding instead of melena, if the bleed is too rapid for digestion of blood to occur. Consideration should be given to

   - If clinical suspicion is high (e.g., hypotensive, elevated urea, known liver disease)— OGD after appropriate resuscitation.

   - If clinical suspicion is low (e.g., previous diverticular bleed, not hypotensive)— either OGD or nasogastric lavage (i.e., insert nasogastric tube and connect to wall suction). Coffee-ground aspirates or fresh blood on nasogastric lavage confirms an upper gastrointestinal source of bleed; however, it may be falsely negative if bleeding arises beyond a closed pylorus (e.g., in a duodenal ulcer). Avoid nasogastric tube insertion if varices are suspected as it may traumatise the varices and cause more bleeding.

2. **CT mesenteric angiogram (CTMA)**: This is particularly useful in ongoing massive bleeding, and allows identification of a bleeding source anywhere in the gastrointestinal tract (including small bowel).

   - **CTMA positive**: An active brisk bleed (>0.3 mL/min) is visualised as an arterial blush (i.e., contrast extravasation from vessels). If CTMA is positive, proceed to catheter angiography, which allows embolisation of the bleeding vessel.

   - **CTMA negative**: A negative CTMA implies either that bleeding has either stopped, or is too slow (<0.3 mL/min) to be visualised. Diverticula may bleed intermittently and elude capture by CTMA. If CTMA is negative, proceed to colonoscopy as in non-massive bleed.

Non-Massive Lower Gastrointestinal Bleed

There are numerous causes of non-massive lower gastrointestinal bleeding. Most patients should be evaluated clinically, and receive colonoscopy.

1. **Clinical evaluation**: Useful information can be obtained on clinical history and examination. As a rule of thumb, proximal bleeding (small bowel and right-sided colon) gives altered (darker) blood mixed with faeces; distal bleeding (left-sided colon and anorectal, e.g., haemorrhoids) gives fresh (red) blood coating faeces, toilet paper or dripping into the toilet bowl after defecation. This is a helpful clinical distinction but, unfortunately, not completely reliable. Three questions are helpful

   (a) Apart from rectal bleeding, are there any other symptoms or concerning history?

   (b) What does rectal exam and proctoscopy find?

   (c) If isolated painless per-rectal bleeding, with normal rectal exam, what can it be?

(a) **Are there any other symptoms or concerning history?**

- **Suspicion of cancer**: Loss of appetite and weight, change in bowel habits (alternating constipation and diarrhoea, decrease in stool calibre), palpable abdominal mass or positive family history of colorectal cancer raises suspicion of cancer. Tenesmus, a persistent, uncomfortable desire to defecate, is worrisome for rectal cancer.

- **Colitis**: Bloody diarrhoea with abdominal colic, tenderness to palpation ± fever, malaise and systemic toxicity. Colitis may be due to

  - Inflammatory bowel disease (Crohn's disease and ulcerative colitis): usually in a young patient, who may also have extra-intestinal manifestations (arthritis, uveitis, erythema nodosum, etc.).

  - Ischaemic colitis: Can arise from atherosclerotic disease or vasculitis. There may be post-meal abdominal colic.

  - Infective colitis: Acute bloody diarrhoea, possibly with a history of travel, or consumption of spoilt food. The amount of blood in stool is usually mild to moderate, and mixed with stools.

- Previous pelvic radiation: In patients with previous pelvic radiation (e.g., for rectal or prostate cancer), consider radiation colitis vs. cancer recurrence.

- Recent endoscopic therapy: Bleeding may occur following endoscopic biopsy or polypectomy, and is self-limited in most cases.

(b) **What does rectal exam and proctoscopy find?**

- **Haemorrhoids**: Dilated submucosal veins (visible on proctoscopy in the 3, 7 and 10 o'clock positions), often with contact bleeding or blood stains. Haemorrhoidal bleeding is usually bright red, of small amount, and may coat faeces or toilet paper. Some haemorrhoids may also prolapse (protrude from the anus during defecation).

- **Other anorectal abnormalities**: For example, anorectal tumour (palpable mass on rectal exam), rectal ulcers and so forth.

(c) **Isolated painless per-rectal bleeding, with normal rectal exam**—conditions in this category include

- **Diverticular bleed**: Diverticuli are outpouchings of the colonic mucosa through weaknesses of the colon wall. Diverticular bleeds are common, can be of rather large amount (can also be small amount), and blood may be red or dark.

- **Angiodysplasia**: Dilated, tortuous submucosal vessels.

- **Colon polyp or tumour** may be asymptomatic.

2. **Colonoscopy**: Most patients (unless medically unfit) should receive colonoscopy after appropriate resuscitation, transfusion and bowel preparation. This is because even if a source of bleeding (e.g., haemorrhoids) can be found on clinical examination, it does not exclude a second source of bleeding, which may be sinister (e.g., colon cancer). Colonoscopy is useful to identify anatomic lesions causing bleeding (e.g., tumour, diverticula, ulcerative colitis), and allows for endoscopic therapeutics.

Initial Evaluation Negative

In a minority of patients, clinical evaluation and colonoscopy fail to reveal a source of per-rectal bleeding. In these patients, consider

- **OGD**: For an upper gastrointestinal source, if not already done.

- **Repeat colonoscopy**: Especially if the first colonoscopy was suboptimal (e.g., poor bowel preparation) and lesions could have been missed.

- **Small bowel evaluation**: Small bowel sources of bleeding include a Meckel's diverticulum, vascular lesions (e.g., Dieulafoy's lesion), small bowel tumour and so forth. There are a variety of methods to evaluate the small bowel. Patients with brisk bleeding should undergo CTMA. Patients with slow bleeding or chronic iron-deficiency anaemia should be considered for capsule endoscopy or push enteroscopy.

  Using what you have learnt, **pen down your approach** to the Clinical Case at the start of the chapter **BEFORE reading the discussion** below.

Case Discussion

This is a middle-aged gentleman with upper gastrointestinal bleeding. He is tachycardic, pale and giddy—suggesting that he has bled sufficiently to cause hypovolaemia and anaemia. He has signs of chronic liver disease (ascites and palmar erythema) and risk factors (heavy drinking), and should be managed as a presumptive variceal bleed. Following resuscitation and blood transfusion, he will require early endoscopy, which may reveal oesophageal varices. Alternatively, it may also find peptic ulceration—he also has risk factors of non-steroidal anti-inflammatory drug (NSAIDs) and alcohol.

Key Lessons	1. Upper gastrointestinal bleeding may be variceal or non-variceal (peptic ulcers, Mallory–Weiss tear, vascular lesions, etc.). Early oesophagogastroduodenoscopy is diagnostic and therapeutic.
	2. In massive per-rectal bleeding, exclude an upper gastrointestinal source, and consider CT mesenteric angiogram (CTMA).
	3. Non-massive per-rectal bleeding is most commonly due to diverticulosis, haemorrhoids and cancer. Following clinical evaluation (including rectal examination and proctoscopy), most patients should receive colonoscopy.
Common Pitfalls	1. Haemoglobin may be normal in acute gastrointestinal bleeding.
	2. The presence of obvious haemorrhoids does not exclude a second cause of gastrointestinal bleeding.
	3. Diverticular bleeding is relatively *painless*, at most, there may be an uncomfortable urge to defecate (as blood is a cathartic). Significant abdominal pain, tenderness or systemic toxicity is inconsistent with diverticular bleeding—suspect colitis.

Questions   1. **REFLECT!** Have you ever had a patient with haemodynamic instability from gastrointestinal bleeding? What were the differential diagnoses, and what was done for the patient?

2. **EXPLORE!** Consent-taking for OGD and colonoscopy is commonly performed by junior physicians. How would you counsel a patient on the procedure, as well as its risks and alternatives?

3. **DISCUSS!** It is not uncommon for patients with poor premorbids to present with gastrointestinal bleeding. Suppose an 80-year-old lady who is bedbound after a cerebrovascular accident presents with per-rectal bleeding and a haemoglobin of 5 g/dL. Should endoscopy be performed? What are the considerations here?

Chapter

12

An Approach to Nausea and Vomiting

Clinical Case

A 29-year-old school teacher complains of a 2-day history of progressively severe vomiting. The contents of his vomitus were initially partially digested food, then yellow-green fluid. He has also been having intermittent abdominal pain. His last bowel output was yesterday, and it was of normal consistency. He has no headache or giddiness. He has no past medical history. On examination, his vitals are: T 37.6, BP 121/59, HR 95. He is alert and orientated. His abdomen is distended with sluggish bowel sounds. How would you approach his complaint?

Vomiting is a forceful expulsion of gastric contents (unlike regurgitation which involves minimal effort). **Nausea** is a sensation of a desire to vomit. Vomiting is a complex reflex involving both the gastrointestinal tract and central nervous system; it is therefore unsurprising that the causes of vomiting are not merely limited to the gut.

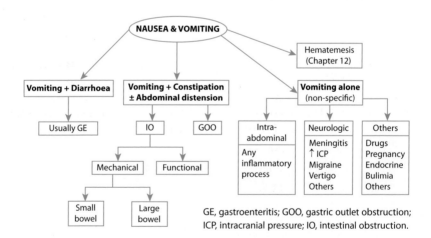

GE, gastroenteritis; GOO, gastric outlet obstruction; ICP, intracranial pressure; IO, intestinal obstruction.

Figure 12.1. Approach to nausea and vomiting.

Using the symptom complex, distinguish between four clinical pictures (Figure 12.1).

1. Vomiting (or nausea) + **Diarrhoea**: Usually gastroenteritis.

2. Vomiting (or nausea) + **Constipation** ± **Abdominal distension**: Gastrointestinal obstruction.

3. Vomiting (or nausea) **without diarrhoea or constipation**: Non-specific, may be due to gastrointestinal or non-gastrointestinal disease.

4. **Hematemesis**: Bloody vomiting or coffee-ground vomitus is a symptom of upper gastrointestinal bleeding (Chapter 11).

1. Vomiting + Diarrhoea

Vomiting with diarrhoea indicates a gastrointestinal tract that is attempting to purge its contents from both ends. Where acute, this is almost always due to gastroenteritis, and further workup is usually unnecessary (see Chapter 13).

2. Vomiting + Constipation + Abdominal Distension

The symptom complex of vomiting, constipation and abdominal distension indicates obstruction of the gastrointestinal tract. This may occur at the gastric or intestinal levels.

- **Intestinal obstruction (IO)**: The cardinal features are abdominal colic, distension, nausea/vomiting and lack of passage of stool or flatus.

- **Gastric outlet obstruction (GOO)**: Post-meal vomiting of undigested food, early satiety and bloating, epigastric pain and weight loss.

Intestinal Obstruction

IO is suspected based on its symptom complex—abdominal colic, distension, nausea/vomiting and lack of passage of stool (and flatus, if obstruction is complete)—although not all four cardinal features may be present. Examination may find abdominal distension, sluggish or tinkling bowel sounds and dehydration. Abdominal X-ray (AXR) shows distended bowel loops. The key questions are:

1. Is this small or large bowel IO?
2. Are there any complications requiring immediate intervention?
3. What is the aetiology of IO?

1. **Small or large bowel IO?**

   (a) **Clinical features**: The dominant clinical features may give a clue. Vomiting is early and constipation late in proximal IO (stools may pass until existing gut contents clear), while constipation is early and vomiting late in distal IO. Bilious vomiting indicates obstruction below the ampulla of Vater in the duodenum, while feculent vomiting indicates distal small bowel or large bowel obstruction (unless there is a gastro-colic fistula).

(b) **Imaging**: Obtain a supine Kidneys–Ureter–Bladder (KUB) X-ray.[1] This confirms the diagnosis of IO and helps to localise the obstruction as small vs. large bowel.

- **Small bowel IO**: Multiple loops in a central location, forming a 'stack of coins' appearance (Figure 12.2a).

- **Large bowel IO**: A single loop in a peripheral location (Figure 12.2b). There may also be distended small bowel loops (which cannot empty into the large bowel).

2. **Are there any complications requiring immediate intervention?**

- **Bowel perforation**: Severe abdominal tenderness and guarding, air under diaphragm on erect chest X-ray (CXR) (Figure 9.2)[2] or Rigler's double-wall sign on KUB.

- **Impending perforation**: For example, small bowel > 3 cm, large bowel > 6 cm, cecum > 9 cm or large bowel obstruction with right iliac fossa tenderness.

- **Closed loop obstruction**: Where a loop of bowel is obstructed both distally and proximally, pressure builds up rapidly without a chance for proximal decompression, and the risk of perforation is high. This may occur in an obstructed hernia, or large bowel obstruction with a competent ileocecal valve (dilated large bowel loops but no dilated small bowel loops).

3. **What is the aetiology of IO?**

The causes of IO are listed (Table 12.1). While it is not always possible to identify the exact aetiology of IO clinically, clinical decision making (trial of conservative management, perform further imaging or proceed to surgery) requires only a limited amount of information.

- **Look for obvious causes**: Always examine for a hernia (in the groin and at incision sites). A sigmoid volvulus, which usually occurs in debilitated elderly patients, may be seen on X-ray as a coffee bean sign (Figure 12.2d).

- **Small bowel IO**: Small bowel IO in a patient with prior abdominal surgery is usually due to adhesions; a trial of conservative therapy is usually offered, and further imaging obtained only if the patient fails to respond. In contrast, small bowel IO in a virgin abdomen generally requires further imaging (CT scan); most patients would require surgery, which may identify lesions such as a congenital band causing obstruction.

---

[1] AXR vs. KUB X-ray: AXR visualizes the diaphragm but may cut off the pubic symphysis, while KUB shows the pubic symphysis but may cut off the diaphragm. The KUB is generally better in IO, as it is useful to visualise rectal gas (which would indicate an incomplete obstruction). Between a supine and erect film, the erect film tends to show air-fluid levels, which are impressive but make the radiologic localisation of IO more challenging.

[2] A loop of large bowel may mimic air under the right diaphragm (Chilaiditi syndrome), but such a bowel loop has haustrations.

Figure 12.2. The KUB X-ray in intestinal obstruction.

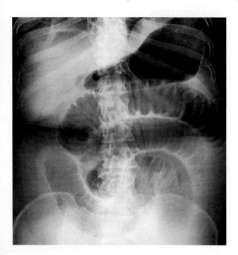

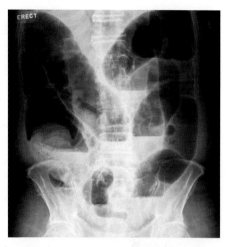

(a) **Small bowel IO**: Multiple, smaller, central loops creating a 'stack of coins' appearance. Note the plicae circulares—lines that transverse the entire bowel width. A distended stomach is also visible in this X-ray. This patient had adhesions from previous abdominal surgery.

(b) **Large bowel IO**: A single, peripheral, larger loop of bowel with haustrations that *do not* transverse the entire bowel width. Air-fluid levels are seen as this is an erect film. There are *no* distended small bowel loops—suggesting a competent ileocecal valve, that is, a closed-loop obstruction. This patient had a stenosing rectal tumour and liver metastases.

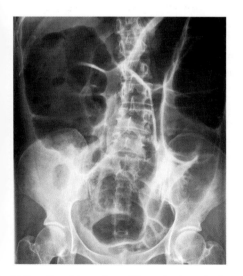

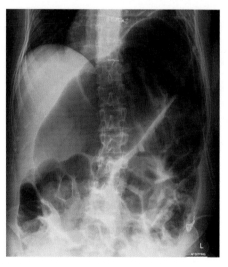

(c) **Functional large bowel ileus**: Again, a single, peripheral loop of large bowel. Unlike Figure 12.2(b), the entire colon is distended and rectal gas is present; these features suggest functional rather than mechanical obstruction. This patient had paralytic ileus from sepsis and severe hypokalaemia.

(d) **Sigmoid volvulus**: The classic 'coffee bean' sign is seen. This was a nursing home resident, bed-bound after a large stroke, who suffered from severe chronic constipation.

Table 12.1. Causes of Intestinal Obstruction

Intestinal obstruction

	Mechanical		Functional
	Small bowel	**Large bowel**	

Extraluminal	Adhesions
	Hernia
	Congenital bands
	Compression by
	  extrinsic mass
		Compression by
		  extrinsic mass
			Electrolyte imbalance
			  especially hypokalaemia
			Post-operative
			Critical illness
			Drugs e.g., opioids
			Neurologic: e.g., Parkinson's
			  and spinal cord disease

Luminal	Small bowel tumour
	Stricture e.g., IBD
	  and radiation
	Intussusception
		Colorectal cancer
		Sigmoid volvulus
		Stricture e.g., IBD and
		  radiation	

Intraluminal	Intraluminal object (foreign body, bezoar, gallstone, parasites)		

IBD, inflammatory bowel disease.

- **Large bowel IO**: The main worry is that of an obstructing colorectal tumour. There may be a suggestive history of weight loss, change in bowel habit, rectal bleeding, anaemia or an abdominal mass. Consider CT scan to look for a mass. Note that colonoscopy with bowel preparation is contraindicated in IO.

- **If CT scan is obtained**: An obstructing mass (e.g., a tumour, intraluminal object or extrinsic compressive mass) may be visualised. Look for a transition point (i.e., bowel dilated proximally but collapsed distally), which suggests mechanical obstruction at that point.

- **Functional (paralytic ileus)**: Clues that obstruction is functional, rather than mechanical, include (i) critical illness, abdominal operation or severe electrolyte imbalance preceding onset of IO, (ii) preserved rectal gas on X-ray, (iii) absence of transition point on CT scan.

Gastric Outlet Obstruction

GOO presents with post-meal vomiting (usually within 1 hour) of undigested food, early satiety and bloating, epigastric pain and weight loss. Examination may find a succession splash, and there is usually cachexia and dehydration.

Aetiologies: The main causes are

- **Malignancy**: Gastric outlet involvement in distal gastric cancer, pancreatic cancer invading the distal stomach or compression by extraluminal cancer.

- **Benign gastric outlet stricture**: For example, due to peptic ulcer disease, Crohn's disease, caustic chemical ingestion.

- **Gastroparesis**: Functional obstruction in longstanding diabetes, neurological disease (e.g., Parkinson's disease) or scleroderma.

Workup:

- CT abdomen/pelvis: Confirms gastric distension, identifies any masses/large cancers.

- Oesophagogastroduodenoscopy: Allows direct visualisation and biopsy of mechanical lesions.

- If suspecting gastroparesis, consider scintigraphic study of gastric emptying (using a radioactive tracer).

3. Vomiting Alone

Vomiting is a non-specific symptom of many illnesses. A careful systematic review should be performed to look for any other localising symptom, which gives further clues on its aetiology.

Intra-Abdominal

Any intra-abdominal inflammatory process can trigger vomiting—including appendicitis, pancreatitis, gallstone disease and so forth. Vomiting is usually not the only symptom—ask about any abdominal pain, jaundice and so forth. Further evaluation is based on the symptom complex.

Neurological

Have a high index of suspicion of neurological disease especially if there are (1) neurological abnormalities including headache, giddiness, drowsiness, seizures, focal weakness or cranial nerve abnormality, unequal pupils, (2) a soft abdomen but a toxic patient, (3) a history of trauma, (4) chronic vomiting of insidious onset and progressive severity. Consider

- Headache with vomiting: Meningitis, raised intracranial pressure, intracranial haemorrhage, migraine (see Chapter 22).

- Giddiness with vomiting: Peripheral vertigo, for example, benign postural positional vertigo, but beware of central causes, for example, posterior circulation cerebral infarction (see Chapter 24).

Other Causes

Look for the following systemic causes, which may present non-specifically with nausea and vomiting.

- **Drugs and toxins**: Especially chemotherapy and general anaesthesia. Take a full drug history including non-prescription drugs.

- **Pregnancy**: Usually early morning vomiting. Consider a pregnancy test in females of the appropriate age group.

- **Endocrine**: Uraemia, diabetic ketoacidosis, adrenal insufficiency, hypercalcemia, thyroid disease. There will usually be other localising symptoms.

- **Bulimia nervosa**: Often adolescent females with post-meal vomiting, especially after binge eating. Clues include distorted body image, anxiety or depressive symptoms, dental enamel erosion, calluses on the dorsum of the hand/fingers and lanugo hair.

- **Other systemic disease**: Geriatric patients with infections, congestive heart failure and other systemic illnesses may have non-specific nausea and vomiting.

If no other cause of chronic nausea and vomiting is identified, functional gastrointestinal disorders (e.g., chronic nausea vomiting syndrome) may need to be considered.

 Using what you have learnt, **pen down your approach** to the Clinical Case at the start of the chapter **BEFORE reading the discussion** below.

Case Discussion

This is a young gentleman with intestinal obstruction (IO). He has bilious vomiting, abdominal pain and abdominal distension with sluggish bowel sounds. Although he passed stools yesterday, that may reflect clearance of existing gut contents distal to the obstruction. No note of his hernia orifices was made; he must be examined for an obstructed inguinal hernia, as well as any abdominal masses. The next step is to perform a KUB X-ray, which is likely to identify small bowel obstruction. Exclude perforation or impending perforation.

If KUB confirms small bowel IO in a virgin abdomen, having excluded hernia, he will probably require further imaging (CT scan) then surgery. It may be prudent to prepare him for surgery at this point (check and correct electrolytes, which are likely deranged from vomiting, and send FBC, coagulation profile and cross-match). The exact diagnosis (e.g., congenital bands or small bowel tumour) will be identified at surgery.

Key Lessons	
	1. Acute vomiting with diarrhoea is usually gastroenteritis.
	2. The cardinal symptoms of IO are vomiting, constipation, abdominal pain and distension. IO may be small or large bowel, mechanical or functional.
	3. Vomiting can be a non-specific symptom of systemic illness. Vomiting with headache, drowsiness, giddiness or focal neurologic deficit should lead to strong suspicion of neurologic disease including meningitis and intracranial haemorrhage. Vomiting can also be a non-specific symptom of intra-abdominal inflammation, pregnancy, drug side effects, endocrine and other systemic illnesses.

Common Pitfalls	1. Non-gastrointestinal causes of vomiting (especially neurologic emergencies and diabetic ketoacidosis) can be missed if not deliberately considered.
Questions	1. **REFLECT!** Have you ever seen a patient who presented with vomiting, but turned out to have non-gastrointestinal disease? What were some clues that the cause of vomiting was non-gastrointestinal?
	2. **EXPLORE!** A systematic approach to reading abdominal X-rays is important to avoid missing abnormalities. What are the pathologies that an Abdominal X-ray (AXR)/KUB may identify, and how would you systemically approach an AXR/KUB film?
	3. **DISCUSS!** In the approach to IO, how would the patient's age and past medical history affect your differential diagnosis?

Chapter 13 An Approach to Diarrhoea

Clinical Case

A 35-year-old Chinese lady presents to primary care with a 5-month history of intermittent diarrhoea. She passes five watery stools every alternate day, associated with crampy abdominal pain, which is relieved by defecation. While she is inconvenienced by her frequent diarrhoea, her appetite remains good and weight is stable. She has no prior medical problems or surgery. Examination is unremarkable. A full blood count (FBC), electrolytes, liver function test and thyroid panel is normal. She requests to be referred for colonoscopy. How would you advise her?

Diarrhoea is the frequent (e.g., ≥ 3/day) passage of loose or watery stools. It may be divided into acute (< 2 weeks) or chronic (> 4 weeks; 2–4 weeks—causes overlap; Figure 13.1).

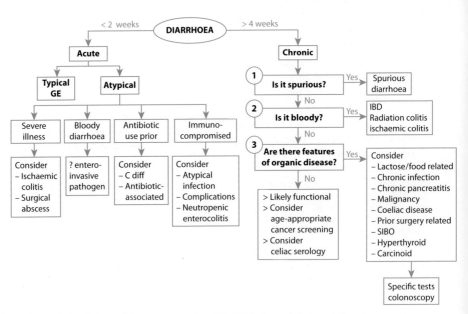

C. diff, Clostridium difficile infection; GE, gastroenteritis; IBD, inflammatory bowel disease; SIBO, small intestinal bowel overgrowth.

Figure 13.1. Approach to diarrhoea.

Acute Diarrhoea

Gastroenteritis is responsible for most episodes of acute diarrhoea.

Typical Gastroenteritis

Typical gastroenteritis presents with mild abdominal colic, diarrhoea, vomiting ± fever and malaise. Patients are well and disease is self-limiting. Most patients should be managed with hydration and symptomatic therapy; further testing would not change management.

Traveller's diarrhoea: While travel to developing countries is associated with a wider range of infective aetiologies, including parasites, most cases are bacterial and self-limiting. Stool ova/cyst/parasite microscopy is usually unnecessary unless diarrhoea persists or there are atypical features.

Atypical Features

The following features are atypical for simple gastroenteritis, and patients may benefit from further workup

1. **Severe illness**: In patients with profuse watery diarrhoea, severe abdominal pain, guarding, severe hypovolaemia or systemic toxicity (tachycardia, hypotension, fever), evaluate for

   Workup

   − Stool cultures
   − Blood cultures
   − Electrolytes and creatinine

   - Complications: For example, electrolyte imbalances, acute kidney injury and systemic sepsis (e.g., *Salmonella* bacteraemia).

   - Ischemic colitis: Acute ischemic colitis may present with abdominal colic and bloody diarrhoea. The diagnosis should be suspected in patients who are systemically ill, especially in those with risk factors including aortic or cardiothoracic surgery, myocardial infarction or thrombophilia.

     − CT abdomen for ischemia (bowel wall oedema and pneumatosis coli) and complications (e.g., colonic necrosis, abscess, perforation)

   - Surgical complications: Intra-abdominal abscess formation, perforation.

2. **Bloody diarrhoea**: Suggests infection with an enteroinvasive pathogen, for example, enterohaemorrhagic *Escherichia coli* or *Entamoeba*.

   − Stool culture with testing for Shiga toxin
   − Stool ova/cyst/parasites for *Entamoeba*

3. **Antibiotic use**, recent hospitalisation or institutionalisation: Consider

   − Stool *C. difficile* polymerase chain reaction

   - *Clostridium difficile* diarrhoea.

   - Antibiotic-associated diarrhoea.

4. **Immunocompromised host** including HIV infection, immunosuppression or chemotherapy. Consider

- Atypical infections: parasites, cytomegalovirus (CMV).

- Invasive disease, severe infection, abscess formation and other complications.

- Neutropenic enterocolitis (typhlitis) in oncology patients on chemotherapy—this is a severe infection precipitated by gut mucosal breakdown and impaired host defences.

- Stool and blood cultures
- Stool microscopy for ova/cyst/parasites
- Consider endoscopic biopsy for CMV
- CT abdomen: bowel wall thickening and dilation, pneumatosis intestinalis, fat stranding

Chronic Diarrhoea

There are many causes of chronic diarrhoea and many tests to hunt for them, but is impossible and imprudent to investigate every possibility. The diagnostic challenge is to assess, based only on clinical features and simple investigations, whether a patient likely has (i) organic pathology that may require treatment, or (ii) functional disease that is best managed symptomatically.

1. Is This Spurious Diarrhoea?

Elderly patients with chronic constipation may develop such severe faecal impaction that only fluid matter is able to pass. This diarrhoea is *spurious* because the real problem is constipation, not diarrhoea. Spurious (overflow) diarrhoea is common and easy to exclude—always do a per-rectal examination ± abdominal X-ray for severe faecal loading.

2. Is Diarrhoea Bloody?

Bloody diarrhoea implies bowel inflammation. There may also be abdominal colic, anaemia and weight loss. Severe disease may come with fever, tachycardia and severe abdominal pain. Differentials include

- **Inflammatory bowel disease** (Crohn's disease, ulcerative colitis): Onset of symptoms is usually gradual, but a few patients present with fulminant disease (including severe colitis, bleeding or perforation). There may be extraintestinal manifestations including arthritis, red eye (uveitis), skin lesions (erythema nodosum) and liver disease. Patients with Crohn's disease may also have perianal abscesses, anal skin tags, oral and oesophageal involvement.

- **Radiation colitis**: Patients who received prior pelvic radiation (e.g., for anal or prostate cancers) may develop radiation colitis weeks to years after.

- **Chronic ischaemic colitis**: Symptoms are usually less severe than in acute ischaemic colitis.

Approach: Apart from general assessment of disease severity and complications (full blood count [FBC], C-reactive protein [CRP], electrolytes).

- Exclude infection—stool culture and microscopy for ova/cyst/parasites, Giardia stool antigen. Consider sending rectal swabs for gonorrhoea and chlamydia in men who have receptive anal intercourse.

- Colonoscopy with terminal ileum intubation and biopsy: This may identify ulcerations, mucosal erythema and friability in inflammatory bowel disease or atrophy and granulation tissue in ischaemic colitis.

- Imaging, for example, CT or MR enterography to evaluate for small bowel involvement in Crohn's disease.

- Supportive tests: Faecal calprotectin (elevated in inflammatory diarrhoea) and antibody testing (antineutrophil cytoplasmic antibodies [ANCA] and anti-*Saccharomyces cerevisiae* antibodies) may be helpful, but not routinely necessary for diagnosis.

Patients with frank per-rectal bleeding should be approached as in Chapter 11.

3. Are There Features of Organic Disease?

Begin with a clinical history, examination and simple investigations (FBC, electrolytes, CRP, thyroid function, liver function test and albumin). Look for features suggestive of organic pathology. Apart from bloody diarrhoea, these include

- **Steatorrhoea**: Greasy, foul-smelling, bulky stools that float in water suggest fat malabsorption. Faecal elastase is low.

- **Secretory diarrhoea**: Diarrhoea which is large volume, nocturnal or continues despite fasting.

- **Consequences of malabsorption**: Iron-deficiency anaemia, weight loss, vitamin deficiency (e.g., B12 or fat soluble vitamins A, D, E, K) and hypoalbuminaemia.

- Features specific of specific aetiologies (below).

(a) Possible Organic Disease

Look for features suggestive of specific aetiologies	Additional Workup
• **Lactose intolerance or other food allergy**: Explore association of diarrhoea with specific food products (e.g., dairy products suggesting lactose intolerance, excessive sorbitol-containing sweets).	− Consider temporary avoidance of suspect foods
• **Chronic infection**: Patients with immunosuppression, HIV infection (or risk of HIV), travel to or residence in developing countries are at risk of chronic infective diarrhoea, including parasitic infection.	− Stool ova/cyst/parasites − Giardia faecal antigen − HIV testing

- **Chronic pancreatitis**: Suspect if there is chronic epigastric pain or a history of recurrent pancreatitis. Cystic fibrosis impairs pancreatic exocrine function.

    - Abdominal X-ray or CT for pancreatic calcifications
    - Amylase/lipase is normal

- **Malignancy**: Loss of weight or appetite, change in stool calibre, family history of colorectal malignancy, advanced age.

- **Coeliac disease**: History of autoimmune disease (e.g., type 1 diabetes or hypothyroidism), dermatitis herpetiformis (a rash with grouped pruritic papules and vesicles).

    - Anti-tissue transglutaminase (TTG) and IgA levels (IgA deficiency results in false negative anti-TTG)

- **Related to prior abdominal surgery**: After cholecystectomy, there is no gallbladder to store and concentrate bile; continuous and excessive bile drainage into the gut may cause diarrhoea. Bowel resection decreases the length and resorptive capacity of the gut, which may lead to diarrhoea from short gut syndrome.

- **Small intestine bacterial overgrowth** (SIBO): Excessive bacterial growth occurs most commonly in patients with intestinal stasis (e.g., surgical blind loops, strictures, scleroderma, chronic pancreatitis); this leads to malabsorption and altered motility.

    - Carbohydrate breath test

- **Hyperthyroidism**: Heat intolerance, tremors, palpitations, lid lag, goitre.

    - Thyroid function tests

- **Carcinoid tumours**: Episodic diarrhoea with flushing and bronchospasm.

    - Urinary 5-Hydroxyindoleacetic acid (5-HIAA)

Colonoscopy: In addition to the specific workup above, if indicated, most patients should be offered colonoscopy. This may identify any mucosal abnormalities or mass. Abnormalities should be biopsied; if there are no abnormalities, blind biopsies should be taken (this may find microscopic colitis, a condition in which the mucosa is grossly normal).

(b) Likely Functional Diarrhoea

In the absence of features of organic disease, a positive diagnosis of functional diarrhoea can be made; it is not a diagnosis of exclusion that first requires extensive testing.

    Irritable bowel syndrome—predominant diarrhoea (IBS-D): Patients complain of chronic abdominal pain and diarrhoea. Pain may be exacerbated by emotional stress and relieved by defecation. Diarrhoea usually does not occur when the patient is asleep. The Rome IV criteria define IBS as recurrent abdominal pain (at least 1×/week in 3 months) with two or more of (1) relationship to defecation, (2) changes in stool frequency or (3) change in stool consistency. IBS may be diarrhoeal-predominant, as in this case, constipation-predominant (see Chapter 14), or mixed (alternating constipation and diarrhoea).

Screening tests: In patients with a positive diagnosis of functional diarrhoea, consider

- Age-appropriate colonoscopic screening for malignancy (e.g., > 50 years old for the general population, younger if there are other risk factors).

- Exploring the possibility of lactose intolerance or other food allergy.

- Celiac disease serology (as earlier) particularly for Caucasian populations, or if diarrhoea does not respond to symptomatic treatment. It may mimic IBS-D well and not present with overt malabsorption (see earlier).

 Using what you have learnt, **pen down your approach** to the Clinical Case at the start of the chapter **BEFORE reading the discussion** below.

Case Discussion

This young lady has a typical presentation of irritable bowel syndrome (IBS) (diarrhoeal subtype). She is young, healthy and has no alarm features (e.g., bloody diarrhoea, weight loss, anaemia, abdominal masses) thus far. After excluding additional features of organic disease (e.g., travel history to developing countries, symptoms of autoimmune disease), a clinical diagnosis of IBS can be made.

Further investigation, such as colonoscopy, is not routinely indicated unless she subsequently develops alarm features, has a family history of inflammatory bowel disease or young colorectal cancer. Colonoscopy can be considered if she fails to respond to symptomatic therapy.

Key Lessons	1. Gastroenteritis is responsible for most episodes of acute diarrhoea. Patients with atypical features (severe illness, bloody diarrhoea, recent antibiotic use, hospitalisation or immunosuppression), may benefit from further workup such as abdominal imaging, stool cultures or stool ova/cyst/parasites.
	2. Chronic diarrhoea in an otherwise well patient is often functional. Features suggestive of organic disease (bloody stools, steatorrhoea, nocturnal diarrhoea, weight loss, nutritional deficiencies) may prompt further workup including colonoscopy. Travel to less-developed settings, prior abdominal surgery, immunocompromise or other autoimmune diseases may prompt consideration of specific aetiologies of diarrhoea.
Common Pitfalls	1. Always exclude spurious diarrhoea, especially in elderly patients.
	2. IBS is a clinical diagnosis; colonoscopy is not mandatory to exclude other causes before a diagnosis can be made.

Questions

1. **REFLECT!** General practitioners and emergency departments see many patients with gastroenteritis each day. What features would prompt you to consider further investigation (e.g., blood tests) or admission instead of symptomatic care?

2. **EXPLORE!** Why is it important to distinguish between Crohn's disease and ulcerative colitis? Compare and contrast their clinical, endoscopic and histological findings.

3. **GO FURTHER!** There are many viral, bacterial and protozoal organisms that cause diarrhoea. Some of them have characteristic presentations (e.g., staphylococcal diarrhoea is rapid onset, < 6 hr), associations with specific foods/exposures (e.g., norovirus and cruise ship outbreaks) or associations with certain complications (e.g., Campylobacter and Guillain–Barre syndrome). What are the important pathogens that cause diarrhoea, and what is unique about each of them?

4. **DISCUSS!** IBS is 'not a diagnosis of exclusion that first requires extensive testing'. In practice, many young patients do undergo colonoscopy even if they meet clinical criteria for IBS and have no red flags. Why might this be the case, and what are your thoughts on it?

Chapter

14 An Approach to Constipation

Clinical Case

A 76-year-old gentleman presents with severe faecal impaction. He has had constipation for many years, but this is his first time requiring manual evacuation. Apart from a stroke 5 years ago which left him wheelchair bound, his past medical history includes diabetes, benign prostatic hyperplasia, congestive cardiac failure and chronic rotator cuff tendinitis. Medications include bisoprolol, furosemide, insulin, metformin, oxybutynin, telmisartan and as-needed tramadol. How would you approach his complaint?

Constipation means different things to different people. It may mean infrequent stools, hard stools or unsatisfactory defecation (e.g., defecatory straining, or a sensation of incomplete evacuation). It is a common complaint and most often functional, although patients should be evaluated for alarm symptoms suggesting structural gastrointestinal disease, as well as secondary causes of constipation (including neurologic disease, endocrine disease and medication side effects; Figure 14.1).

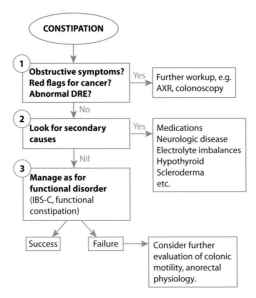

AXR, abdominal X-ray; DRE, digital rectal examination; IBS-C, irritable bowel syndrome, constipation predominant.

Figure 14.1. Approach to constipation.

Evaluation

1. Is There Structural Gastrointestinal Disease?

Obstructive gastrointestinal lesions, including colorectal cancer, may present with constipation. Look for alarm symptoms:

- Acute onset of severe constipation.

- Obstructive symptoms: Association with abdominal pain, increasing abdominal distension and/or nausea/vomiting. See further workup, for example, abdominal X-ray, discussed in Chapter 12.

- Red flags for cancer: Rectal bleeding, decrease in stool calibre, weight loss, anaemia or a strong family history of colorectal cancer. This should prompt further evaluation including colonoscopy.

Anorectal disorders: A rectal examination should be performed in all patients with constipation. Identify

- Painful anal disorders, for example, anal fissure, thrombosed haemorrhoids. These can be the result of constipation or exacerbate it (because defecation becomes painful).

- Rectal prolapse—this may be more obvious when the patient bears down.

2. Look for Secondary Causes

These diseases rarely first present with constipation, but commonly contribute.

	Workup
1. **Medications**: Especially opioid analgesia and anticholinergics (antihistamines, antipsychotics, tricyclic antidepressants). Other culprit drugs include iron supplements and calcium channel blockers.	– Go through drug list
2. **Neurologic disease**	
• Autonomic neuropathy including longstanding diabetes, Parkinson's disease and related syndromes.	– Clinical examination – Screen for diabetes
• Upper motor neuron lesions including spinal cord injury, multiple sclerosis.	
3. **Metabolic and other disease**	
• Electrolyte disturbance especially hypokalaemia, hypercalcemia.	– Screen electrolytes and thyroid
• Hypothyroidism.	
• Scleroderma: Examine for clinical features including sclerodactyly, Raynaud's phenomenon and so forth.	

- Psychiatric disease, for example, anorexia: It's hard to have significant bowel output if there is little food intake.

3. Manage As for Functional Disorder

Excluding the structural and secondary causes of constipation leaves us with its idiopathic/functional causes. This may be

- **Irritable bowel syndrome**, constipation predominant (IBS-C): Some patients have a syndrome of constipation with abdominal pain and/or bloating and may fulfil diagnostic criteria for IBS-C—recurrent abdominal pain (at least 1×/week in 3 months) with two or more of (1) relationship to defecation, (2) changes in stool frequency or (3) change in stool consistency. There may be alternating periods of diarrhoea (IBS-mixed).

- **Functional constipation**: Other patients do not have abdominal pain symptoms, and are simply termed to have functional constipation. Some (but not all) patients have decreased colonic motility or pelvic floor dysfunction (failure to relax pelvic floor muscles during defecation).

An approach:

- Begin with a trial of diet modification (increase fibre) and symptomatic therapy (laxatives).

- Colonoscopy is not necessary for every patient, but offer age-appropriate screening (e.g., above 50 years old for the general population).

4. If Unacceptable Outcome with Symptomatic Management

Consider further specialist evaluation in patients with severe constipation who do not respond to simple measures. Apart from colonoscopy, this may include studies of colonic motility and anorectal physiology.

 Using what you have learnt, **pen down your approach** to the Clinical Case at the start of the chapter **BEFORE reading the discussion** below.

Case Discussion

This is an elderly gentleman with multiple comorbids. His constipation is probably multifactorial; modifiable contributors include medications (oxybutynin and tramadol), and possible electrolyte imbalances (furosemide), non-modifiable factors include diabetic autonomic neuropathy, immobility and age. Nonetheless, given that his constipation is so severe, and this is the first time he has had such severe constipation, it would be imperative to rule out intestinal obstruction (mechanical or functional).

Look for obstructive symptoms, and examine for abdominal distension. Perform a rectal examination. An abdominal X-ray is likely to reveal faecal loading, and would be helpful to rule out obstruction or sigmoid volvulus. In view of his premorbids, the role of further investigation including colonoscopy may be limited (even in the presence of poor appetite or anaemia).

Key Lessons	1. Structural gastrointestinal disease including obstruction, malignancy and anorectal disorders may present with constipation.
	2. Secondary causes of constipation include medication side effects, neurologic disease, electrolyte disturbances, hypothyroidism and scleroderma. These should be sought and addressed, before constipation is managed as a purely functional disorder.
	3. Functional constipation is common. Patients with recurrent abdominal pain and constipation may have irritable bowel syndrome.
Common Pitfalls	1. Failure to offer age-appropriate colonoscopy. A complaint of constipation is an opportunity to offer screening.
Questions	1. **EXPLORE!** It is said that 'the pen that prescribes an opioid should also write a laxative'. What is the mechanism by which opioids, anticholinergics and other drugs lead to constipation? How would you manage this unwanted side effect?
	2. **DISCUSS!** A patient sees you in clinic for constipation. What are the questions you would ask to screen for non-functional constipation? What are the important points in physical examination you would perform?
	3. **GO FURTHER!** How might the digital rectal examination clue you in to the presence of dyssynergic defecation?

Chapter

15

An Approach to Dysphagia

Clinical Case

A 62-year-old man presents with a 4-month history of difficulty swallowing. This started as difficulty swallowing hard food (e.g., steak), which tends to get 'stuck' in his chest. He has switched to a porridge-based diet, but in the last 2 weeks, found swallowing even porridge difficult. He has lost 7 kg in the last 4 months, and feels generally lethargic. He has a past medical history of chronic reflux symptoms, and is a heavy smoker. Physical examination is unremarkable apart from dehydration. How would you approach his complaint?

Dysphagia is a sensation of difficulty swallowing. It is never normal (Figure 15.1).

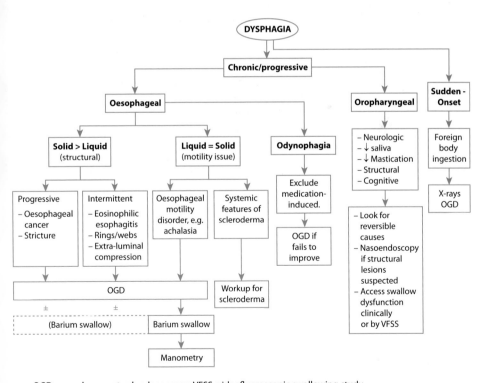

OGD, oesophagogastroduodenoscopy; VFSS, videofluoroscopic swallowing study.

Figure 15.1. Approach to dysphagia.

Initial Approach

The first division is between

- **Oropharyngeal dysphagia**: Difficulty initiating a swallow, especially if associated with coughing, choking, regurgitation and drooling. Patients sometimes use their fingers to help position food, and there may also be abnormalities with speech.

- **Oesophageal dysphagia**: A sensation of food getting stuck a few seconds after initiating a swallow. Patients are often able to point to the location in the neck or chest where they feel the food is getting stuck.

- **Acute-onset dysphagia**: Suggests foreign body ingestion. Ask for relevant history. Consider neck and chest X-rays to identify radio-opaque foreign bodies (not all foreign bodies are visible on X-ray), as well as endoscopy (urgent if obstruction is complete, i.e., unable to swallow even secretions, or the suspected foreign body is dangerous, e.g., caustic, sharp-pointed or large).

Oesophageal Dysphagia

The symptomology of oesophageal dysphagia correlates with its mechanism

- **Structural obstruction**: Causes greater difficulty swallowing solids than liquids, as the larger the food particle, the more difficult to pass down a narrow oesophagus. Patients may have dysphagia to solids only, or to solids first before liquids are involved later.

- **Motility disorder**: Causes equal difficulty swallowing both solids and liquids from the start.

- **Odynophagia** (painful swallowing): Suggests oesophagitis.

Patients with severe dysphagia are often unable to maintain adequate food and water intake, becoming cachexic and dehydrated.

Dysphagia to Solids > Liquids

Aetiologies—progressively worsening dysphagia:

- **Oesophageal cancer**: Progressive solid dysphagia in an elderly patient is worrisome, especially if accompanied with severe weight loss, anaemia, hoarseness of voice and cervical lymphadenopathy.

- **Stricture**: Patients may have a history of heartburn or reflux symptoms (peptic stricture from gastroesophageal reflux disease), neck radiation (radiation stricture) or caustic chemical ingestion.

Aetiologies—intermittent dysphagia:

- Intra-luminal oesophageal abnormalities including eosinophilic oesophagitis, rings and webs.

- Extra-luminal compression of the aorta by congenital aortic arch abnormalities, enlargement of the left atrium or thoracic aorta, thyroid nodules or mediastinal lymph nodes.

Approach: The first consideration is oesophageal cancer, especially in an older patient. Most patients should receive oesophagogastroduodenoscopy (OGD) to visualise the abnormality. Barium swallow is an alternate diagnostic modality in patients who are unfit for OGD, or if severe anatomical distortion is suspected (OGD carries higher risk of perforation).

Dysphagia to Liquids = Solids

(a) **Suspect systemic disorder—scleroderma**: Oesophageal dysmotility is a key feature of scleroderma. Look for other features including Raynaud's phenomenon, skin tightening (especially of the hands and mouth, or diffuse), puffy swollen fingers, calcinosis and telangiectasia. There may be systemic organ involvement including interstitial lung disease, renal impairment and so forth.

(b) **Suspect oesophageal motility disorder**: In achalasia, a motility disorder of unknown cause, oesophageal peristalsis is lost, and the lower oesophageal sphincter does not relax. Other oesophageal motility disorders include distal oesophageal spasm, ineffective oesophageal contractility and so forth. Approach:

- OGD should be performed to exclude structural aetiologies of dysphagia.
- Barium swallow: This may reveal specific findings in achalasia (dilated oesophagus with a bird beak's narrowing at the gastroesophageal junction) or oesophageal motility disorders (e.g., corkscrew oesophagus).
- Oesophageal manometry: This further characterises abnormalities of oesophageal motility and diagnoses motility disorders.

Odynophagia

Odynophagia suggests oesophagitis. This may be medication-induced (i.e., swallowed tablets stuck in the oesophagus) or infective. An approach would be to

- Take a history for medications known to cause oesophagitis (e.g., bisphosphonates, tetracyclines, clindamycin and non-steroidal anti-inflammatory drugs [NSAIDs]); discontinue these medications.
- Examine for oral candidiasis; if present test for HIV and look for other immunodeficiencies.
- If odynophagia fails to resolve 1 to 2 weeks after discontinuing culprit medications, consider OGD. This may reveal a discrete ulcer (medication-induced oesophagitis), white plaques (candidiasis) or multiple ulcers (HSV). Biopsies confirm aetiology.

Oropharyngeal Dysphagia

Oropharyngeal dysphagia is often multifactorial. The goal of evaluation is to identify reversible causes and minimise complications such as aspiration pneumonia.

Aetiologies

- **Neurologic disease**: Coordination of swallowing is a complex process. Dysphagia can be prominent in a number of neurological diseases including upper motor neuron lesions (e.g., stroke), extrapyramidal lesions (Parkinson's disease) and lower motor neuron lesions (myopathies and myasthenia gravis). A careful neurologic examination will be able to identify these diseases (Chapters 25 and 26).

- **Decreased saliva production**: Due to medication side effects (anticholinergics and antihistamines) or as an autoimmune process (Sjogren's syndrome).

- **Inadequate mastication**: Poor dentition and mucosal lesions (e.g., ulcers and viral mucositis).

- **Structural abnormalities**: Oropharyngeal malignancies, Zenker's diverticulum (pharyngeal pouch) and so forth.

- **Cognitive overlay**: Cognitive dysfunction (delirium or dementia) is a significant contributor to dysphagia and aspiration risk in many elderly patients.

Approach

- If a possibly reversible aetiology (e.g., myasthenia gravis and Sjogren's syndrome) is identified, pursue specific workup and diagnosis for that aetiology.

- Bedside swallowing tests to confirm oropharyngeal dysfunction and assess aspiration risk. If in doubt, videofluoroscopic swallowing study (VFSS), a modified barium swallow, can assist.

- **Nasoendoscopy** assists in looking for structural lesions, if the patient does not already have a good cause for dysphagia (e.g., large stroke).

 Using what you have learnt, **pen down your approach** to the Clinical Case at the start of the chapter **BEFORE reading the discussion** below.

Case Discussion

This is a middle-aged man with oesophageal dysphagia, affecting solids more than liquids. Switching from a solid to a soft diet is a telling behavioural modification in many patients with dysphagia. In spite of this, dysphagia has worsened progressively and there is associated weight loss. These symptoms are concerning for oesophageal cancer, especially in a patient with risk factors (GERD, smoking). He should receive oesophagogastroduodenoscopy (OGD) with biopsy, and subsequent cancer staging.

Key Lessons	1. Oesophageal dysphagia is a sensation of 'food getting stuck in neck/chest after initiating a swallow'. A structural cause, most notably oesophageal cancer, affects solids more than liquids. A motility disorder affects solids and liquids equally. Most patients should receive OGD ± barium swallow. Add oesophageal manometry if a motility disorder is suspected.
	2. Oropharyngeal dysphagia is difficulty initiating the swallow. Contributory factors include neurologic disease, decreased saliva production, structural abnormalities and impaired cognition. Apart from looking for reversible aetiologies, consider videofluoroscopic swallowing studies and nasoendoscopy.
Common Pitfalls	1. Dysphagia is abnormal and should not simply be attributed to old age.
Questions	1. **REFLECT!** Have you ever encountered geriatric patients on nasogastric tube feeding due to severe dysphagia? What were the common underlying diseases leading to dysphagia, and to what extent are they reversible?
	2. **EXPLORE!** The barium swallow may be abnormal in oesophageal cancer, strictures and achalasia. How would you distinguish between the appearance of these disorders on barium swallow?
	3. **GO FURTHER!** A patient has oesophageal dysphagia to both solids and liquids. What features of scleroderma would you look for, on both history and physical examination? How is a diagnosis of scleroderma made?

Kidneys and Urinary Tract

Chapter

16

An Approach to Acid-Base Disorders

Clinical Case

A 65-year-old gentleman presents to the emergency department with fever and drowsiness. His blood pressure is 88/40 mmHg. Blood gases and electrolytes on arrival are:

pH 7.18   pO$_2$ 120 mmHg (on 50% oxygen)   pCO$_2$ 68 mmHg   HCO$_3^-$ 24 mmol/L

Na$^+$ 143 mmol/L   K$^+$ 3.5 mmol/L   Cl$^-$ 95 mmol/L   Albumin 30

Chest X-ray reveals hyperinflated lung fields and a right sided patch. He has a history of chronic obstructive pulmonary disease (COPD) with a baseline blood gas of pH 7.36, pO$_2$ 55 mmHg, pCO$_2$ 53 mmHg, HCO$_3^-$ 29 mmol/L.

What are his acid-base abnormalities?

The clinical features of acid-base disturbances vary with their aetiology and chronicity. Patients with uncompensated **acidosis** are unwell, with respiratory distress, anxiety, confusion and eventual circulatory arrest. **Alkalosis** can cause paraesthesia, muscle cramps, dizziness and confusion. An arterial blood gas (ABG) is fast and helpful in any sick patient.

ABG Interpretation

ABG interpretation is simple and logical. Characterise the acid-base derangement fully. Disorders may be mixed, for instance, diabetic ketoacidosis (DKA; acidosis) with vomiting (alkalosis), severe pneumonia (respiratory acidosis) with hypotension and lactic acidosis (metabolic acidosis). A stepwise approach:

Normal ABG Values:

pH	7.35–7.45
pO$_2$	70–100 mmHg (room air)
pCO$_2$	35–45 mmHg
HCO$_3^-$	22–26 mmol/L

1. **Is this acidosis or alkalosis?** Look at the pH: < 7.4 (acidosis) or > 7.4 (alkalosis). *There is never overcompensation.*

   - Normal pH with abnormal pCO$_2$ or HCO$_3^-$ suggests a mixed disorder (respiratory acidosis + metabolic alkalosis, or respiratory alkalosis + metabolic acidosis).

   - Severe pH derangement (< 7.2 or > 7.6) often arises in combined respiratory and metabolic acidosis, or combined respiratory and metabolic alkalosis.

2. **Is the primary pathology respiratory or metabolic?** CO_2 is acidic and HCO_3^- is alkaline—look at which explains the pH derangement. For example, $\downarrow$pH with $\uparrow CO_2$ and $\uparrow HCO_3^-$ is a primary respiratory acidosis ($\uparrow CO_2$ explains the $\downarrow$pH), while $\downarrow$pH with $\downarrow CO_2$ and $\downarrow HCO_3^-$ is a primary metabolic acidosis ($\downarrow HCO_3^-$ explains the $\downarrow$pH).

3. **Is compensation appropriate?** The expected compensation is

   Respiratory

acidosis:	acute:	*for every*	$pCO_2 \uparrow 10$,	*then*	$HCO_3^- \uparrow$ ***1***
	chronic:	*for every*	$pCO_2 \uparrow 10$,	*then*	$HCO_3^- \uparrow$ ***4***
alkalosis:	acute:	*for every*	$pCO_2 \downarrow 10$,	*then*	$HCO_3^- \downarrow$ ***2***
	chronic:	*for every*	$pCO_2 \downarrow 10$,	*then*	$HCO_3^- \downarrow$ ***5***

   Metabolic

acidosis:		*calculate*	$pCO_2 = 1.5 \times HCO_3^- + 8$	
alkalosis:		*for every*	$HCO_3^- \uparrow 1$, *then*	$pCO_2 \uparrow$ ***0.75***

   (pCO_2 in mmHg, HCO_3^- in mmol/L)

   - Inappropriate compensation suggests a mixed disorder. For example, in metabolic acidosis, if pCO_2 > predicted, there is a concomitant respiratory acidosis; conversely, if pCO_2 < predicted, there is a concomitant respiratory alkalosis.

4. **In metabolic acidosis, what is the anion gap (AG)?**

   - The AG measures unmeasured anions (e.g., lactate and ketones). A high anion gap metabolic acidosis (HAGMA) arises when unmeasured anions are produced. Conversely, a normal anion gap metabolic acidosis (NAGMA) arises from bicarbonate loss, and *not* production of unmeasured anions.

   - Normal AG is 8 to 12 mmol/L, if albumin is normal (there may be slight differences based on the lab). As albumin is also an 'unmeasured anion', the expected AG falls when albumin falls.

   - Calculate AG and compare with expected AG:

     Calculated AG = $Na^+ - (HCO_3^- + Cl^-)$ (all units in mmol/L)

     Expected AG = 10 – 2.5 [(40 – albumin)/4]
                   (for every albumin $\downarrow$10, expected AG $\downarrow$ by 2.5)

     If calculated AG > expected AG, this is a HAGMA.

   - Look for a concomitant disturbance by comparing the change in AG (Δ AG) with the change in bicarbonate (Δ HCO_3^-).

     Δ **AG** = calculated AG – expected AG

     Δ **HCO_3^-** = current HCO_3^- – normal HCO_3^-

     In a pure HAGMA, each $\uparrow$1 mmol acid is buffered by $\downarrow$1 mmol HCO_3^-, so Δ AG = Δ HCO_3^-. Therefore,

     Δ AG = Δ HCO_3^- = pure HAGMA (a difference of ±6 is acceptable)

$$\Delta\,AG > \Delta\,HCO_3^- = HAGMA + metabolic\ alkalosis$$
$$\Delta\,AG < \Delta\,HCO_3^- = HAGMA + NAGMA$$

(You can also use the delta ratio, i.e., $\Delta\,AG/\Delta\,HCO_3^-$, which operates on the same principles.)

The internal consistency of an ABG can be verified using the Henderson–Hasselbalch equation:

$$[H^+]\ in\ nmol/L = 24\ (pCO_2/HCO_3^-)$$
$$pH = -\log[H^+].$$

Having fully characterised the acid-base disturbance, proceed based on the primary derangement.

Metabolic Acidosis

Metabolic acidosis arises from (a) accumulation of unmeasured anions, causing a high AG, or (b) bicarbonate losses, causing a normal AG (Figure 16.1).

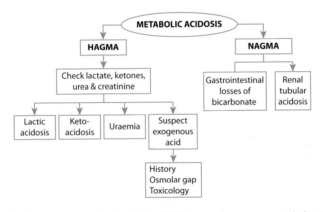

HAGMA, high-anion gap metabolic acidosis; NAGMA, normal-anion gap metabolic acidosis.

Figure 16.1. Approach to metabolic acidosis.

High-Anion Gap Metabolic Acidosis

First check lactate, ketones and creatinine:

- **Lactic acidosis**: Lactate is produced from anaerobic metabolism.
  - **Type A**: Due to tissue hypoperfusion, for example, in septic shock, cardiac failure. Unexplained lactic acidosis, especially with abdominal pain, raises concern for mesenteric ischemia.
  - **Type B**: With normal oxygen delivery to tissue. This occurs due to drugs (e.g., metformin), leukaemia and in inborn errors of metabolism.

- **Ketoacidosis:**
  - DKA presents with hyperglycaemia[1] (glucose $\geq$ 14 mmol/L), acidosis (pH $\leq$ 7.3 or HCO_3^- $\leq$ 18) and ketosis (urine ketones +ve or serum beta-hydroxybutyrate $\geq$ 3).
  - Alcoholic ketoacidosis: Due to increased lipolysis in chronic alcoholics who suddenly stop drinking.
- **Uremic acidosis:** Normal metabolism generates a daily acid load. In acute or severe chronic kidney disease (CKD), diminished excretion of organic acids results in HAGMA (see Chapter 18).[*]

Is cause uncertain, or exogenous acid ingestion suspected? History is key to suspect poisoning with exogenous acids, for example:

- **Methanol, ethylene glycol:** These are metabolised to organic acids. If suspected, measure serum osmolality. A difference between measured and calculated serum osmolarity ($2Na^+$ + glucose + urea) suggests toxic alcohol ingestion.
- **Salicylic acid:** For example, aspirin and some medicated oils. Serum salicylate can be measured.
- **Oxoproline:** Chronic paracetamol use (at therapeutic doses) in malnourished elderly females can result in accumulation of an acidic metabolite, oxoproline.

Normal-Anion Gap Metabolic Acidosis

- **Gastrointestinal bicarbonate loss:** Gastrointestinal contents distal to the duodenum are alkaline. Diarrhoea, ileostomy losses or drainage of pancreatic or biliary secretions causes NAGMA. These disorders would be apparent from the clinical history.
- **Renal tubular acidosis:** Suspect renal loss of HCO_3^- if there is NAGMA but no history of gastrointestinal HCO_3^- loss.[2]
  - Hypokalaemic renal tubular acidosis—Type 1 (distal) or 2 (proximal): An inability to acidify urine, either congenital or acquired (associated with autoimmune disease, myeloma or certain drugs).
  - Hyperkalaemic renal tubular acidosis (Type 4): Decreased K^+ and NH_4^+ excretion in a hypoaldosteronimic state (e.g., diabetic nephropathy, ACE-inhibitors, potassium-sparing diuretics; patients with mild to moderate renal impairment are particularly predisposed.[*]

[*]**Which type of metabolic acidosis occurs in CKD?** Acidosis usually develops by stage 4 of CKD (eGFR 15–29 mL/min). Initially, the loss of ammonium excretory capacity leads to a NAGMA. As CKD progresses towards end-stage renal disease (eGFR < 15), uremic toxins accumulate and the AG widens, leading to HAGMA ± NAGMA.

---

[1] Rarely, glucose may not be elevated (*euglycemic ketoacidosis*) in patients on sodium/glucose cotransporter 2 (SGLT-2) inhibitors (e.g., empagliflozin).

[2] The urinary anion gap (Na_{urine}^+ + K_{urine}^+ − Cl_{urine}^-) can be helpful. It is negative in causes of gastrointestinal HCO_3^- loss, and usually positive in renal HCO_3^- loss.

Metabolic Alkalosis

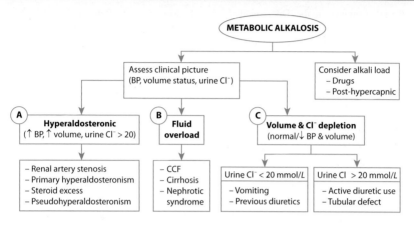

CCF, congestive cardiac failure.

Figure 16.2. Approach to metabolic alkalosis.

The approach to metabolic alkalosis (Figure 16.2) begins by **excluding exogenous alkali loads**, including

- **Drugs**, for example, excess bicarbonate administration.

- **Post-hypercapnic metabolic alkalosis:** In respiratory acidosis, a compensatory metabolic alkalosis develops. When the lung pathology resolves, respiratory acidosis can correct rapidly. The metabolic component takes longer to normalise, leading to transient metabolic alkalosis.

Next, assess blood pressure, clinical volume status and urinary chloride. This will identify one of three clinical pictures:

(a) **Hyperaldosteronic state:** Hypertension, mildly increased volume status and elevated urine Cl^- (> 20 mmol/L).

(b) **Overt fluid overload**.

(c) **Volume and chloride depleted state:** A history of volume loss, normo- or hypotension, clinical eu- or hypovolaemia and usually a low urine Cl^- (< 20 mmol/L).

Note that hypokalaemia is tightly linked with alkalosis, as K^+ competes with H^+ for renal excretion and exchange across cell membranes.

(a) Hyperaldosteronic State

Physiologically, aldosterone stimulates the renal collecting tubules to reabsorb Na^+ with water, and excrete K^+ and H^+; aldosterone excess therefore results in hypertension, hypernatremia, hypokalaemia and alkalosis. Urinary Cl^- is not low (unlike in volume-depletion).

Aetiologies of a hyperaldosteronic state include	Workup
• **Renal artery stenosis**: Decreased renal perfusion stimulates the juxtaglomerular apparatus and activates the renin–angiotensin–aldosterone system.	– Renal artery Doppler ultrasound
• **Primary hyperaldosteronism** (Conn's syndrome): Aldosterone overproduction by an adrenal tumour or adrenal hyperplasia.	– Plasma aldosterone to renin ratio ($\uparrow$ aldosterone, $\downarrow$ renin) – Confirmatory: salt loading or saline suppression test – CT adrenal gland for adrenal tumour
• **Steroid excess**: Including exogenous steroid ingestion (take a history) and Cushing's syndrome (look for its characteristic appearance—central obesity, dorsocervical and supraclavicular fat pads, thin skin, proximal muscle weakness).	– Screen for Cushing's syndrome, for example, dexamethasone suppression test (see Chapter 38)
• **Pseudohyperaldosteronism**: Rare genetic syndromes[3] and chronic liquorice ingestion mimics the effect of aldosterone, but with suppressed aldosterone levels.	

(b) Overt Fluid Overload

Metabolic alkalosis occurs in heart failure, cirrhosis and nephrotic syndrome. These patients appear fluid overloaded (e.g., pedal oedema and pleural effusion), but actually have decreased effective arterial blood volume as much of the excess fluid is in third spaces. There is low-normal blood pressure and decreased renal perfusion, which activates the renin–angiotensin–aldosterone system, resulting in elevated aldosterone levels and consequent alkalosis.

The aetiology of fluid overload should be clinically apparent; workup of unexplained fluid overload is discussed in Chapter 47.

(c) Volume and Chloride Depletion

Check urine Cl⁻.

(i) **Urine Cl⁻ < 20 mmol/L**: This reflects reabsorption of almost all available Cl⁻, as occurs in

- **Vomiting** (or nasogastric tube suction): Metabolic alkalosis, along with volume and chloride depletion, is *generated* by loss of acid and Cl⁻ rich gastric secretions. The metabolic alkalosis so created is *perpetuated* by the kidneys, which attempt to conserve water (given volume depletion) by reabsorbing electrolytes. Because

[3] Liddle syndrome, syndrome of apparent minerocorticoid excess.

of Cl⁻ depletion, the kidneys have to reabsorb more HCO_3^- (as an anion to match each cation reabsorbed, to maintain charge balance); increased HCO_3^- reabsorption results in persistence of metabolic alkalosis.

- **Contraction alkalosis**: Rapid recovery from a fluid overloaded state, usually via administration of IV diuretics, causes a metabolic alkalosis due to chloride loss during diuresis, as well as contraction of body fluid volume around a relatively constant amount of bicarbonate.

(ii) **Urine Cl⁻ > 20 mmol/L**: On the other hand, urine Cl⁻ is paradoxically elevated in

- **Active diuretic use**: Inhibition of tubular reabsorption leads to loss of volume and Cl⁻, generating metabolic alkalosis.
- **Renal tubular genetic defects** which mimic the effect of diuretics.[4]

Respiratory Acid-Base Disorders

Respiratory Acidosis

Respiratory acidosis occurs in hypercapnic (type 2) respiratory failure, often with concomitant hypoxia. Two pointers

- Metabolic compensation for respiratory acidosis (i.e., a rise in bicarbonate concentration) takes time to occur; therefore, patients with acute respiratory acidosis have near-normal bicarbonate, while elevated bicarbonate indicates a chronic component (patients with stable chronic obstructive pulmonary disease [COPD] can have a relatively normal pH in spite of markedly elevated pCO_2, due to metabolic compensation).

- Marked acidosis (pH < 7.3) indicates a failure of metabolic compensation, as occurs in acute respiratory acidosis, or decompensated chronic respiratory acidosis.

Hypercapnic respiratory failure may arise from pulmonary disease (e.g., pneumonia and COPD), neurological or thoracic cage disorders causing hypoventilation, and pulmonary vascular diseases. The approach to respiratory failure is discussed in Chapter 4.

Respiratory Alkalosis

Respiratory alkalosis occurs in hyperventilation ('blowing off' excess CO_2), due to

- As a response to hypoxia (i.e., type 1 respiratory failure), as may occur in pulmonary disease (asthma, pneumonia, pulmonary embolism), cardiac disease (see Chapter 4).
- Stimulation of the respiratory centre by pain, fever or sepsis.
- Voluntary hyperventilation by patient (e.g., anxiety) or iatrogenic by physician (mechanical ventilation).

---

[4] Bartter and Gitelman syndromes.

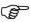 Using what you have learnt, **pen down your approach** to the Clinical Case at the start of the chapter **BEFORE reading the discussion** below.

Case Discussion

The patient has an infective exacerbation of chronic obstructive pulmonary disease (COPD). At baseline, he has type 2 respiratory failure (respiratory acidosis + compensatory metabolic alkalosis), but now presents hypoxic (P/F 120/0.5 = 240) and drowsy (likely from hypercapnia).

Have a closer look at his admission blood gases. Going step-by-step,

1. *Is this acidosis or alkalosis—acidosis (pH 7.18).*

2. *What is the primary pathology?—respiratory (pCO$_2$ 68 mmHg while HCO$_3^-$ is not low).*

3. *Is compensation appropriate?—No, we expect a compensatory metabolic alkalosis, but HCO$_3^-$ is inappropriately normal (and in fact lower than baseline). This suggests a concomitant metabolic acidosis.*

4. *What is the anion gap (AG)?*

   Calculated AG = Na$^+$ – Cl$^-$ – HCO$_3^-$ = 143 – 95 – 24 = 24 (elevated)

   Expected AG = 10 – 2.5 (as albumin is 30) = 7.5

   Δ AG = Calculated AG – Expected AG = 24 – 7.5 = 16.5

   Δ HCO$_3^-$ = 0

There is an elevated AG, implying high AG metabolic acidosis. The elevation in AG is not met by a fall in HCO$_3^-$, suggesting a concomitant metabolic alkalosis.

Therefore, he has respiratory acidosis (from pneumonia and COPD), metabolic alkalosis (compensation for chronic hypercapnia in COPD), and a high-anion gap metabolic acidosis (HAGMA). The HAGMA is likely due to lactic acidosis as he is in septic shock; this can be confirmed by testing lactate and ketones.

Key Lessons	
	1. Four questions help in interpreting arterial blood gases: (1) is this acidosis or alkalosis, (2) is the primary pathology respiratory or metabolic, (3) is compensation appropriate and (4) in metabolic acidosis, what is the anion gap? There may be a mixed disorder.
	2. Metabolic acidosis may be either HAGMA or NAGMA. HAGMA may be due to lactic acidosis, ketoacidosis, uremic acidosis and exogenous acids. NAGMA may be due to gastrointestinal loss of bicarbonate, or renal tubular acidosis.
	3. Metabolic alkalosis occurs in volume/chloride depletion, hyperaldosteronic states, fluid overloaded states and in exogenous alkali loads (drugs or post-hypercapnia). Determination of blood pressure, volume status and urinary chloride helps to distinguish between these causes.

Common Pitfalls

1. Pay attention to the bicarbonate value in the renal panel. Low bicarbonate often indicates a sick patient—this has been missed.

2. The blood gas *never* overcompensates. For example, if you suspect a primary respiratory acidosis with compensatory metabolic alkalosis, but pH is 7.5, please reconsider which is the primary acid-base disturbance.

Questions

1. **REFLECT!** Recall your last patient with a single digit bicarbonate value. Did the patient look unwell? What was the cause of metabolic acidosis, and how did the patient do?

2. **EXPLORE!** Metabolic alkalosis due to volume and chloride depletion is also termed 'saline-responsive metabolic alkalosis'. Why does administering normal saline correct alkalosis?

3. **GO FURTHER!** In NAGMA, the urinary anion gap ($U_{Na} + U_K - U_{Cl}$) can be helpful to distinguish gastrointestinal bicarbonate loss from renal bicarbonate loss. What is the principle behind the urinary anion gap and how is it interpreted?

An Approach to Electrolyte Imbalances

Clinical Case

A 75-year-old lady with a history of diabetes was admitted for a 3-day history of cough, fever, lethargy and poor oral intake. In the last 24 hr, she had also become increasingly confused. Her admission labs were significant for a white cell count of 19 and sodium of 120 mmol/L. She was given antibiotics and 2 L of normal saline over 24 hr.

You review her the next morning. She is still confused. Her blood pressure is 120/80 mmHg and HR 70/min. Examination findings are consistent with a right-sided pneumonia. Her tongue is moist. Jugular venous pressure is not elevated, and she has no pedal oedema. A repeat sodium is 118 mmol/L. How would you approach her hyponatremia?

With routine blood tests, the *diagnosis* of an electrolyte abnormality is almost never in question. Apart from correcting the abnormality, it is important to *find and treat the underlying cause*. The aetiology is at times apparent from the clinical context, but may at other times be more obscure and often multifactorial. This approach discusses the aetiological workup of electrolyte imbalances, including:

- Sodium disorders: hypo- (1) and hypernatremia (2)
- Potassium disorders: hyper- (3) and hypokalaemia (4)
- Calcium disorders: hyper- (5) and hypocalcaemia (6)
- Phosphate disorders (7)
- Magnesium disorders (8).

Normal Electrolyte Values
[check laboratory reference range]

Na^+	135–145 mmol/L
K^+	90–105 mmol/L
Cl^-	2.2–2.6 mmol/L*
Ca^{2+}	0.8–1.6 mmol/L
PO_4^{3-}	0.7–1.0 mmol/L
Mg^{2+}	0.7–1.0 mmol/L

*Corrected Ca^{2+} = Measured Ca^{2+} + 0.02 (40 – Albumin)

Understanding the regulatory physiology helps to make sense of the disorders. Particularly, remember that Na^+ excretion (by the renin–angiotensin–aldosterone system [RAAS]) is coupled to water excretion and hence controls extracellular fluid volume, not osmolality. Osmolality is controlled by free water excretion, under antidiuretic hormone (ADH) control.

1. Hyponatremia

In **acute hyponatremia**, water moves via osmosis from hypotonic serum into cerebral neurons, causing cerebral oedema. This presents with *neurological symptoms—* headache, nausea/vomiting, altered mental state and seizures. Given time, cerebral neurons can adapt to hyponatremia by losing organic osmoles, reducing cerebral oedema. Therefore, **chronic hyponatremia** presents with more *subtle cognitive and gait changes.*

If chronic hyponatremia is corrected too rapidly, water moves via osmosis out of the cells that form the blood–brain barrier (as serum is now hypertonic relative to the neurons), and the cells shrink. The blood–brain barrier loses its integrity and allows immune cells to enter. This causes demyelination of certain pontine neurons, leading to permanent neurological deficits including paralysis, cranial nerve palsies and locked-in syndrome—this is the **osmotic demyelination syndrome**. Therefore, *a key management concern is to avoid overly rapid correction of chronic hyponatremia.* Risk factors for osmotic demyelination include $Na^+ < 105$ mmol/L, alcoholism, malnutrition, liver disease and hypokalaemia.

The diagnostic approach to hyponatremia involves (Figure 17.1):

1. Is this true (hypotonic) hyponatremia?

2. Is hyponatremia acute or are symptoms severe?

3. What is the aetiology? If not clinically obvious, paired serum and urine osmolality and sodium are helpful.

1. Is It True (Hypotonic) Hyponatremia?

Measure serum osmolality. This is correspondingly reduced (< 275 mOsm/kg) in true hyponatremia. Several conditions lead to hyponatremia with normal or elevated serum osmolality:

- Hyperglycaemia
  (glucose $\uparrow$ 3 mmol/L, Na $\downarrow$ 1 mmol/L)

- Mannitol
  (given to patients with raised intracranial pressure)

- Glycine
  (irrigation fluid in urologic surgery)

Translocational hyponatremia: These effective osmoles raise serum osmolality and attract water from the intracellular compartment, hence reducing serum Na^+.

- Severe hyperlipidaemia

- Hyperproteinaemia (e.g., in myeloma)

Pseudohyponatremia: A lab measurement artefact due to reduced plasma water in these conditions.

If serum osmolality measurements are not available, proceed as per hypotonic hyponatremia, if the causes of translocational and pseudohyponatraemia are excluded clinically.

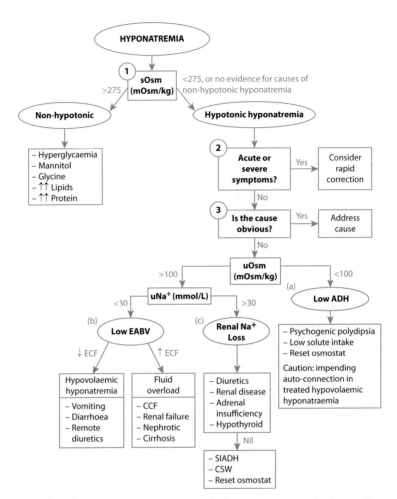

ADH, antidiuretic hormone; CCF, congestive cardiac failure; CSW, cerebral salt wasting; EABV, effective arterial blood volume; SIADH, syndrome of inappropriate diuretic hormone; sOsm, serum osmolality (mOsm/kg); uNa, urine sodium (mmol/L); uOsm, urine osmolality (mOsm/kg).

Figure 17.1. Approach to hyponatremia.

2. Is Hyponatremia Acute or Are There Severe Symptoms?

- Rapid correction of hyponatremia may be considered if hyponatremia developed acutely (< 48 hr). This is because cerebral neurons would not have had the time to lose organic osmoles, therefore there is reduced risk of osmotic demyelination. One must be confident that hyponatremia is acute (e.g., if it develops inpatient and a recent sodium < 48 hr ago was normal); avoid rapid correction if unsure. Patients from the community usually have chronic hyponatremia.

- Severe symptoms (e.g., coma and seizures) may prompt the use of hypertonic saline (e.g., aiming ↑Na^+ 4–6 mmol/L in 6 hr), before any further workup for aetiology.

3. What Is the Aetiology

The causes of hyponatremia can be classified (1) by volume status (hypovolaemic, hypervolaemic and euvolaemic) or (2) biochemically (using paired serum and urine sodium and osmolality). Clinical volume assessment can be insensitive.

If volume status is clinically apparent, the aetiology of hyponatremia may be clear:

- Overt hypovolaemia: With a good history of recent vomiting or diarrhoea, hypovolaemic (depletional) hyponatremia is likely.

- Overt hypervolaemia: In a clinically fluid overloaded state (pedal oedema, pulmonary congestion, elevated jugular venous pressure), hyponatremia may be blamed on low effective arterial blood volume from the underlying cause of fluid overload (e.g., cardiac failure, renal failure, cirrhosis or nephrotic syndrome; see below).

If the cause of hyponatremia is not clinically overt, look at urine osmolality and sodium, taken with a paired serum osmolality and sodium.

(a) Low Urine Osmolality (< 100 mOsm/kg)

Low urine osmolality (< 100 mOsm/kg) indicates suppressed ADH secretion, that is, the kidneys are excreting large volumes of free water, which is an appropriate response to hyponatremia. Hyponatremia in spite of low ADH levels is seen in:

- **Psychogenic polydipsia**: Usually patients with psychiatric disease, who ingest so much free water (exceeding renal excretory capacity) such that serum osmoles are diluted by excess free water.

- **Low solute intake**: Classically described in malnourished alcoholics ('beer potomania') or a low-salt, low-protein ('tea and toast') diet. The inadequate solutes from these diets is diluted by high water intake.

- **Reset osmostat syndrome**: Some patients maintain sodium balance (intake = output) at a chronically stable Na^+ of 125 to 135 mmol/L. These patients respond to fluids normally by suppressing ADH secretion and excreting dilute urine, hence urine sodium and osmolality is low if measured soon after water ingestion.

- **(Caution) Treated hypovolaemic hyponatremia with impending auto-correction**: In patients with hypovolaemic hyponatremia (page 160), fluid repletion corrects hypovolaemia and removes the stimulus for ADH release, resulting in dilute urine (< 100 mOsm/kg). This biochemical picture mimics psychogenic polydipsia but is a dangerous scenario; once ADH secretion is turned off, dilute urine is secreted in large amounts, causing rapid and perilous Na^+ rise ('auto-correction'). *Bottom line: if urine osmolality is measured after fluid repletion is given, consider treated hypovolaemic hyponatremia with impending auto-correction as a differential.*

(b) High Urine Osmolality (> 100 mOsm/kg), Low Urine Na$^+$ (< 30 mmol/L)

Concentrated urine indicates the presence of ADH effect. Low urine Na$^+$ suggests active Na$^+$ reabsorption via a stimulated RAAS, which occurs in conditions with low effective arterial blood volume. Assess for clinical hypo- or hypervolaemia:

(i) **Reduced extracellular fluid—hypovolaemic (depletional) hyponatremia**:
- Gastrointestinal losses: Diarrhoea, vomiting, stoma losses.
- Renal losses: Remote diuretic use (prescribed or covert).

(ii) **Increased extracellular fluid (fluid overload state)**: Patients with cardiac failure, renal failure, cirrhosis or nephrotic syndrome may have low effective arterial blood volume due to translocation of fluid from the intravascular space into third spaces, which in turns lead to pedal oedema, pulmonary congestion and elevated jugular venous pressure. If the aetiology of fluid overload is unclear, review the approach in Chapter 47.

(c) High Urine Osmolality (> 100 mOsm/kg), High Urine Na$^+$ (> 30 mmol/L)

This biochemical pattern indicates renal sodium loss. There is ADH effect without renin–angiotensin–aldosterone stimulation.

(i) **Consider**:	**Workup**
• **Active diuretic use**: Diuretics inhibit tubular sodium absorption. Thiazides, in particular, cause significant hyponatremia.	
• **Renal disease**: Free water excretion is impaired in advanced kidney disease (eGFR < 20 ml/min), recovery from acute kidney injury, renal tubular acidosis and other tubulopathies.	− Serum creatinine
• **Adrenal insufficiency**: Causes hyponatremia via hypovolaemia or via removal of ADH inhibition by cortisol.	− 8 am cortisol, short synacthen test
• **Severe hypothyroidism**: Can cause hyponatremia (mechanism unclear). Mildly abnormal thyroid function in hospitalised patients (sick euthyroid) should not preclude a diagnosis of syndrome of inappropriate ADH secretion (SIADH) (below).	− Thyroid function tests

(ii) **If the earlier are unrewarding**, consider:
- **Syndrome of inappropriate ADH secretion (SIADH)**: Inappropriate ADH secretion results in hypotonic hyponatremia (serum osmolality < 275 mOsm/kg), high urinary osmolality (uOsm) (> 100 mOsm/kg) and inappropriately high urine Na$^+$ (> 30 mmol/L) in a clinically euvolaemic state. SIADH is a diagnosis

of exclusion, after the diagnoses in (i) are excluded. There are multiple causes of SIADH, including:

- Tumours: Small cell lung cancer, lymphoma, squamous cell cancers and others.
- Pulmonary: Pneumonia, tuberculosis and so forth.
- Neurological: Meningitis, intracranial haemorrhage, tumours, trauma and so forth.
- Drugs: Psychiatric drugs (selective serotonin reuptake inhibitors, anti-psychotics, tricyclics), ecstasy, carbamazepine and others.

Workup (e.g., thorax and brain scans) should be considered in unexplained SIADH.

(iii) **Two rare mimics** of SIADH:

- **Cerebral salt wasting (CSW)**: CSW is a syndrome where central nervous system disease (classically subarachnoid haemorrhage) impairs sodium reabsorption, leading to hyponatremia. Unlike SIADH, which is a euvolaemic state, there is patients with CSW are hypovolaemic (although this may not be clinically apparent) and volume expansion may improve hyponatremia.

- **Reset osmostat syndrome**: These patients maintain sodium balance (intake = output) at a chronically stable Na^+ of 125 to 135 mmol/L, and are able to concentrate and dilute urine appropriately. If their free water intake is low, these patients have serum and urine biochemistries resembling SIADH. However, once a fluid bolus is administered, dilute urine is produced; this is unlike SIADH, in which fluid administration does not change urine osmolality, because ADH secretion (and hence urine osmolality) has become independent of serum osmolality.

2. Hypernatremia

Hypernatremia, like hyponatremia, manifests with neurological symptoms—altered mental state, lethargy, nausea—as the cells that are the most sensitive to osmotic fluid shifts are in the brain.

Hypernatremia is a result of too little water relative to the amount of solutes (of which sodium is the most important). It arises in severely dehydrated patients, often those who are too debilitated to drink to thirst.

Pre-Requisite: Inadequate Water Intake

Alert patients with an intact thirst mechanism and access to water should be able to compensate for water losses and *not* develop hypernatremia. Inadequate water intake is seen in:

- Delirium or cognitive impairment.
- Hospitalised patients given inadequate free water.

- Impaired thirst mechanism, for example, in some cases of central diabetes insipidus.

Contributory Factors

Patients may also have:

(a) **Renal water losses**:
- Osmotic diuresis (glycosuria in diabetic ketoacidosis and mannitol).
- Diuretic use.
- Diabetes insipidus: Failure of the renal concentrating mechanism (see Chapter 19).

(b) **Extra-renal water losses**: For example, diarrhoea and vomiting.

(c) **High salt intake without adequate water**: For example, salt poisoning and seawater ingestion.

Workup

- In most cases, the aetiology of hypernatremia is apparent from the clinical history.

- **Check urine osmolality**: The appropriate renal response to hypernatremia is to concentrate urine, raising urine osmolality. Therefore, high urine osmolality (> 600 mOsm/kg) implies that hypernatremia is *not* due to renal water loss (i.e., it may be due to extra-renal water loss, high salt or inadequate water intake). Conversely, inappropriately low urine osmolality (< 300 mOsm/kg) in spite of high serum osmolality (> 295 mOsm/kg) suggests renal water losses.

- **Diabetes insipidus**: Suspect diabetes insipidus if large amounts of dilute urine are being produced despite hypernatremia. Water deprivation test is *not* necessary (and in fact dangerous) if serum Na^+ > 145 mmol/L or osmolality > 295 mOsm/kg. Desmopressin administration distinguishes central diabetes insipidus from nephrogenic diabetes insipidus (see Chapter 19).

3. Hyperkalaemia

Hyperkalaemia results in weakness, and most critically, cardiac arrhythmias including ventricular fibrillation and asystole. Assess (1) is this true hyperkalaemia, (2) the severity of hyperkalaemia and (3) what is its aetiology? (Figure 17.2.)

1. Is This True Hyperkalaemia?

Pseudohyperkalaemia (i.e., measured K^+ > serum K^+) is common, most often due to haemolysed blood from traumatic sampling. Most labs report the degree of haemolysis. Consider repeating K^+ if a haemolysed sample shows borderline hyperkalaemia, it is often worth repeating; but do not discount profound hyperkalaemia simply because of mild haemolysis.

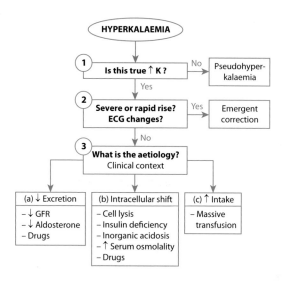

Figure 17.2. Approach to hyperkalaemia.

Figure 17.3. ECG changes in hyperkalaemia.

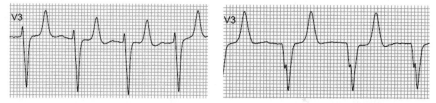

(a) Hyperkalaemia, K^+ = 7.0 mmol/L. Recognise the tall tented T waves.

(b) As K^+ rises further to 9.0 mmol/L, the QRS complex widens, a bundle brunch block develops and P waves disappear.

2. Stratify Severity of Hyperkalaemia

Factors prompting emergent correction include:

- Severe hyperkalaemia (K^+ > 6.0 mmol/L) and rapid rate of rise.
- **ECG changes**: Initially tall tented T waves, flat P waves, widened QRS and ultimately ventricular fibrillation (Figure 17.3).

3. What Is the Aetiology?

Hyperkalaemia may be due to (a) impaired excretion, (b) release of intracellular K^+ or (c) increased intake. This can usually be determined from the clinical context and available blood tests (creatinine and bicarbonate); unlike in hypokalaemia, urine K^+ is generally not helpful.

(a) **Impaired renal excretion of K^+**: This may occur via:

- **Decreased glomerular filtration**: Acute kidney injury and chronic kidney disease (CKD) from various causes (Chapter 18), usually when eGFR < 20 mL/min.

- **Hypoaldosteronism**:
  - Adrenal insufficiency, whether primary (Addison's, congenital adrenal hyperplasia) or secondary. This causes hyperkalaemia, hyponatremia and hypotension. Consider 8 am cortisol, synacthen test and renin/aldosterone testing if suspected.
  - Hyperkalaemic (type 4) renal tubular acidosis: Relative aldosterone deficiency causes reduced K^+ and H^+ excretion (hyperkalaemia and normal anion gap metabolic acidosis). This occurs in diabetes with mild nephropathy (mild volume expansion inhibits aldosterone release) and with drugs like NSAIDS (inhibit prostaglandin-dependent renin secretion).
  - Rare genetic syndromes:[1] Consider in young patients with otherwise unexplained hyperkalaemia.

- **Drugs**: Most commonly in renin–angiotensin–aldosterone axis inhibitors (angiotensin-converting enzyme inhibitors, angiotensin receptor blockers, spironolactone), drugs impairing renal function (e.g., NSAIDs) and others directly impairing tubular excretion (cyclosporine and bactrim).

(b) **Shift of intracellular K^+ into extracellular space**: This occurs in:

- **Cell lysis**: For example, rhabdomyolysis (crush injury, heat stroke, etc.), tumour lysis syndrome (e.g., upon initiation of chemotherapy in leukaemia with high tumour burden) or in burns.

- **Insulin deficiency**: Insulin drives cellular uptake of K^+, so insulin deficiency especially in diabetic ketoacidosis results in hyperkalaemia.

- **Inorganic acidosis**: Excess H^+ enters cells to buffer acidosis, but in exchange for K^+ (this tends not to occur in lactic acidosis).

- **Increase in serum osmolality**: IV hypertonic mannitol, IV intravenous globulin and hyperglycaemia causes water efflux out of cells along an osmotic gradient, 'dragging' along K^+.

- **Drugs**: Succinylcholine (depolarises muscles, causing K^+ efflux), digoxin overdose and fluoride poisoning (inhibits K^+ uptake via Na/K pump).

(c) **Increased intake of K^+**:

- Large-volume red cell transfusion.

- High dietary intake of K^+ alone should not result in hyperkalaemia, except in patients with CKD and impaired renal K^+ excretion.

---

[1] Pseudohypoaldosteronism, Gordon syndrome and so forth.

4. Hypokalaemia

Mild hypokalaemia is common and frequently asymptomatic. Severe hypokalaemia may affect cardiac (ECG changes, arrhythmias; Figure 17.4) and skeletal muscle (weakness, constipation, leg cramps). The approach to hypokalaemia is given in Figure 17.5.

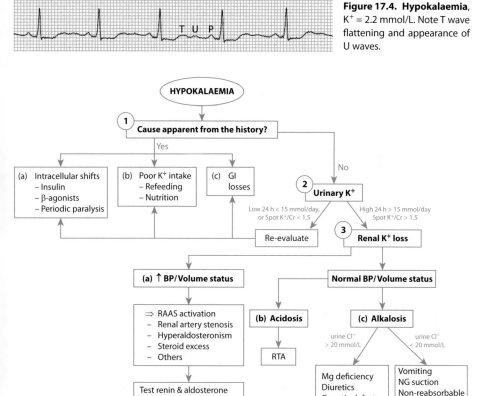

Figure 17.4. Hypokalaemia, K+ = 2.2 mmol/L. Note T wave flattening and appearance of U waves.

GI, gastrointestinal; RAAS, renin–angiotensin–aldosterone system; RTA, renal tubular acidosis.

Figure 17.5. Approach to hypokalaemia.

1. Is It Apparent From This History?

The clinical context may lead to a suspicion of hypokalaemia due to intracellular–extracellular shifts, inadequate K+ intake, or K+ loss.

(a) **Intracellular–extracellular shifts**:

- Intensive insulin therapy for diabetic ketoacidosis.
- Increased beta-adrenergic activity: Bronchodilators (e.g., acute asthma), stress-induced catecholamine release (e.g., myocardial infarction).

- Periodic paralysis: Hypokalaemic (due to a genetic calcium channel mutation) or thyrotoxic (acquired). Episodes of marked generalised weakness, associated with low potassium levels, characteristically occurs after exercise, stress or a high-carbohydrate meal.

(b) **Poor potassium intake:**

- **Refeeding syndrome**: Severe hypokalaemia, hypomagnesaemia and hypophosphatemia when malnourished patients with low body K^+ stores are fed, stimulating insulin release.

- **Chronic poor nutrition**: Mild chronic hypokalaemia is common in elderly patients with poor nutrition, but this is rarely the only cause of hypokalaemia. Search for another cause especially if hypokalaemia is severe.

(c) **Gastrointestinal potassium loss**: For example, diarrhoea, vomiting, ileostomy losses.

2. Test Urinary Potassium

If the aetiology of hypokalaemia is not apparent from the history, test urinary K^+. This should be suppressed in a hypokalaemic patient (so as to conserve K^+).

- **Urine potassium low** (24-hr urine K^+ < 15 mmol/day or spot urine K^+/creatinine < 1.5): Suggests appropriate renal reabsorption of potassium. Look again for a cause of potassium loss, transcellular shift or inadequate intake. Intermittent surreptitious diuretic use can present with low urinary K+ between doses.

- **Urine potassium high** (24-hr urine K^+ > 15 mmol/day or spot urine K^+/creatinine > 1.5): Suggests renal K^+ wasting. These disorders may be occult.

Check magnesium: At this juncture, it is usually worth screening serum magnesium as hypomagnesaemia is associated with refractory hypokalaemia.

3. Workup of Renal K^+ Losses

The causes of renal potassium wasting can be differentiated on (i) blood pressure and extracellular volume status, and (ii) acidosis or alkalosis.

(a) **Hypertension, hypervolaemia + metabolic alkalosis**: Suggests RAAS activation driving hypokalaemia. These can be differentiated based on renin and aldosterone levels. Some causes:

Workup

- **Renal artery stenosis**: Decreased renal perfusion stimulates the juxtaglomerular apparatus and activates the RAAS.

  − Renal artery Doppler ultrasound: decreased flow

- **Primary hyperaldosteronism** (Conn's syndrome): Aldosterone overproduction by an adrenal tumour or adrenal hyperplasia.

  − Plasma aldosterone to renin ratio (↑ aldosterone, ↓ renin)

- Confirmatory: salt loading or saline suppression test
- CT adrenal gland for adrenal tumour

- Low-dose dexamethasone suppression test if suspecting Cushing's syndrome
- See Chapter 38

- **Steroid excess**: Including exogenous steroid ingestion (take a history) and Cushing's syndrome (look for its characteristic appearance—central obesity, dorsocervical and supraclavicular fat pads, thin skin, proximal muscle weakness).

- **Pseudohyperaldosteronism**: Various genetic syndromes[2] and chronic liquorice ingestion mimic the effect of aldosterone, but with suppressed renin and aldosterone levels.

(b) **Normo/hypotension, eu/hypovolaemia + Metabolic acidosis**: Most causes of hypokalaemia cause alkalosis; apart from severe diarrhoea (which should be apparent from history, as discussed earlier), acidosis occurs in:

- **Renal tubular acidosis**, type 1 (distal) or 2 (proximal): An inability to acidify urine, which may be congenital or acquired (associated with autoimmune disease, myeloma or certain drugs). K^+ loss is a result of increased distal sodium delivery, which enhances K^+ excretion.

(c) **Normo/hypotension, eu/hypovolaemia + Metabolic alkalosis**: A urine Cl^- is helpful.

(i) **High urine chloride** (> 20 mmol/L)

- **Magnesium deficiency**: Magnesium is required in the distal nephron to block K^+ wasting via the ROMK channel. Test and treat hypomagnesaemia, as hypokalaemia is often refractory to replacement until magnesium levels are corrected.

- **Active diuretic therapy**: Diuretics inhibit renal K^+ and Cl^- reabsorption.

- Renal tubular genetic defects, which mimic the effect of diuretics.[3]

(ii) **Low urine chloride** (< 20 mmol/L)

- **Vomiting or nasogastric tube suction**: Loss of K^+-rich upper gastrointestinal secretions. Furthermore, vomiting also results in metabolic alkalosis (page 152), in response, the kidney may reabsorb H^+ in exchange for K^+ (to maintain electrical neutrality), perpetuating hypokalaemia.

- **Non-reabsorbable anions**: For example, ketoanions and salicylate. Excretion of these anions also requires excretion of accompanying cations (Na^+ and K^+) to maintain electroneutrality.

---

[2] Liddle syndrome, syndrome of apparent minerocorticoid excess, congenital adrenal hyperplasia (increase in non-aldosterone mineralocorticoid) and others.

[3] Bartter and Gitelman syndromes.

5. Hypercalcaemia

The clinical features of moderate to severe hypercalcaemia are aptly captured in the maxim *stones* (calcium precipitation leading to nephrolithiasis), *bones* (osteopenia, erosions, fractures), *groans* (abdominal pain, constipation, nausea/vomiting, as hypercalcaemia depresses gut contractility) and *moans* (depression, lethargy, fatigue). There can be cardiac effects (short QT and arrhythmias). On the other hand, hypercalcaemia may be a coincidental finding in an asymptomatic patient, and may herald occult malignancy (*take it seriously!*)

Initial Steps

1. **Calculate corrected calcium** = Ca^{2+} + 0.02 (40 – albumin). Measured Ca^{2+} includes protein-bound and free Ca^{2+}, but only free Ca^{2+} is biologically active. Hence, in hypoalbuminaemic states, total Ca^{2+} is falsely low.

2. **Classify into three clinical pictures**: If aetiology is not obvious, do serum creatinine and parathyroid hormone (PTH) to distinguish (Figure 17.6):

   (a) Hypercalcaemia in CKD.

   (b) Hypercalcaemia with normal/↑ PTH and normal kidney function.

   (c) Hypercalcaemia with ↓ PTH and normal kidney function.

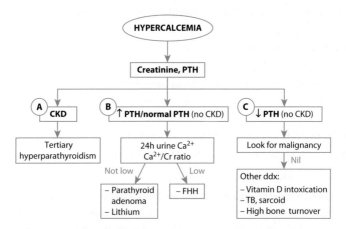

CKD, chronic kidney disease; FHH, familial hypocalciuric hypercalcaemia; PTH, parathyroid hormone.

Figure 17.6. Approach to hypercalcaemia.

Hypercalcaemia + CKD

Hypercalcaemia in late CKD (eGFR < 30 mL/min) implies tertiary hyperparathyroidism.

It is helpful to understand the biochemical picture of primary, secondary and tertiary hyperparathyroidism (Table 17.1). In CKD, Ca^{2+} is initially low, due to deficient

Table 17.1. Biochemical Pictures in Hyperparathyroidism

Aetiology	Ca^{2+}	PO_4^{3-}	PTH
Primary hyperparathyroidism (e.g., parathyroid adenoma)	↑	↓	↑
Secondary hyperparathyroidism	↓	↑	↑
Tertiary hyperparathyroidism	↑	↑	↑
Malignancy	↑	Variable	↓

PTH, parathyroid hormone.

hydroxylation of vitamin D to active vitamin D (performed by the kidneys). Low Ca^{2+}, coupled with PO_4^{3-} retention due to reduced renal clearance, stimulates PTH secretion (its action being to raise Ca^{2+} and lower PO_4^{3-})—this is *secondary hyperparathyroidism*. With time, however, PTH secretion becomes autonomous and decoupled from Ca^{2+} levels; if this causes hypercalcaemia, it is termed *tertiary hyperparathyroidism*.

Other causes of hypercalcaemia, especially myeloma, remain possible and should be considered if there are atypical features (e.g., if PTH is suppressed).

Hypercalcaemia + Normal/High PTH (No CKD)

Hypercalcaemia should suppress PTH; normal or high levels are inappropriate and suggest that PTH is driving the hypercalcaemia. The diagnoses to consider in this situation are:

Workup

- **Parathyroid adenoma**: Primary hyperparathyroidism due to a solitary adenoma or diffuse hyperplasia.

  – ^{99m}Tc sestamibi scan

- **Lithium therapy**: Lithium, used in bipolar disorder, can stimulate PTH secretion.

- **Familial hypocalciuric hypercalcaemia (FHH)**: A genetic mutation in the calcium-sensing receptor results in Ca^{2+} levels being maintained at a mildly higher-than-normal set-point. This is a benign disorder.

  – Low 24 hr urine Ca^{2+} (< 100 mg/day) and calcium/creatinine ratio

Hypercalcaemia + Low PTH (No CKD)

This indicates suppression of PTH by an extrinsic cause of hypercalcaemia—usually malignancy. Cancer can cause hypercalcaemia via bone invasion, production of PTH-related protein as a paraneoplastic syndrome (which can be measured), and high vitamin D levels in lymphoma. The clinical course is usually rapid, with other clinical features of malignancy developing soon after onset of hypercalcaemia if not already present. Hypercalcaemia > 1 year with no other symptoms tends not to be due to cancer.

The main concern in approaching these patients is to search for malignancy.

Look for a malignancy: This is essentially an approach to a cancer of unknown primary. Consider:

- Clinical features: Attempt to localise the cancer based on symptoms and physical exam.
- Imaging: CT chest, abdomen, bone scan. Squamous cell cancers (lung, head and neck, renal and urogenital) are particularly prone to causing hypercalcaemia.
- Look for haematological anomalies (see Chapter 34). In particular, hypercalcaemia is a classical feature in multiple myeloma (look for anaemia, consider serum protein electrophoresis).
- Consider direct endoscopic visualisation, especially age-appropriate screening not yet done (e.g., pap smear and colonoscopy).

Other differentials: If cancer is excluded, consider:

- **Vitamin D intoxication**: Due to chronic overdose of vitamin D supplements. Serum 25(OH)D proves to be severely elevated (caution: vitamin D levels are also elevated in lymphoma).
- **Granulomatous disease**: Sarcoidosis or tuberculosis can cause vitamin D activation and hypercalcaemia. Imaging and biopsy may reveal these causes.
- **High bone turnover**: Hyperthyroidism, Paget's disease and other disorders of bone turnover may cause mild hypercalcaemia.

6. Hypocalcaemia

Hypocalcaemia causes neuromuscular excitability, which affects the sensory nerves (circumoral numbness and paraesthesia), muscles (muscle cramps, twitching, dystonias), brain (irritability, psychosis) and heart (long QT and arrhythmias). Classic signs include the Trousseau (BP cuff inflation causes carpal spasm) and Chvostek sign (tapping facial nerve causes facial twitching). In severe cases, there can be seizures and laryngospasm leading to respiratory arrest.

Initial Steps

1. **Calculate corrected calcium** = $Ca^{2+} + 0.02$ (40 – albumin). Albumin is a negative acute phase reactant and falls in acute illness; in hypoalbuminaemia, measured (total) calcium apparently falls due to the fall in albumin-bound calcium, although active (ionised) calcium levels remain normal.

2. **Approach**: Look for an overt cause of Ca^{2+} loss from circulation. Measure PTH, PO_4^{3-} and Mg^{2+} levels. This classifies hypocalcaemia into three clinical pictures (Figure 17.7).

   (a) Hypocalcaemia with overt source of Ca^{2+} loss.

   (b) Hypocalcaemia with high PTH.

   (c) Hypocalcaemia with low PTH.

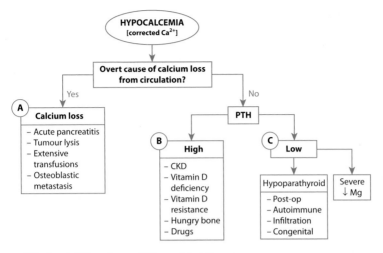

CKD, chronic kidney disease; PTH, parathyroid hormone.

Figure 17.7. Approach to hypocalcaemia.

(a) Calcium Loss

These situations are generally clinically overt

- **Acute pancreatitis**: Released pancreatic enzymes autodigest fat, forming free fatty acids, which bind Ca^{2+} (saponification). Ca^{2+} deposition causes hypocalcaemia (with variable PTH levels depending on the time elapsed). The degree of hypocalcaemia is a severity marker for pancreatitis.

- **Cell lysis**—in tumour lysis and rhabdomyolysis, large quantities of intracellular PO_4^{3-} are released, causing calcium phosphate deposition, and a fall in Ca^{2+} levels.

- **Extensive transfusions**: Citrate in blood chelates Ca^{2+}.

- **Osteoblastic metastases**: Patients with widespread osteoblastic metastases (e.g., prostate or breast cancer) can have hypocalcaemia due to Ca^{2+} deposition around the tumour.

(b) Hypocalcaemia with High PTH

High PTH implies that the parathyroid glands are responding appropriately to low Ca^{2+}, but PTH is ineffective in increasing serum Ca^{2+}. This occurs in:

- **CKD**: Impaired 1-hydroxylation of vitamin D hinders Ca^{2+} absorption, leading to hypocalcaemia and secondary hyperparathyroidism.

- **Vitamin D deficiency**: Measured vitamin D and PO_4^{3-} is low (as vitamin D is required for both Ca^{2+} and PO_4^{3-} absorption). This may occur in poor sunlight exposure (reduced vitamin D synthesis), nutritional deficiency and gastrointestinal disease leading to malabsorption of fat-soluble vitamins.

- **Genetic vitamin D or PTH resistance**: These are rare disorders. In vitamin D resistance (vitamin D dependent rickets), there is a biochemical picture of vitamin D deficiency ($\downarrow Ca^{2+}$, $\downarrow PO_4^{3-}$) but with high vitamin D levels. In PTH resistance (pseudohypoparathyroidism), there is apparent hypoparathyroidism ($\downarrow Ca^{2+}$, $\uparrow PO_4^{3-}$) but with high PTH levels, and there may be phenotypic features of Albright's hereditary osteodystrophy (short stature, round facies, obesity, short forth metacarpal bones, developmental delay).

- **Hungry bone syndrome**: Longstanding vitamin D deficiency or hyperparathyroidism (which stimulates Ca^{2+} release from bone) depletes bone Ca^{2+}. When these disorders are corrected, 'hungry' bones may take up Ca^{2+} rapidly, leading to hypocalcaemia.

- **Drugs**: Especially the inhibitors of bone resorption used in osteoporosis (bisphosphonates and denosumab).

Biochemical distinction: Test serum creatinine, PO_4^{3-}, and vitamin D levels (Table 17.2). Remember that the effect of vitamin D is to raise Ca^{2+} and PO_4^{3-} by increasing their absorption, while that of PTH is to raise Ca^{2+} but lower PO_4^{3-}.

Table 17.2. Biochemical Pictures in Hypocalcaemia

Aetiology	Ca^{2+}	PO_4^{3-}	PTH	25(OH)D
CKD (secondary hyperparathyroidism)	↓	↑	↑	
Vitamin D deficiency	↓	↓	↑	↓
Vitamin D resistance	↓	↓	↑	↑
PTH resistance	↓	↑	↑	
Hypoparathyroidism	↓	↑	↓	

Hungry bone syndrome and drugs need to be excluded clinically.

(c) Hypocalcaemia with Low PTH

Low PTH is inappropriate in hypocalcaemia and indicates failure to respond to hypocalcaemia. This occurs in:

- **Hypoparathyroidism**: Various causes—inadvertent parathyroid gland damage during thyroid surgery, autoimmune disease (e.g., polyglandular autoimmune syndrome), infiltration (hemochromatosis) or congenital syndromes.

- **Hypomagnesaemia**: This impairs PTH secretion.

7. Phosphate Disorders

Acute hypophosphatemia causes ATP depletion, ruining oxidative cellular metabolism. Tissue dysfunction manifests with neuromuscular symptoms (limb or cranial nerve weakness, altered mental state), rhabdomyolysis and cardiac dysfunction.

Chronic hypophosphatemia causes bone pain, osteomalacia and rickets. Patients with **hyperphosphatemia** may be asymptomatic or present with symptoms of an associated hyper- or hypocalcaemia.

Isolated PO_4^{3-} imbalances are rare as PO_4^{3-} homeostasis is closely tied to K^+ and Ca^{2+} balance. Hence, the following scenarios can be discerned (check electrolytes including Ca^{2+}):[4]

(a) Phosphate disorder in renal impairment.

(b) Phosphate disorder with concomitant K^+ derangement.

(c) Phosphate disorder with concomitant Ca^{2+} derangement.

(d) Phosphate disorder with normal K^+, Ca^{2+} and creatinine: consider renal phosphate wasting.

(a) Phosphate Disorder in Renal Impairment

- Hyperphosphatemia occurs due to impaired PO_4^{3-} excretion; this drives secondary hyperparathyroidism. Other factors may contribute to hyperphosphatemia—most commonly an ill-advised fleet enema, which has a high PO_4^{3-} load.

- Hypophosphatemia can occur if excess phosphate binders are used or phosphate is rapidly removed via dialysis (usually in patients who are newly initiated on dialysis).

(b) Phosphate Disorder with Abnormal Potassium

PO_4^{3-} usually moves in the same direction as K^+.

Hypokalaemia with hypophosphatemia:

- **Increased excretion**: Gastrointestinal or renal losses. These can be distinguished by the 24-hr urinary phosphate, which is appropriately low (< 100 mg/day) in gastrointestinal losses but high in renal losses (> 100 mg/day). A proximal tubular defect (e.g., Fanconi syndrome) may cause renal wasting of K^+, PO_4^{3-}, HCO_3^- (renal tubular acidosis), glucose and amino acids.

- **Increased cellular uptake**: Insulin therapy (diabetic ketoacidosis [DKA]) and beta agonist therapy.

- **Refeeding syndrome.**

Hyperkalaemia with hyperphosphatemia:

- **Release of intracellular ions**: Rhabdomyolysis, tumour lysis, severe haemolytic anaemia and so forth.

(c) Phosphate Disorder with Abnormal Calcium

This is less straightforward as Ca^{2+} and PO_4^{3-} do not always move in the same direction. However, this can also be deduced by working through the causes of hypo- or hypercalcaemia and their pathophysiology (Table 17.3).

---

[4] This is an unconventional strategy, but it saves learning yet another approach.

Table 17.3. Phosphate Disorder with Abnormal Calcium

	$\uparrow Ca^{2+}$	$\downarrow Ca^{2+}$
$\uparrow PO_4^{3-}$	Vitamin D excess TB, sarcoidosis	Hypoparathyroidism Pseudohypoparathyroidism
$\downarrow PO_4^{3-}$	Primary hyperparathyroidism Malignancy	Vitamin D deficiency Vitamin D resistance Hungry bone syndrome

See the sections on K^+ and Ca^{2+} disorders for a further discussion of aetiologies and workup.

(d) Primary Renal Phosphate Wasting Syndromes

The renal phosphate wasting syndromes exhibit inappropriately high 24-hr urinary PO_4^{3-} in spite of low serum PO_4^{3-}. Examples include hereditary hypophosphatemia rickets (a genetic defect) or oncogenic osteomalacia (excess fibroblast growth factor-23 production by a tumour). These syndromes are rare, and will not be discussed in further detail.

8. Magnesium Disorders

The clinical features of magnesium disorders parallel that of calcium derangements. **Hypomagnesaemia** causes neuromuscular irritability affecting peripheral nerves (tetany, weakness, tremor), brain (seizure, vertigo, ataxia, delirium) and cardiac muscle (tachyarrhythmias and long QT). **Hypermagnesaemia** causes neuromuscular blockade (weakness, coma, areflexia, bradycardia, heart block) and vasodilation (hypotension).

Mg^{2+} homeostasis is closely tied to K^+ and Ca^{2+} balance, with many overlapping causes. Hypomagnesaemia is associated with refractory hypokalaemia (renal K^+ wasting via ROMK channel) and hypocalcaemia (PTH resistance and decreased PTH secretion).

Hypomagnesaemia

Hypomagnesaemia with hypokalaemia:

- Increased excretion: Gastrointestinal losses or renal losses (e.g., diuretics, genetic defects which mimic diuretics, proximal tubular defects, e.g., Fanconi syndrome). 24-hr urinary magnesium is low in gastrointestinal losses, and high in renal losses.
- Increased cellular uptake: Insulin or beta-agonist therapy.
- Reduced intake: Alcoholism, starvation and re-feeding syndrome.

Hypomagnesaemia with hypocalcaemia:

- Deposition: In acute pancreatitis.
- Vitamin D deficiency.

- Hungry bone syndrome.

Normal K$^+$ and Ca^{2+}: Rare genetic tubular defects (not discussed further).

Hypermagnesaemia

The main causes are a subset of the causes of hyperkalaemia:

- Reduced excretion: Renal impairment is the most common reason of hypermagnesaemia; normal kidneys can easily excrete excess Mg^{2+}.
- Release of intracellular Mg^{2+}: Rhabdomyolysis, trauma, tumour lysis or burns.
- Increased intake: Mg^{2+}-containing antacids and laxatives, iatrogenic administration of intravenous Mg^{2+}.

Refer to the sections on K$^+$ and Ca^{2+} disorders for further workup.

 Using what you have learnt, **pen down your approach** to the Clinical Case at the start of the chapter **BEFORE reading the discussion** below.

Case Discussion

This is a 75-year-old lady with pneumonia and hyponatremia; she is clinically euvolaemic. The managing team seems to have thought that she had hypovolaemic hyponatremia (perhaps prompted by her poor oral intake) and treated her with IV fluids, but this had resulted in a further fall in her sodium levels. This behaviour suggests that she has high urinary osmolality (uOsm).

Isotonic fluids may lower sodium in patients with obligate high uOsm and urine sodium (especially SIADH). Consider a patient who has SIADH with urine osmolality fixed at 600 mOsm/kg, regardless of serum sodium. Suppose he is given 1 L of normal saline (Na$^+$ 154 mmol/L, Cl$^-$ 154 mmol/L), which contains 308 mOsm of solutes and 1 L of water. He will excrete this 308 mOsm of solutes in only ~0.5 L of water (to make a urine osmolality of 600 mOsm/kg), leaving behind 0.5 L of free water, which further worsens hyponatremia.

Our patient likely has SIADH from pneumonia, although other aetiologies (diuretics, renal disease, adrenal insufficiency, hypothyroidism) should also be considered. The next step is to measure serum osmolality (exclude non-hypotonic hyponatremia), urine osmolality (likely high) and urine sodium (likely high), thyroid function and 8 am cortisol (exclude adrenal insufficiency and hypothyroidism). She should not receive any further isotonic fluid, but will instead require fluid restriction, sodium tablets and/or hypertonic saline (if symptoms are severe).

| **Key Lessons** | 1. The causes of true (hypotonic) hyponatremia can be divided by clinical volume status (euvolaemic, hypovolaemic or hypervolaemic) or by urinary osmolality (uOsm) and urinary sodium (uNa)—(a) uOsm < 100 mOsm/kg in excess free water or low solute intake, (b) uOsm > 100 mOsm/kg and |

uNa < 30 mmol/L in conditions with low effective arterial blood volume and (c) uOsm > 100 mOsm/kg and uNa > 30 mmol/L in SIADH and related disorders.

2. Hypernatremic patients always have inadequate water intake, and may also have free water losses or high salt intake.

3. The cause of hyperkalaemia is usually clinically overt, and includes conditions with decreased excretion (reduced GFR and hypoaldosteronism), cellular shifts (e.g., cell lysis) and increased intake.

4. Hypokalaemia occurs in cellular shifts, reduced potassium intake and increased losses either from gastrointestinal (urine K < 20 mmol/L) or renal tracts (urine K > 20 mmol/L). Measuring blood pressure, serum bicarbonate and urine chloride helps to distinguish the causes of renal potassium loss.

5. Creatinine and PTH levels differentiate the causes of hypercalcaemia— (a) chronic kidney disease (CKD) with tertiary hyperparathyroidism, (b) dysregulated PTH secretion as in parathyroid adenoma and (c) an extrinsic cause of hypercalcaemia with PTH suppression, usually malignancy.

6. Hypocalcaemia occurs in (a) situations with overt calcium loss, for example, pancreatitis, (b) in spite of high PTH levels, as in CKD and vitamin D deficiency or resistance, (c) due to low PTH, as in hypoparathyroidism and hypomagnesaemia.

7. Disorders of phosphate and magnesium tend to occur with concomitant potassium and calcium derangements.

Common Pitfalls

1. Before jumping to correct an abnormal electrolyte, always check that the abnormal result is true—that is, pseudohyponatremia is excluded, hyperkalaemia is not due to gross haemolysis and calcium is corrected for albumin.

2. Beware of the patient who has been hydrated for presumptive hypovolaemic hyponatremia, and is now found to have low urine osmolality. Low urine osmolality in this context may herald impending autocorrection and rapid sodium rise, with its attendant risk of osmotic demyelination.

Questions

1. **REFLECT!** Have you ever seen a patient with severe hyponatremia? What are the challenges in the aetiological diagnosis and management of hyponatremia, and how may they be overcome?

2. **DISCUSS!** Hyperkalaemia is a common 'abnormal lab result' on-call. Suppose you are called to review a patient, whom you have never seen before, for hyperkalaemia. How would you search through the clinical notes/patient charts/lab results, so as to rapidly identify the cause of hyperkalaemia? Most clinicians develop an efficient routine after a while.

3. **EXPLORE!** Revise the physiology of sodium, potassium and calcium homeostasis. Write down the various hormonal regulators and their roles.

kidney. Patients with AoCKD are more likely to develop volume and electrolyte complications, and are more likely to require dialysis, which may be long-term. Every episode of AKI accelerates CKD progression; many patients are initiated on dialysis during an episode of AKI and are never weaned off.

Chronic Kidney Disease

CKD is defined as kidney damage ≥ 3 months, as evidenced by glomerular filtration rate (GFR) < 60 mL/min/1.73 m^2 or structural or functional abnormalities (e.g., proteinuria, imaging changes or biopsy findings, with or without ↓GFR). It is staged according to the intersection of estimated GFR (eGFR) (lower is worse) and proteinuria (higher is worse). CKD is not a singular disease, but the common endpoint of a variety of disease processes. The goal in approaching a patient with CKD is to (a) identify the aetiology, and (b) identify complications.

Causes of CKD

Begin with a clinical history, examination, UFEME and ultrasound. Identify:

Pre-renal:

- **Renal artery stenosis** (as discussed in AKI).

Post-renal:

- **Urinary obstruction**, for example, benign prostatic hyperplasia, neurogenic bladder, pelvic tumours. If untreated, these aetiologies result in irreversible parenchymal injury.
- **Childhood reflux nephropathy** can lead to long-term renal scarring.

Intrinsic renal:

- **Diabetic nephropathy**: This is the most common cause of CKD, and usually occurs in long-standing poorly controlled diabetics, many of whom also have retinopathy.
- **Hypertensive nephrosclerosis**: In patients with long-standing, poorly controlled hypertension. There is typically also retinopathy and left ventricular hypertrophy.
- **Glomerulonephritis** (GN): Active GN presents with haematuria, proteinuria, hypertension ± systemic features. Other times, GN is insidious and first presents as late CKD—too late to undo the damage done.

Workup

- Renal artery Doppler ultrasound

- Renal ultrasound: severe hydronephrosis and/or scarring

- Screen fasting glucose, HbA1c
- Exclude other causes

- Exclude other causes

- Other GN workup (page 194)
- Renal biopsy (may not change management in established, irreversible GN)

- **Myeloma**: Presents with hypercalcaemia, *r*enal impairment, *a*naemia and *b*one lesions. Myeloma should be considered in any older person with any combination of the 'CRAB' features.

  – Myeloma screen (serum/urine protein electrophoresis, serum free light chains)

- **Cystic kidney diseases** including autosomal dominant polycystic kidney disease.

  – Usually clinically palpable if causing late CKD
  – Renal ultrasound: large cysts

Patients with Presumed Diabetic Nephropathy/Hypertensive Nephrosclerosis

Many patients with long-standing diabetes or hypertension are presumed to have CKD due to diabetic nephropathy or hypertensive nephrosclerosis, without renal biopsy or extensive investigations to rule out other causes. This is fair as these causes are so common.

Red flags that would cast doubt on this diagnosis include:

- Young patient, or short-duration and well-controlled diabetes/hypertension.

- Rapid progression of CKD. This is inconsistent with the natural history of diabetic nephropathy or hypertensive nephrosclerosis, which are expected to progress slowly (e.g., maximum eGFR drop ~5 mL/min/1.73 m^2 per year).

- Abnormal UFEME (e.g., haematuria).

- Known systemic autoimmune disease, or features suggestive of autoimmune disease, for example, rashes, joint pain, sclerodactyly and so forth.

- Anaemia out of proportion to degree of CKD or pre-dating CKD, severe hypercalcaemia, weight loss (consider myeloma).

- Abnormal renal ultrasound.

These red flags should prompt further investigation, possibly including renal biopsy. Missing diagnoses such as GN or myeloma is problematic because disease-modifying treatment is available, and these conditions can affect other organs if not addressed.

Other Issues in CKD

CKD is often a management problem rather than a diagnostic dilemma. While these considerations are not strictly diagnostic issues, a brief mention is in order:

- In addition to identifying the aetiology of CKD, **look for complications**:
  - *A*naemia: Normocytic anaemia due to decreased erythropoietin production (but rule out iron deficiency).
  - *B*lood pressure: Hypertension from volume overload.
  - *C*alcium, vitamin D and bone metabolism: Hyperphosphataemia (reduced clearance) and hypocalcaemia (activated vitamin D deficiency) leads to elevated PTH and mineral bone disease (see page 168).

- *E*lectrolyte derangements: hyperkalaemia, acidosis.
- *F*luid status: volume overload.

- Management priorities differ based on the severity of CKD. For instance, in CKD 3 (eGFR 30–59 mL/min), the goal is to retard disease progression and avoid further renal damage (e.g., optimise diabetic control); complications are usually mild. Conversely, patients with late CKD (eGFR < 15 mL/min) inevitably progress to dialysis, and dialysis planning should be undertaken early; they are also very vulnerable to complications and often crash-land into emergent dialysis. As for patients already on dialysis, a new set of dialysis issues will need to be cared for.

- Pay attention to the patient's comorbids. In these patients, cardiac death is a far more common cause of mortality than CKD itself.

 Using what you have learnt, **pen down your approach** to the Clinical Case at the start of the chapter **BEFORE reading the discussion** below.

Case Discussion

This young lady has 'crash-landed' into emergent dialysis. At this point, it is uncertain whether she has AKI or CKD. The short duration of symptoms favours AKI, while low haemoglobin favours CKD; it is best to keep an open mind. She is young—which makes diagnoses like diabetic nephropathy or myeloma less likely, and aetiologies like glomerulonephritis (GN) more likely.

There are many possibilities in this scenario (think pre-renal, renal and post-renal)

- *If there is multi organ dysfunction, consider:*
  - *Overwhelming sepsis, cardiac or hepatic failure causing AKI as one of many organ failures.*
  - *A systemic autoimmune disease with GN.*
  - *Thrombotic thrombocytopenia purpura (TTP).*

- *Look for any suggestion of GN on UFEME and autoimmune serology.*

- *Obtain renal ultrasound looking for post-renal obstruction or structural kidney diseases, and use Doppler to look for bilateral renal artery stenosis (fibromuscular dysplasia in this age group).*

- *Ensure that she is not pregnant (send beta hCG); if pregnant, entities like pre-eclampsia must be considered.*

She will require renal biopsy, after initial stabilisation.

Key Lessons

1. The best way to distinguish between acute kidney injury (AKI) and chronic kidney disease (CKD) is looking at a baseline creatinine value. Failing this, features favouring CKD include: chronic symptoms, lack of acute illness, anaemia, raised parathyroid hormone (PTH) and shrunken kidneys on ultrasound.

2. AKI may be classified as pre-renal, renal and post-renal. Clinical history, chart review (including medication history), clinical examination (exclude post-renal) and a UFEME is usually able to identify the aetiology of AKI. Some patients benefit from further workup.

3. The most common causes of CKD are diabetic nephropathy and hypertensive nephrosclerosis. Red flags (including rapid progression, haematuria and systemic features) should prompt consideration of other causes such as glomerulonephritis, myeloma and chronic urinary obstruction.

Common Pitfalls	1. Drug history includes asking for non-prescribed medication and traditional supplements. 2. CKD in patients with diabetes should not be automatically assumed to be diabetic nephropathy.
Questions	1. **REFLECT!** If you have seen a number of patients with AKI or CKD, you will notice that some patients are remarkably asymptomatic, while others present in extremis (like the young lady in our clinical case). Why do the patients present so differently? What does it depend on? 2. **EXPLORE!** The interaction between drugs and the kidney is two-way. Read up on drugs and the kidney: (a) what drugs have high risk of causing renal injury, and by what mechanisms (often more than one)? (b) which commonly used drugs require dose adjustment in renal impairment, and why? 3. **DISCUSS!** When can CKD be managed in the community, and when should patients be referred to a renal physician? 4. **GO FURTHER!** CKD used to be staged according to GFR alone, but recent staging systems incorporate both GFR and albuminuria. Why was this change made? What is the significance of albuminuria in CKD?

Chapter

19

An Approach to Polyuria

Clinical Case

A 40-year-old lady, who is on psychiatric follow up, complains of the frequent passage of large volumes of urine which started a week ago. She also complains of always feeling thirsty. How would you approach her complaint?

Polyuria is an increase in urine output (> 3 L). This is quite distinct from urinary frequency (frequent passage of small volumes of urine, see Chapter 21)—so always clarify what a patient means by 'frequent urination'. To maintain water balance, patients with polyuria also develop **polydipsia** (excessive drinking); if thirst is impaired or water intake restricted, hypernatraemia can develop (page 161).

There are only a few major causes of polyuria (Figure 19.1).

- **Osmotic diuresis**, as in uncontrolled diabetes mellitus.

- **Diabetes insipidus** (DI): Inappropriate passage of large volumes of dilute urine. This is a disorder of antidiuretic hormone (ADH) secretion or effect:

  (a) Central (neurogenic) DI: Failure of ADH secretion by the posterior pituitary in response to rising plasma osmolality.

  (b) Peripheral (nephrogenic) DI: Failure of the kidneys to concentrate urine in response to ADH.

- **Psychogenic polydipsia**: Excessive and inappropriate fluid intake, most commonly seen in patients with psychiatric illness (e.g., schizophrenia).

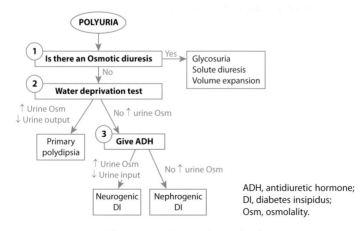

Figure 19.1. Approach to polyuria.

1. Is There an Osmotic Diuresis?

First, exclude an osmotic diuresis by considering the clinical history and doing a urine dipstick.

- **Glycosuria**: Diabetes was named after the production of large volumes of urine ('diabetes'), which tasted sweet ('mellitus'). In uncontrolled diabetes, glomerular filtration of glucose exceeds tubular reabsorption capacity, leading to glycosuria; in turn, glycosuria results in water loss via osmosis. Always do a capillary glucose and urine dipstick for glucose.

- **Solute diuresis**: This occurs (a) in the recovery phase of acute kidney injury, when tubules have not regained their concentrating ability, (b) post-obstructive diuresis after a urinary obstruction is released, for example, catheterisation for acute urinary retention and (c) due to diuretic use. This would have been apparent in the clinical history.

- **Volume expansion**: Ongoing large volume IV fluids results in polyuria, as the body attempts to maintain euvolaemia.

2. Is the Response to Water Deprivation Normal?

Next, test the patient's response to water deprivation, *unless there is already hypernatraemia* ($Na^+ > 145$ mmol/L); hypernatraemia provides sufficient evidence of a water deprived state, and further water deprivation would be dangerous.[1]

   Water deprivation test: Stop oral fluid intake, strictly measure urine output and test urine and plasma sodium and osmolality every 2 hr. Two outcomes:

- **Primary polydipsia—Urine osmolality rises significantly** (to ~600 mOsm/kg) and urine output falls: This reflects normal ADH secretion (in response to a rise in plasma osmolality) and effect (to concentrate urine). The likely diagnosis is primary polydipsia.

- **DI—Urine osmolality rises inadequately**[2] in spite of increasing plasma osmolality (> 295 mOsm/kg) or sodium (> 145 mmol/L); this reflects a failure of ADH secretion or effect. There is DI. In this scenario, proceed to administer ADH (see the following).

---

[1] If there is already hypernatremia, proceed directly to evaluate the response to ADH administration (step 3).

[2] What exactly is 'adequate rise'? This is not clear-cut, because DI can be partial (so urine osmolality may paradoxically rise in DI), and maximum urinary concentrating ability is not always normal in primary polydipsia (so urine osmolality may not rise as much as predicted in primary polydipsia). For our purposes, it will be profitable to learn the principles and not sweat these details.

3. If There Is Diabetes Insipidus, Is Neurogenic or Nephrogenic?

ADH response: Continuing from the water deprivation test (when urine osmolality does not rise in spite of rising plasma osmolality or sodium) administer synthetic ADH (ddAVP/desmopressin).

(a) **Neurogenic DI—Urine output falls and osmolality rises**: This is a normal renal response to ADH, implying that the defect is in ADH secretion. This is neurogenic DI. There are a number of causes:

- Idiopathic: Thought to be autoimmune destruction of ADH-secreting cells in the hypothalamus.

- Trauma: Trauma to the pituitary or hypothalamus, neurosurgery including transsphenoidal pituitary surgery.

- Infiltration: Brain tumour (e.g., craniopharyngioma), Langerhans cell histiocytosis and sarcoidosis.

- Familial and congenital defects: Ask about a family history and look for other abnormalities (optic atrophy, cerebral midline malformations, etc.).

(b) **Nephrogenic DI—No change in urine output and osmolality**: Abnormal renal response to ADH signifies nephrogenic DI. Causes:

- Drug induced: Most commonly lithium toxicity (measure lithium levels), and a number of other drugs.

- Hypercalcaemia (Ca^{2+} > 2.75 mmol/L) interferes with renal concentrating ability (see page 168).

- Renal disease: Acute kidney injury (especially during recovery), early chronic kidney disease (if tubular reabsorption affected disproportionately compared to glomerular filtration), cystic kidney disease and amyloidosis.

- Congenital: Inherited defects in ADH receptor or aquaporin genes. Onset of polyuria is usually in childhood.

 Using what you have learnt, **pen down your approach** to the Clinical Case at the start of the chapter **BEFORE reading the discussion** below.

Case Discussion

Please do not assume that polyuria in a patient with psychiatric disease is primary polydipsia (this is a cognitive bias—framing effect, page 12). She may well be thirsty because polyuria had led to hypovolaemia and hypernatraemia. Apart from primary polydipsia, she is at increased risk of nephrogenic diabetes insipidus (DI) (if on lithium for bipolar disorder) and osmotic diuresis from glycosuria (some antipsychotics increase risk of diabetes).

Begin by testing urine glucose and serum electrolytes. Perform a water deprivation test; if water deprivation results in a rise in urine osmolality and a fall in urine volume, diagnose primary polydipsia. If urine osmolality remains low in spite of rising plasma osmolality, diagnose DI. In that case, continue to administer ADH to differentiate neurogenic from nephrogenic DI.

Key Lessons	1. Polyuria may be due to osmotic diuresis, as in glycosuria, or a true water diuresis, as in primary polydipsia and diabetes insipidus (DI).
	2. In primary polydipsia, water deprivation test results in a normal rise in urine osmolality; conversely, in DI, urine osmolality fails to rise even with water deprivation.
	3. Administration of exogenous antidiuretic hormone (ADH) restores urinary concentrating ability in neurogenic DI, but not in nephrogenic DI.
Common Pitfalls	1. A water deprivation test should not be performed if the patient is already hypernatraemic ($Na^+ > 145$ mmol/L), as sodium will rise further.
Questions	1. **REFLECT!** Have you ever met a patient whose first presentation of diabetes mellitus was with symptomatic polydipsia and polyuria? How else can diabetes mellitus present; ideally, would patients present with symptomatic hyperglycaemia?
	2. **DISCUSS!** It is uncommon for patients with diabetes insipidus to develop frank hypernatraemia ($Na^+ > 145$ mmol/L). Why might this be so?

Chapter **An Approach to Haematuria**
20 **and Proteinuria**

Clinical Case

A 30-year-old nurse is referred for haematuria. She has had intermittent episodes of haematuria for the last 1 to 2 years, with no other symptoms. In particular, she has no dysuria, loin pain, fever, joint pains or rash. On examination, her blood pressure is 152/94 mmHg. The examination is otherwise normal, with no skin or joint abnormalities. Blood tests reveal a creatinine of 123 umol/L, with normal full blood count, electrolytes and liver function. Urine investigations show 35 red cells (75% dysmorphic) and three white cells per high powered field, with no casts, and a urine protein creatinine ratio of 0.2 g/mmol. What is the most likely diagnosis, and what further investigations would you perform?

Macroscopic haematuria presents as visible red or brown urine. **Microscopic haematuria** is detectable only on urine examination; urine is not discoloured but microscopy reveals ≥ 3 red blood cells (RBC) per high power field. **Proteinuria** is the presence of urinary protein above physiological limits, which may present as frothy urine, frank nephrotic syndrome, or be asymptomatic and detected on urine dipstick.

Clinical Syndromes

It is clinically helpful to first identify the clinical picture:

a. **Isolated haematuria**: Without proteinuria, oedema, hypertension or renal insufficiency.

b. **Nephritic syndrome**: Haematuria ± pyuria ± casts, with hypertension and impaired renal function (raised creatinine). There may be varying degrees of proteinuria and oedema.

c. **Rapidly progressive glomerulonephritis** (RPGN, crescentic glomerulonephritis [GN]): Acute-onset nephritic features quickly leading to acute kidney injury (AKI) and oliguria over a short duration (days–months). This corresponds to a histological picture of crescent formation on renal biopsy.

d. **Isolated proteinuria**: Proteinuria less than nephrotic range (< 3 g/day), without haematuria, oedema, hypertension or renal insufficiency.

e. **Nephrotic syndrome**: Nephrotic-range proteinuria (> 3 g/day), hypoalbuminaemia, oedema, ± hyperlipidaemia, with minimal haematuria and urinary casts.

f. **Chronic kidney disease** (CKD): The end stage of renal damage, which not uncommonly is the first presentation of renal disease (see Chapter 18).

Each syndrome is discussed in turn, considering both renal and urological aetiologies. Yet these syndromes are closely related and cannot always be clearly distinguished. At times the clinical picture is an overlap (e.g., a mixed nephritic–nephrotic pattern). Other times the syndromes are a spectrum—for instance, a GN may begin as isolated haematuria, progress through nephritic syndrome, and end as CKD. Finally, one aetiology (esp. lupus nephritis) may present with different syndromes. CKD is the common end-stage for untreated progressive GN.

A. Isolated Haematuria

The approach to isolated haematuria is given (Figure 20.1).

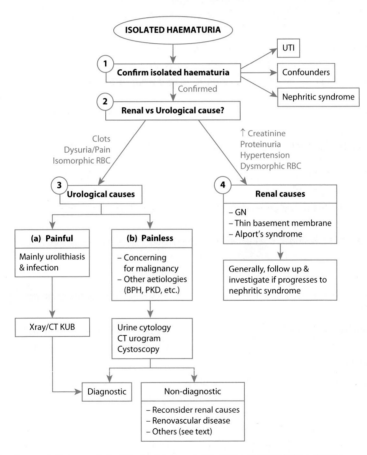

BPH, benign prostatic hyperplasia; GN, glomerulonephritis; PKD, polycystic kidney disease; UTI, urinary tract infection.

Figure 20.1. Approach to isolated haematuria.

1. Confirm Isolated Haematuria

Ensure that the clinical picture is an otherwise well patient with nothing more than isolated haematuria. In particular:

(a) **Rule out urinary tract infection (UTI)**: Acute onset dysuria, frequency or cloudy urine suggests infection (Chapter 21). Look at the dipstick for nitrite and leukocyte esterase, and urine full examination microscopy (UFEME) for pyuria.[1]

(b) **Exclude confounders**: Haematuria in an asymptomatic patient may not be true haematuria.

- **Menstrual blood contamination**: Repeat a sample after menstruation ceases; consider menarche or post-menopausal bleed in non-reproductive age groups.

- **Benign trauma**: For example, preceding sports, sex, recent cystoscopy, traumatic catheterisation. Repeat the sample.

- **Obstructive jaundice**: 'Tea-coloured' urine mimics haematuria; look for scleral icterus, biliary symptoms (Chapter 10).

Where urine is red but UFEME shows no RBCs, centrifuge the urine. In true haematuria, RBCs settle into a red sediment, and the supernatant remains clear. A red supernatant is not haematuria, and should be tested for heme with a dipstick. Interpretation:

- **Supernatant clear, sediment red**: True haematuria.

- **Supernatant red, dipstick heme positive**: Haemoglobinuria (e.g., haemolysis, see Chapter 32), myoglobinuria (rhabdomyolysis).

- **Supernatant red, dipstick heme negative**: Porphyria, red beets, drugs (e.g., rifampicin, phenolphthalein, phenytoin, quinine).

(c) **Nephritic syndrome**: If there is grossly elevated creatinine, hypertension and peripheral oedema, approach as for nephritic syndrome (page 194).

2. Consider If Renal vs. Urological

At times, either a renal or urological aetiology is apparent, other times, both workups may have to proceed in parallel. Certain clinical features favour one but are not absolute:

- **Urine**: Clots or bright red gross haematuria favour urological disease; microscopic haematuria may be of either urological or renal origin. Frothy urine suggests proteinuria and hence renal disease.

- **Urinary symptoms**: Lower urinary symptoms (e.g., dysuria, frequency, hesitancy, dribbling) suggest urological causes. On the other hand, their absence does not rule out urological disease.

---

[1] Note that pyuria with negative urine cultures (sterile pyuria) may be seen in partially treated UTI, infection with fastidious organisms or tuberculosis (TB), prostatitis and other causes of urologic inflammation (urolithiasis, bladder tumour).

- **Systemic features**: Hypertension, raised creatinine, oliguria, fluid overload, prominent lethargy and a known autoimmune disease favours renal differentials.

Urinalysis provides further clues:

- **UTI**: Should be ruled out in all patients.

- **Proteinuria**: Suggests a renal cause.

- **Casts**: These cylindrical structures take the shape of the renal tubular lumen in which they form, and are reasonably specific for renal disease.
  - **Muddy brown granular casts**: Acute tubular necrosis (ATN).
  - **Tubular epithelial cell casts**: Desquamation of tubular epithelium, for example, proliferative GN, ATN, acute interstitial nephritis (AIN).
  - **RBC casts**: Glomerular damage, for example, GN.
  - **WBC casts**: Inflammatory (e.g., proliferative GN, AIN) vs. infective (pyelonephritis).

- **Crystalluria**: Urate nephropathy.

- **Phase contrast microscopy**: This exploits the observation that passage through glomeruli and tubules may deform RBCs. Hence, > 80% dysmorphic RBC is likely of glomerular origin, implying a renal disease. > 80% isomorphic RBC is more likely non-glomerular. This test depends on the availability of skilled lab personnel; 20% to 80% dysmorphic is a grey zone.

3. Urological Aetiologies and Workup

Divide the urological aetiologies into those with loin pain, and those without.

(a) Painful Haematuria

The main considerations are:

- **Urolithiasis**: Episodes of loin-to-groin colic are classic (page 94).

- **Infection**: There will also be flank pain, fever and potentially systemic toxicity. Rule out complications, for example, pyonephrosis, emphysematous pyelonephritis (Chapter 21).

- **Recent instrumentation** including catheterisation can cause traumatic haematuria.

Workup:

- Imaging may begin with a kidneys–ureter–bladder (KUB) X-ray or CT KUB. These non-contrast studies are appropriate in a history typical for stone disease with low suspicion of cancer; consider CT urogram instead if there is concern of malignancy.

- Recurrent stone formers may benefit from an evaluation to identify aetiologies of stone formation. Consider lifestyle factors (fluid intake), systemic disease (e.g., gout and hyperparathyroidism), 24 hr urine collection and metabolic workup (pH, Ca^{2+}, Mg^{2+}, citrate, oxalate, PO_4^{3-}, uric acid, cysteine) with paired serum electrolytes.

(b) Painless Haematuria

The timing of haematuria may be valuable: Initial haematuria suggests a urethral origin, terminal haematuria indicates bladder outlet, neck or prostatic urethra and haematuria occurring throughout micturition suggest upper urinary tract or upper bladder. Aetiologies include:

- **Malignancy**, including renal cell, urothelial and bladder cancers. This is the main concern in painless haematuria, and suspicion increases with age. Look for risk factors (e.g., smoking, occupational chemical exposure, pelvic radiation, schistosomiasis), and constitutional symptoms.

- Causes of painful haematuria (e.g., urolithiasis) may present atypically without pain; these will be revealed on imaging.

- **Benign prostatic hyperplasia (BPH)**: Haematuria is an atypical presentation, lower urinary tract symptoms being more common. See Chapter 21.

- **Papillary necrosis**: In patients with chronic analgesia use, diabetes or ischaemic risk factors (e.g., vasculitis).

- **Polycystic kidney disease**: A patient with known polycystic kidneys, presenting with haematuria, may have bled into his cyst.

Workup: The aim of workup is to rule out malignancy. Perform:

- **Urine**: Cytology, as well as UFEME and culture if not already done.

- **Imaging**: CT urogram is ideal. This is a triphasic contrast CT (plain, parenchymal and excretory phases) which allows identification of stones, masses, filling defects and urinary system dilation proximal to an obstruction.

- **Cystoscopy**: This directly visualises and biopsies bladder tumours, it is necessary as imaging is less sensitive for bladder cancers, and should be done even if CT urogram finds an upper tract tumour (there is a 50% risk of synchronous bladder tumour).

Further workup—consider if the above are negative:

- Reconsider glomerular causes, for example, IgA nephropathy (see the following).

- Hypercalciuria, hyperuricosuria: May predispose to formation of small calculi.

- Renovascular diseases: For example, renal artery embolism, renal vein thrombosis, nutcracker syndrome, AV malformation.

- Bleeding diathesis: But do not ascribe haematuria simply to coagulopathy, without excluding sinister causes.

- Follow up for resolution of haematuria, especially in older patients at higher risk of malignancy.

4. Renal Aetiologies

These aetiologies may present with isolated haematuria and no other worrisome features (proteinuria, raised creatinine, hypertension).

- **Mild glomerulonephritis**, for example, IgA nephropathy (see Section 'Nephritic Syndrome').

- **Thin basement membrane disease (familial benign haematuria)**: Intermittent episodes of haematuria with a positive family history of haematuria without renal failure. This is a benign disease.

- **Alport's syndrome**: A genetic syndrome of haematuria, bilateral sensorineural hearing loss ± ocular changes. There may be a positive family history.

The majority of patients with asymptomatic isolated haematuria and normal renal function (and who have been urologically cleared) do not develop progressive renal disease. Autoantibodies may be performed (see Section 'Nephritic Syndrome'), but renal biopsy is usually deferred and performed only if there is progression to frank nephritic syndrome.

B. Nephritic Syndrome

In the nephritic syndrome, inflammatory glomerular damage makes itself known with haematuria ± pyuria ± casts, and mild-moderate proteinuria. As glomerular damage progresses, glomerular filtration rate (GFR) falls and creatinine rises; hypertension and mild-moderate oedema develops. Clinical features and serological results may suggest a diagnosis; renal biopsy is usually performed in most patients.

Aetiologies and Clinical Features

(a) **Known history of infection**

Workup

- **IgA nephropathy** (synpharyngitic haematuria): This is the most common cause of nephritic syndrome. Clinically, it presents as one or several episodes of haematuria, each < 5 days after a viral respiratory illness. Haematuria may persist between episodes. Progressive proteinuria and renal insufficiency can develop over time, especially if the patient already has proteinuria or raised creatinine. Henoch–Schonlein purpura is a closely related IgA deposition disease, which develops in children and teenagers, classically with a purpuric rash on lower limb extensors, arthralgia, abdominal pain ± nephritic syndrome.

  − Evidence of streptococcal infection, for example, anti-streptolysin O titre
  − Complement levels: low C3 with normal C4

- **Infection-associated GN**: This used to be called *post-infectious* GN, where skin or throat infection with a nephritogenic *Streptococcus pyogenes* strain results in haematuria 1 to 3 weeks later. Recently, it was recognised that GN can occur concomitantly with staphylococcal and streptococcal infection. Prognosis is good, typically with complete resolution of haematuria.

  − Normal complement levels
  − No serology available, no role for IgA levels

- **Subacute endocarditis**: Medical students memorise that this may cause immune complex phenomena including Osler nodes and haematuria. Keep in mind especially if blood cultures are positive for typical organisms that cause endocarditis, or there are risk factors (e.g., IV drug use, prosthetic valves).
  - Blood cultures
  - Echocardiogram

(b) **Multiorgan involvement** suggests a rheumatologic disease, for example,

- **Lupus nephritis**: There may be other manifestations involving the skin (alopecia, malar rash, ulcers), serosa (pleuritis, pericarditis), joints (arthritis), bone marrow (cytopenias), nerves and other organs.
  - Antibodies: ANA, dsDNA, ENA (anti-Sm, anti-Ro anti-La)
  - Complement consumption: low C3, C4

- **Antineutrophil cytoplasmic antibody (ANCA) vasculitis**:
  - **Granulomatosis with polyangiitis** (Wegener's granulomatosis): Causes fever, otolaryngological (otitis media, hearing loss, nasal discharge, ulcers), lung (cough, dyspnoea, haemoptysis, CXR nodules and infiltrates), nerve (mononeuritis multiplex), joint (polyarthritis) and skin (purpura) involvement.
    - ANCA
    - Test for other organ involvement, for example, liver function

  - **Microscopic polyangiitis**: As for Wegener's, but with less profound otolaryngological or lung disease.

  - **Eosinophilic granulomatosis with polyangiitis** (Churg–Strauss syndrome): Asthma, eosinophilia, otolaryngological disease (allergic rhinitis, nasal polyposis, otitis media with effusion, etc.), tender subcutaneous granulomas, heart disease (failure, arrhythmia, pericarditis); also involves nerves (mononeuritis multiplex), gut and other organs.

- **Anti-GBM disease (Goodpasture's syndrome)**: Glomerulonephritis and alveolar haemorrhage (haemoptysis, infiltrates on CXR).
  - anti-GBM antibody

(c) **No symptoms other than nephritic syndrome itself**: Most commonly IgA nephropathy, also consider lupus nephritis (renal disease may precede or be separate from other manifestations). Serology and biopsy would be necessary for diagnosis.
  - Antibodies above

Workup

In practice, the following workup is standard:

- All of the earlier antibodies are sent.
- Screening tests for hepatitis B, C and HIV (these can present with glomerulone-phritis, but positive serology does not prove that glomerulonephritis is due to these viruses).
- Ultrasound of the kidneys.

Renal biopsy is performed in most patients to establish the diagnosis, determine prognosis (activity, scarring) and guide therapy. One exception is a clear-cut infection-associated nephritis, in which prompt recovery of glomerulonephritis would be expected. Biopsy may reveal:

- **Immune complex deposition**: Granular staining pattern as glomeruli are marked by deposited immune complexes for autoimmune attack. Specific immunoglobulin/complement types are deposited in each disease, for example, IgA in IgA nephropathy, 'full house' pattern in lupus.
- **Linear staining** of glomerular capillary walls is found in anti-GBM disease.
- **Pauci-immune pattern**: No immunofluorescence on biopsy—classically in ANCA vasculitis.

C. Rapidly Progressive GN

This is essentially an extreme presentation of nephritic syndrome; aetiologies are that of nephritic syndrome. On the other hand, aetiologies of nephrotic syndrome tend not to present this dramatically. Some notes:

- A biopsy is necessary. This will show crescents and identify the aetiology.
- In the presence of lung haemorrhage, consider the pulmonary–renal syndromes including ANCA vasculitis, anti-GBM disease and lupus.

D. Isolated Proteinuria

Proteinuria may be detected in a number of ways. The gold standard, 24-hr urine protein, is very inconvenient. The spot protein–creatinine ratio is a more convenient test, but may be unreliable in AKI, or in a very muscular or cachectic patient (Table 20.1).

Table 20.1. Detection of Proteinuria

	24 hr urine[a]	Protein/creatinine ratio (PCR)[b]
Microalbuminuria	30–300 mg/day	> 2.5 (male), > 3.5 (female) mg/mmol
Proteinuria	> 0.3 g/day	> 30 mg/mmol
Nephrotic range	> 3 g/day	> 300 mg/mmol

[a] For a 1.73 m^2 person; adjust value for children or very large/small. Microalbuminaemia is only of value in diabetic nephropathy.
[b] To convert PCR from mg/mmol to mg/g, multiple values by 10.

In asymptomatic patients with isolated proteinuria, the focus is to verify sustained proteinuria, and consider secondary causes. Patients with concomitant haematuria, nephrotic-range proteinuria, renal insufficiency or oedema should be considered for primary glomerular disease.

1. Verify Sustained Proteinuria

- Ensure that the patient is not having a UTI: This may cause falsely elevated protein.

- **Do not use dipstick alone**: Patients are commonly referred for proteinuria after positive dipstick testing. This is less reliable; false positives are seen with iodinated contrast, haematuria and pyuria. On the other hand, microalbuminaemia and non-albumin proteinuria (e.g., myeloma) are missed on dipstick.

- **Repeat urinary protein screening**. Transient proteinuria is common (e.g., due to exercise, fever, stress). A single result showing proteinuria of < 1 g/24 hr, with a negative repeat screen, is of no clinical significance.

- **Test first urine sample after overnight rest**: Orthostatic proteinuria is a phenomenon of increased protein excretion when upright but normal when supine, and is also clinically unimportant.

2. Consider Secondary Causes of Proteinuria

- **Diabetic nephropathy**: Microvascular damage from sustained hyperglycaemia occurs in diabetes. Nephropathy begins as microalbuminaemia, progresses into proteinuria, and CKD sets in over many years. Diabetic nephropathy is usually diagnosed presumptively, but other aetiologies should be considered (and biopsy pursued) if GFR declines rapidly, if there is an active urinary sediment with haematuria and casts, or if there are signs and symptoms of a multi-system disease (e.g., suspect autoimmune disease).

- **Myeloma cast nephropathy**: The excreted protein in myeloma is actually immuno-globulin light chains. Suspect the diagnosis in older patients with features of hyper**c**alcaemia, **r**enal impairment, **a**naemia and **b**one pain (the 'CRAB' features). If suspicious, do a myeloma screen (serum and urine protein electrophoresis, plus serum free light chains).

- **Amyloidosis**: Primary in underlying plasma cell disorders (e.g., myeloma), or secondary to chronic inflammatory states (e.g., rheumatoid arthritis and ankylosing spondylitis). There may be multi-organ involvement and this is usually confirmed on biopsy (usually of abdominal fat pad or rectum, rather than kidney).

- **Hypertension**: Uncontrolled hypertension causes hypertensive nephrosclerosis. In the setting of renal failure or other target organ damage (chest pain, pulmonary oedema, aortic dissection, papilloedema, etc.), this is treated as a hypertensive emergency. In the pregnant lady, consider pre-eclampsia.

- **Structural renal causes**: For example, reflux nephropathy, polycystic kidney disease.

3. Consider Primary Glomerular Disease

Almost all causes of nephrotic syndrome can present with sub-nephrotic proteinuria. Consider a basic autoimmune screen (ANA, ANCA) and hepatitis serologies. Discuss renal biopsy should proteinuria become nephrotic, or should haematuria or renal insufficiency develop on subsequent follow up.

E. Nephrotic Syndrome

In the nephrotic syndrome, there is increased filtration of macromolecules and heavy proteinuria (> 3 g/day), leading to hypoalbuminaemia and therefore oedema. There is minimal haematuria. Creatinine is normal or only slightly elevated at first presentation, but with persistent hyperfiltration, renal function declines over months to years.

Adults with nephrotic syndrome should receive (1) renal biopsy, (2) serology to look for secondary causes and (3) workup for complications of nephrotic syndrome. Some patients with diabetic nephropathy progress into nephrotic-range proteinuria over many years; biopsy is often omitted if there is a clear long-standing history of poorly controlled diabetes, and there are no atypical features leading to suspicion of other differentials.

1. Biopsy

Biopsy may reveal the following entities. They generally have little intra-glomerular immune complex deposition, and therefore little inflammation and haematuria. These are histological pictures and not in themselves diseases; each histological picture may be primary (idiopathic) or secondary to another disease.

- **Minimal-change disease** (nil lesion): The majority are idiopathic.
- **Focal segmental glomerulosclerosis** (FSGS): May be primary or secondary; secondary causes include drugs, infection and any entity that decreases nephron mass.
- **Membranous glomerulonephritis** (MGN): Primary vs. secondary due to lupus, malignancy, drugs, hepatitis B and C. 70% to 80% of primary MGN are positive for anti-phospholipase A2 receptor (anti-PLA2R) antibodies, while secondary MGN is rarely positive; therefore, positive anti-PLA2R suggests primary MGN, negative anti-PLA2R may be either primary or secondary MGN and workup for secondary causes would be indicated.
- **Membranoproliferative glomerulonephritis** (MPGN): Classify based on immunofluorescence findings into:
  - Immune complex mediated: Due to infections, autoimmune disease and monoclonal gammopathy of unknown significance (MGUS).
  - Complement mediated, due to dense deposit disease or C3 glomerulonephritis.
  - Neither: For example, healing thrombotic thrombocytopenic purpura.
- **Lupus nephritis** (Class V).

2. Consider Secondary Causes

The histological pictures may be secondary to other disease. Consider workup for:

- **Infection**: A non-exhaustive list includes HIV (FSGS), Hep B (MGN), Hep C (MPGN, MGN), parvovirus (FSGS), syphilis (MGN), malaria and schistosomiasis. As a minimum, do HIV and hepatitis serology.

- **Autoimmune**: Most often systemic lupus erythromatosis (SLE) (MPGN, MGN). Do lupus serology.

- **Malignancy**: MGN with negative anti-PLA2R is strongly associated with cancers, most commonly breast, lung and colon; this histological picture requires a malignancy workup. Minimal-change disease is associated with Hodgkin lymphoma.

- **Myeloma**: As discussed earlier.

- **Drugs**: For example, heroin, analgesics and pamidronate (FSGS); gold, penicillamine, NSAIDs, probenecid (MGN).

- **Diseases that decrease nephron mass**: May force remaining nephrons to hyperfiltrate, causing injury and FSGS. Aetiologies include—hydronephrosis, hypertensive nephrosclerosis or anatomical abnormalities. It is important to identify this group of patients as they are usually not given immunosuppression. It may be apparent on past medical history; also obtain renal imaging (usually ultrasound kidneys and bladder).

3. Look for Complications

Protein loss in nephrotic syndrome may result in systemic complications that should be evaluated. This includes:

- **Severity of oedema**: May require management, e.g., diuresis.

- **Lipids**: Urinary loss of lipoproteins may lead to hyperlipidaemia.

- **Clotting risk**: Urinary loss of antithrombin may lead to hypercoagulability (PT/PTT may be normal but deep vein thrombosis [DVT]/pulmonary embolism [PE] risk is nonetheless increased).

- **Infection risk**: Due to immunoglobulin loss.

 Using what you have learnt, **pen down your approach** to the Clinical Case at the start of the chapter **BEFORE reading the discussion** below.

Case Discussion

This young lady has nephritic syndrome, evidence of which includes microscopic haematuria with renal insufficiency and hypertension (the phase contrast microscopy is technically not > 80% dysmorphic but it is suspiciously high). The history of intermittent haematuria suggests IgA nephropathy that is epidemiologically also the most common. If specifically asked, she may reveal a history of viral upper respiratory tract infection around each episode of haematuria. Lupus nephritis is the other aetiology to consider in a young lady; at present she has no suggestive systemic features, nonetheless it should be considered and definitively ruled out on biopsy and antibody testing. Elicit any history of haemoptysis, which would suggest anti-GBM disease.

Workup should include an anti-streptolysin titre (if currently having haematuria), complement levels, autoantibodies (ANA, dsDNA, ENA profile, ANCA, anti-GBM antibody), hepatitis B and C as well as HIV screening. Renal biopsy should be pursued.

Key Lessons	1. Isolated haematuria may be due to renal or urological causes. Urological causes may be painful (e.g., urolithiasis) or painless (main concern is malignancy). Dysmorphic RBCs, proteinuria, renal insufficiency, hypertension and the presence of systemic autoimmune disease suggests a renal cause.
	2. In patients with proteinuria, first exclude transient and orthostatic proteinuria. The causes of persistent proteinuria include diabetic nephropathy, myeloma and glomerular disease (especially in nephrotic-range proteinuria, or if there is haematuria or renal insufficiency).
	3. Patients presenting with nephritic or nephrotic syndrome generally require renal biopsy. Each histological pattern may be secondary to a systemic cause, or a primary glomerular disease. Consider workup for infection (especially hepatitis, HIV), autoimmune disease (e.g., systemic lupus erythromatosis [SLE], ANCA vasculitis), malignancy and other causes as appropriate.
Common Pitfalls	1. Not all patients with haematuria should be referred to a urologist—first consider if haematuria might be of a renal aetiology!
	2. Not every diabetic with chronic kidney disease has diabetic nephropathy—be alert for suspicious features, which suggest glomerulonephritis.
Questions	1. **REFLECT!** Have you ever encountered a patient with primary glomerulonephritis? How did the patient first present, and what did the investigations show?
	2. **DISCUSS!** Many cases of haematuria or proteinuria can be managed by a non-specialist. What are the indications for urological or renal referral?
	3. **EXPLORE!** Look up how a renal biopsy is performed. What are the complications and contraindications of this procedure?
	4. **GO FURTHER!** Renal involvement is common in lupus. What are the different types of renal disease in lupus?

Chapter 21 An Approach to Difficulty Urinating

Clinical Case

A 70-year-old gentleman presents with lower abdominal pain and a large, palpable bladder. He has not passed urine in the last 12 hr. In the past year, he has had increasing difficulty passing urine, and describes his urine coming out 'very slowly' with much straining. How would you help him?

A young lady with urinary tract infection (UTI), an elderly gentleman with benign prostatic hyperplasia (BPH) and a gentleman on long-term urinary catheterisation after spinal cord injury all have 'difficulty urinating'. Begin by stratifying the patient into one of these clinical pictures (Figure 21.1):

1. **Acute dysuria**: Dysuria is a painful or burning sensation on micturition. Acute-onset dysuria, urgency, frequency and pyuria are most commonly due to UTI.

2. **Acute urinary retention**: An acute inability to empty a distended bladder, which usually causes lower abdominal discomfort.

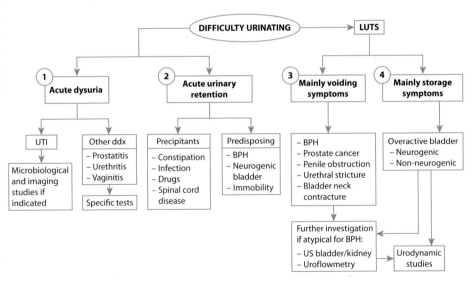

BPH, benign prostatic hyperplasia; LUTS, lower urinary tract symptoms; US, ultrasound; UTI, urinary tract infection.

Figure 21.1. Approach to difficulty urinating.

3. **Chronic lower urinary tract symptoms (LUTS), dominant *voiding* symptoms:**[1]
Voiding symptoms include hesitancy, slow stream, intermittency, straining to void, terminal and post-micturition dribble, incomplete emptying and double voiding. The prototypical disease with this presentation is benign prostatic hyperplasia.

4. **Chronic LUTS, dominant *storage* symptoms:** Frequency, urgency ± urge incontinence. This is a syndrome of overactive bladder (OAB).

1. Acute Dysuria

Acute onset dysuria, urgency, frequency and cloudy urine are most commonly a UTI. Simple UTIs are common but do appreciate a number of subtleties—(a) there are differentials to UTI, (b) UTIs range in severity from cystitis to pyelonephritis to septic shock, with some patients being prone to complications and (c) simple UTIs are common in females due to the short urethra, but cystitis in males, pregnant females or immunosuppressed individuals is potentially more serious.

Differentials in Acute Dysuria

UTI: In cystitis, an infection of the lower urinary tract, patients are well apart from dysuria and frequency. In pyelonephritis, in contrast, patients have flank pain, positive renal punch and may be systemically septic (fever, even hypotension).

Other differentials:	Workup if suspected
• **Prostatitis (males):** In addition to symptoms of UTI (dysuria, frequency, urgency), patients are febrile and unwell, with perineal pain or backache and pain on ejaculation. Rectal examination finds a tender, boggy prostate. This can lead to systemic urosepsis or formation of a prostatic abscess.	− Urine cultures − Ultrasound prostate if suspecting prostate abscess
• **Urethritis**[2] **(both sexes):** Dysuria without frequency or urgency. There may be a non-bloody urethral discharge, or pyuria without bacteriuria. Urethritis is usually sexually transmitted (gonorrhoea, chlamydia and others), so a sexual history should be sought. Inspect the genitals for discharge and other lesions of sexually transmitted disease (STD; ulcers, vesicles, etc.).	− Urethral swab for gram stain − Urine polymerase chain reaction for gonorrhoea and chlamydia − Workup for other STD

---

[1] The clinical features of LUTS do not always fall nicely into these two dichotomous categories; there may be overlaps (see 'GO FURTHER' question at the end of this chapter).

[2] While the urethra is technically a part of the urinary tract, 'UTI' traditionally refers to cystitis and pyelonephritis, not including urethritis.

- **Vaginitis (females)**: Dysuria without frequency or urgency, but instead with abnormal vaginal discharge and pruritus. Perform speculum examination for abnormal vaginal discharge and cervical erythema. There are multiple causes of vaginitis, most commonly vaginal candidiasis, bacterial vaginosis and trichomonas.

 − Empiric treatment, or
 − High vaginal swab and nucleic acid tests for microbiological diagnosis (e.g., 'VP3' test)

Which UTIs Require Investigation?

Young females with uncomplicated cystitis should be diagnosed clinically and treated empirically without further testing. At most, a dipstick can be performed; positive nitrite and leukocyte esterase is consistent with UTI.

- **Urine formed element microscopy (UFEME)** can demonstrate pyuria, which supports a diagnosis of UTI (ensure that the sample is not contaminated, i.e., without abundant epithelial cells).

- **Urine cultures** for microbiological diagnosis should be obtained if there is an increased risk of failing empiric antibiotics (recurrent UTI, catheter-associated UTI, hospital-acquired UTI), or if treatment is high-stakes (pyelonephritis, immunocompromised or pregnant patients).

- **Blood cultures** are of value in pyelonephritis as patients may be bacteraemic.

- **Urinary imaging** (ultrasound or CT) should be considered:

  (a) To identify structural urologic abnormalities in patients at higher risk of structural disease—males, children, patients with recurrent UTIs, symptoms or known history of ureteric stones or a history of pelvic disease (e.g., colorectal cancer and complicated diverticulitis).

  (b) To exclude complications of UTI (abscesses, pyonephrosis and emphysematous pyelonephritis) in diabetics, immunocompromised patients and those with severe illness. Infection of an obstructed urinary tract (i.e., pyonephrosis) is a urological emergency that requires source control.

2. Acute Urinary Retention

The diagnosis of acute urinary retention (ARU) is rarely in doubt. It is usually a distressed elderly gentleman with a palpable suprapubic mass. In doubt, ultrasound confirms the bladder; but far better to catheterise immediately—a large output of urine is diagnostic, and there are no patients happier to be catheterised than these!

ARU usually reflects precipitating insults superimposed on various predisposing factors. Identifying the aetiology of ARU facilitates intervention to prevent future episodes.

Precipitating Factors

- **Constipation**: Faecal impaction worsens urinary obstruction.

- **Infective**: UTI (see earlier); also consider prostatitis. When catheterising patients with ARU, send urine for UFEME and culture.
- **Drugs**: A large number of drugs including those with anticholinergic side-effects (antihistamines, antipsychotics, tricyclic antidepressants, hyoscine), opioids and alpha agonists (e.g., pseudoephedrine).
- **Acute spinal cord syndrome**: This is rare but dangerous and requires emergent intervention. Cauda equina syndrome (e.g., by a prolapsed intervertebral disc) and spinal cord compression (e.g., by malignancy) can present acutely with urinary retention, back pain and lower limb weakness. See Chapter 51.

Predisposing Factors

- **Urinary tract obstruction**: Most commonly benign prostatic hypertrophy, but also others (see next section).
- **Neurogenic bladder dysfunction**: For example, autonomic neuropathy (diabetes, multiple system atrophy), stroke, Parkinson's disease and so forth.
- Immobility, post-operative state.

3. Chronic Voiding Symptoms

In elderly gentleman with longstanding progressive voiding symptoms (hesitancy, slow stream, intermittency, straining to void, terminal dribble, incomplete emptying, etc.), the diagnosis is almost always benign prostatic hyperplasia (BPH). On rectal examination, the prostate should be smooth, enlarged and non-tender, with a palpable median sulcus and mobile overlying rectal mucosa. The severity of symptoms may be quantified using the international prostate symptom score.

Consider Differentials

A number of differentials should be ruled out, initially with history and simple investigations:

	Workup if suspected
Infection: UTI should be ruled out by asking about symptoms (acute onset dysuria) and sending a UFEME. A tender prostate on rectal examination suggests prostatitis.	− See earlier
Prostate cancer: Painless hematuria, weight loss or suspicious rectal exam (hard, irregularly nodular prostate with loss of median sulcus and non-mobile overlying rectal mucosa) should prompt suspicion of cancer. While prostate cancer tends to affect the peripheral prostate and neither cause urethral compression nor present with LUTS, most urologists offer prostate specific antigen (PSA) testing after a discussion of pros and cons.	− PSA > 4 µg/L would prompt further investigation − Transrectal ultrasound and biopsy

- **Penile causes**: For example, phimosis and paraphimosis. These would be obvious on examination of the penis.

- **Urethral stricture**: Suspect stricture in patient with previous urinary instrumentation or STD.
  - Retrograde urethrogram
  - Cystoscopy

- **Bladder neck contracture**: Usually due to prior urologic surgery or pelvic radiation therapy (e.g., for prostate cancer).

Workup in Selected Patients

Straightforward, classical BPH may be diagnosed clinically (the only investigations being a UFEME ± PSA). Further workup may be useful in patients who present with atypical symptoms, in younger patients who are not expected to have BPH, and in those who are considering surgical management. A number of investigations may be helpful:

- **Bladder ultrasound**: Measures intravesical prostatic protrusion (correlates with BPH symptoms), prostatic volume and post-void residual urine.

- **Uroflowmetry**: Reduced peak flow rate (< 10 mL/s) is consistent with BPH (study is valid if volume voided > 150 mL).

- **Urodynamic studies**: If there are prominent storage symptoms (see next section).

- **Creatinine and kidney ultrasound**: To detect hydronephrosis and post-renal renal insufficiency as a consequence of BPH.

4. Chronic Storage Symptoms

Overactive bladder (OAB) describes a syndrome of urinary frequency (both daytime and nocturia) and urgency, with or without urge incontinence.

Causes of OAB

Neurogenic: Usually an upper motor neuron lesion, which decreases cortical inhibition of the micturition reflex, leading to uncontrolled spontaneous contractions of the detrusor muscle. The lesion may be in the brain (stroke and multiple sclerosis), spinal cord (spinal cord injury and cervical myelopathy) or extrapyramidal tracts (Parkinson's disease). Examine the neurological system (see Chapter 25).

Non-neurogenic:

- Bladder outlet obstruction, for example, due to BPH.
- Bladder irritation by bladder calculi or after pelvic surgery.
- Idiopathic detrusor instability.

Workup

Apart from the workup for BPH, which should be performed, a **urodynamic study** is valuable. In OAB, urodynamic studies demonstrate detrusor contractions while the bladder is being filled and poor bladder capacity.

 Using what you have learnt, **pen down your approach** to the Clinical Case at the start of the chapter **BEFORE reading the discussion** below.

Case Discussion

This is an elderly gentleman with acute urinary retention (ARU) on a background of chronic voiding symptoms, most likely due to benign prostatic hyperplasia (BPH). Apart from relieving his urinary obstruction, it would be important look for acute precipitants of ARU, and evaluate for a diagnosis of BPH.

First, insert a urinary catheter, sending urine for UFEME and culture. Perform rectal examination, looking out for an enlarged prostate and faecal impaction (a common precipitant of ARU). Red flags on rectal exam include prostate tenderness (prostatitis), a hard nodular prostate (cancer) and lax anal tone (? cauda equina syndrome). Review his medication list for any drugs that might contribute to ARU, and medical history for any other cause of voiding symptoms (see text). PSA testing should not be offered acutely as ARU (and digital rectal examination) results in falsely elevated PSA.

Key Lessons	1. Acute dysuria and frequency is usually due to urinary tract infection (UTI), and less commonly from prostatitis, urethritis and vaginitis. Uncomplicated female UTIs require no further investigation, but outside this patient profile, consider microbiological diagnosis and structural workup.
	2. Acute urinary retention may be precipitated by infection, constipation, drugs or spinal cord disease, and usually occurs on a background of predisposing factors, for example, benign prostatic hyperplasia (BPH) or immobility.
	3. Chronic voiding symptoms are almost always due to BPH. UTI, prostate cancer and other structural causes of urinary obstruction should be ruled out.
Common Pitfalls	1. PSA levels should not be sent if there is no intention to pursue further testing or treatment of prostate cancer (e.g., patient refusal, poor premorbids). Discuss with the patient *before* doing the test.
Questions	1. **REFLECT!** You are likely to have encountered many patients with UTI. Why do some patients have only mild symptoms, while others turn so sick? (think of disease factors and patient factors).

2. **EXPLORE!** What are the causes of vaginitis, and how might they be differentiated?

3. **DISCUSS!** In patients with BPH, 'most urologists offer prostate specific antigen (PSA) testing after a discussion of pros and cons'. What are the pros and cons you would discuss with a patient? Why is PSA testing controversial?

4. **GO FURTHER!** Lower urinary tract symptoms (LUTS) do not always fit nicely into two dichotomous categories (storage vs. voiding). How does one approach a patient with mixed symptoms? How does clarifying the underlying pathophysiology of LUTS (in the specific patient) aid management?

Brain, Nerves and Senses

An Approach to Headache

Clinical Case

A 50-year-old office manager presents with a severe headache (pain score 10/10). She was having a bad day in the office when a severe headache suddenly started 6 hr ago. She has had headaches in the past but none this bad. Her only other past medical history is hypertension, for which she had defaulted medications. A CT Brain, performed 1 hr ago in the Emergency Department, is normal. She feels much better after having been given paracetamol and diclofenac in the Emergency Department, and asks if you could discharge her now. Would you agree?

Many people have occasional headaches, and live with them, with little consequence. Yet some headaches can be life-threatening. Begin by characterising the headache's time course. A patient who has had a particular episodic headache for years probably won't be harmed by that headache. Conversely, the patient with his first-ever severe headache, or the patient who has a headache 10 times worse than his usual migraine, is far more likely to have a sinister cause of headache. Figure 22.1 provides an approach.

New Acute Headache

A number of neurologic emergencies present as a new acute headache. As patients with known migraine can also develop an unrelated neurologic emergency, any unusually severe headache or headache of a different character should also be investigated as a 'new' headache.

History and Examination

The clinical picture is often characteristic.

Intracranial causes:

- **Meningitis:** An unwell patient with fever, neck stiffness and photophobia. Examination reveals nuchal rigidity (resistance to passive flexion), Kernig's and Brudzinski's signs, and may show a non-blanchable purpuric rash (in meningococcaemia). Bacterial meningitis presents over hours to a day, while fungal and tuberculous meningitis may present in a more subacute fashion.

- **Subarachnoid haemorrhage (SAH):** Classically, 'the worst headache in my life'— sudden onset with pain maximal within seconds to minutes, but improving after.

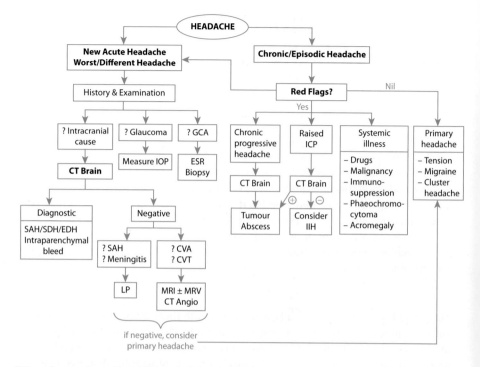

CVA, cerebrovascular accident; CVT, cerebral venous thrombosis; EDH, extradural haemorrhage; ESR, erythrocyte sedimentation rate; GCA, giant cell arthritis; IIH, idiopathic intracranial hypertension; IOP, intraocular pressure; LP, lumbar puncture; MRV, magnetic resonance venogram; SAH, subarachnoid haemorrhage; SDH, subdural haemorrhage.

Figure 22.1. Approach to headache.

Patients may misleadingly be pain-free by the time of consult, or still have nuchal rigidity. It is important to diagnose SAH—catastrophic rupture of an intracranial aneurysm is imminently preventable.

- **Subdural haemorrhage (SDH):** Typically, an elderly patient who sustains head trauma and subsequently develops headache within days (acute SDH) or weeks (chronic SDH). There may also be drowsiness or subtle confusion, localising neurological deficits and vomiting (due to raised intracranial pressure). The history of trauma may be remote and minor, especially in the elderly.

- **Extradural haemorrhage (EDH):** Usually a younger patient who suffered head trauma (e.g., a road traffic accident).

- **Cerebrovascular accident:** While most strokes do not present with headache, headache can occur in (a) some haemorrhagic strokes, (b) occipital strokes and (c) carotid dissection. A history of headache on exertion, or the presence of any neurological deficit (including an isolated Horner's syndrome, which may occur in carotid dissection) increases the suspicion for stroke.

- **Cerebral venous thrombosis (CVT):** Usually occurs in females with a hypercoagulable state (including pregnancy and oral contraceptive pills). Presentation is variable;

in addition to headache, there may be symptoms of raised intracranial pressure (ICP) (e.g., vomiting), seizure or neurological deficit.

Referred pain: Two causes of referred pain require emergent treatment—these must be identified on history and examination, not CT brain.

Workup

- **Acute closed-angle glaucoma**: Unilateral headache ± vomiting with severe eye pain, blurring of vision and halos around lights. Eye is red with a fixed, mid-dilated pupil. A relative afferent pupillary defect can be seen if the optic nerve is damaged. Urgent treatment prevents blindness.

  – Measure intra-ocular pressure, for example, Goldmann tonometry

- **Giant cell arteritis (temporal arteritis)**: Unilateral headache with jaw claudication (jaw pain when chewing), transient visual loss or visual field defect and scalp tenderness. There may be systemic symptoms of polymyalgia rheumatica (joint pains, peripheral synovitis, constitutional symptoms). Examination may find visual field defect and optic disk swelling. This is an autoimmune disease usually in > 50 year olds; early treatment prevents visual loss.

  – ESR: usually high
  – Confirmation via temporal artery biopsy (but do not wait to start treatment, and beware of a falsely normal biopsy due to skip lesions)

Intracranial Causes: Upfront CT Brain

Suspicion of a dangerous intracranial process generally justifies a plain CT brain upfront. This provides important diagnostic information and facilitates further investigations (e.g., excludes mass lesions so that lumbar puncture can be performed safely).

- **Positive CT Brain**: CT brain is particularly sensitive for intracranial haemorrhage, which appears white on CT (Figure 22.2).
- **Negative CT Brain**: CT brain is generally negative in meningitis, and may be negative in CVT, small SAH and early or minor stroke. Proceed based on the likely working diagnosis (a) suspected SAH or meningitis, or (b) suspected stroke or CVT.

Further Investigation: (a) Suspect SAH or Meningitis

Lumbar puncture is the next test if SAH or meningitis is suspected.

In suspected SAH: The sensitivity of CT brain performed within the first 12 hr exceeds 95%. However, this is not good enough to exclude SAH if clinical suspicion is high, because of its potentially catastrophic consequences.

- Lumbar puncture: Best performed > 12 hr after the onset of pain. Look for xanthochromia (yellow discolouration of the CSF, due to haemoglobin breakdown); this is a more reliable finding than red cells in CSF, which may be a traumatic tap.
- If patients refuse lumbar puncture, consider CT or MR angiography as the next-best test.

Figure 22.2. Intracranial haemorrhage.

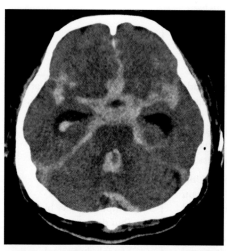

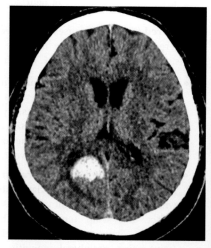

(a) **Subarachnoid haemorrhage (SAH)**: Blood in the basal cisterns and fissures (where the circle of Willis is). This CT shows massive SAH; the patient was comatose from a posterior communicating aneurysm rupture. Most SAH are much subtler.

(b) **Intraparenchymal haemorrhage**: A hyperdense (white) spot seen in the right occipital region. This patient had a haemorrhagic stroke.

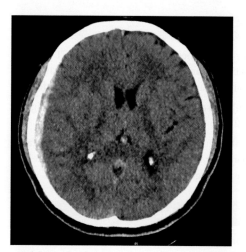

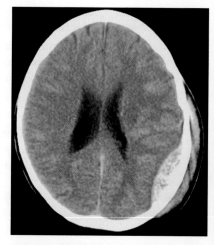

(c) **Subdural haemorrhage (SDH)**: A crescent-shaped opacity in the right frontal-parietal region, with mild midline shift.

(d) **Extradural haemorrhage (EDH)**: A lens-shaped opacity in the left parietal region, with ventricular effacement (it 'looks squashed'). This young man was flung off a motorcycle.

In suspected meningitis: Perform

- Lumbar puncture: Confirms meningitis and allows for microbiological diagnosis. Send for microscopy, protein, glucose (with a paired serum glucose) and microbiological testing as suspected (Table 22.1). Lumbar puncture should not delay prompt administration of antibiotics, and can be performed after antibiotics are dosed.
- Septic workup: Blood inflammatory markers and cultures (which may often be positive).

Table 22.1. Interpretation of Cerebrospinal Fluid in Suspected Meningitis

	Normal	Bacterial meningitis	Viral meningitis	TB or fungal meningitis
Appearance	Clear	Turbid	Clear	Turbid
WBC count	< 5/mm³	↑↑	↑	↑
Differential		Neutrophilic	Lymphocytic	Lymphocytic
Protein	0.2–0.4 g/L	↑	Usually normal	↑
Glucose	> ½ plasma	< ½ plasma	> ½ plasma	< ½ plasma
Microbiological tests to send		Gram stain and culture PCR for pneumococcus and meningococcus	Viral PCR: HSV, VZV, CMV, EBV	AFB smear, culture, PCR India ink stain Fungal culture

AFB, acid-fast bacilli; CMV, cytomegalovirus; EBV, Epstein–Barr virus; HSV, herpes simplex virus; PCR, polymerase chain reaction; TB, tuberculosis; VZV, varicella zoster virus; WBC, white blood cells.

Further Investigation: (b) Suspect Stroke or CVT

Further neuroimaging would be warranted, including:

- MRI brain with MRI venography: Detects strokes not visible on CT scan, as well as CVT.
- CT angiography (beginning from the aortic arch) if carotid dissection is suspected.

Further Investigations Negative

Common things being common, new-onset headache or an unusually severe migraine attack is still more commonly migraine than SAH. Nonetheless, many patients receive CT scans and lumbar puncture, and rightfully so. When these investigations are negative, consider:

- Primary headache disorder (migraine and tension headache) (page 217).
- Hypertensive urgency: Severe hypertension (e.g., systolic ≥ 180 mmHg and/or diastolic ≥ 120 mmHg) alone may present with headache ± giddiness (see Chapter 6).
- Headache associated with acute upper respiratory tract infection.

Chronic/Episodic Headache

Episodic recurrences of the same character and intensity of headache is very suggestive of a primary headache disorder. However, these are diagnoses of exclusion—sinister causes of headache must first be considered and excluded.

Red flags: The following red flags are inconsistent with a primary headache disorder and require further evaluation for a sinister cause:

- New, worst or change in character of headache.
- Neurological deficit: Altered mental status, seizure, focal deficit.
- Visual complaint: Red eye, blurring of vision.   see previous section
- Meningeal irritation: Photophobia, neck stiffness, fever.
- Trauma.
- **Chronic progressive headache**.
- **Raised ICP**: Early morning headache, headache worse on lying supine, coughing or straining, papilloedema.
- **Systemic illness**: Weight loss, history of malignancy, immunosuppression including HIV, drugs including anticoagulants.

Chronic Progressive Headache

A chronic progressive headache is worrisome for a space occupying lesion. Perform a contrasted CT or MRI brain, which may reveal a brain tumour (primary or metastatic) or abscess.

Raised ICP Headache

Symptoms suggestive of raised ICP include headache worse in the early morning, worse on lying down, coughing or straining. Examination may find papilloedema, false localising sixth nerve palsy or unequal pupils. The next step is to perform a CT/MRI brain with contrast. This may find:

- Space occupying lesion, for example, tumour and abscess.
- Normal: Consider **idiopathic intracranial hypertension** (formerly benign intracranial hypertension): usually an obese woman of childbearing age who presents with signs and symptoms of raised intracranial pressure, visual changes (transient visual obscuration when changing posture) and pulsatile tinnitus (in the absence of a structural cause of raised intracranial pressure). Lumbar puncture confirms increased opening pressure. This is not as 'benign' as its old name suggests as it may lead to permanent visual loss.

Headache Associated with Systemic Illness

	Workup
• **Suspect malignancy**: If headache occurs in a patient with history of malignancy, metastatic disease must be ruled out.	− Contrasted CT/MRI brain
• **Immunosuppression**: If there is an immunosuppressed state, including HIV infection, consider opportunistic infection and other HIV CNS syndromes.	− Contrasted MRI brain
• **Pheochromocytoma**: Paroxysmal episodes of headache, palpitations, tachycardia and hypertension. Have a high index of suspicion if the patient is hypertensive or has other endocrine tumours (think of multiple endocrine neoplasia).	− Urinary metanephrines
• **Acromegaly**: This can present as headache. Clinical signs should be apparent to the trained observer: coarsening of facial features (ask for an old photo), soft tissue overgrowth (tongue, hands, rings that do not fit). Examine for visual loss.	− Serum IGF-1, if positive, oral glucose tolerance test − MRI brain for pituitary tumour

Other secondary causes of headache: Apart from overt systemic illnesses, the history may lead to a diagnosis of headache due to these secondary causes:

• **Drugs**: Vasodilators (nitrates), overuse of analgesia (use more than 8 days in a month can lead to medication overuse headache), alcohol, recreational drugs or withdrawal, recent smoking cessation (nicotine withdrawal).

• **Post-concussion syndrome**: Trauma involving the meninges can trigger a headache lasting years.

• **Post lumbar puncture headache**: Some headache is expected due to low CSF pressure.

• **Viral illnesses**: Mild headache occurs in many viral illnesses, such as upper respiratory tract infections, gastroenteritis and dengue.

• Headache may be associated with poorly controlled hypertension/hypertensive urgency; however, in these patients the imperative is to exclude stroke and intracranial bleeds, which are associated with hypertension.

No Red Flags—Consider Primary Headache Disorders

The primary headache disorders are clinical diagnoses. In the absence of any red flags, and a typical history, neuroimaging is not necessary (although often performed for no reason other than reassurance).

- **Tension headache**: A bilateral tight band-like (non-pulsatile) discomfort which builds slowly, fluctuates in severity and may persist for days. There may also be muscular neck pain. Accompanying features of migraine are absent.

- **Migraine**: Episodes of unilateral, pulsating headache with additional features, for example, sensitivity to triggers (light, sound, movement), nausea/vomiting or neurologic dysfunction (even numbness, weakness). Some patients report an aura, for example, visual (flashing lights, zigzag lines), sensory, motor or speech changes that may mimic a transient ischaemic attack. Patients prefer to keep still during attacks. Most patients with disabling headache probably have migraine.

- **Cluster headache**: Short-lasting bouts of explosive pain, up to 8 times a day, occurring daily for a few weeks, interspersed with months of pain-free periods. This headache is associated with ipsilateral autonomic signs such as tearing, rhinorrhoea, miosis and ptosis. Patients tend to move about during attacks. There are other trigeminal autonomic cephalgias with different clinical features, but those are rare.

 Using what you have learnt, **pen down your approach** to the Clinical Case at the start of the chapter **BEFORE reading the discussion** below.

Case Discussion

You should not agree to discharge her right now. This lady gives a history of 'the worst headache in her life'—a red flag worrisome for subarachnoid haemorrhage (SAH). Do not be fooled by her history of previous headaches (this is a new type of headache), her current lack of pain or the normal CT brain (not sensitive enough to exclude SAH). The history of sudden-onset 'thunderclap' headache, pain maximal on onset and improving thereafter, is rather suggestive of SAH. She has hypertension which is a risk factor. She should be counselled for lumbar puncture; if she declines the procedure, consider MRI with MR angiography.

If the lumbar puncture is positive for xanthochromia, the next step will be to identify a cerebral aneurysm on either catheter or MR angiography. Aneurysms can be treated via endovascular clipping or surgical methods to mitigate the future risk of catastrophic rupture. Non-aneurysmal aetiologies of SAH are possible, but less common.

If the lumbar puncture is normal, she can be managed as a case of migraine, after exclusion of other causes of headache (see text).

Key Lessons	1. Evaluate any new acute headache with care. Consider meningitis, subarachnoid haemorrhage, acute closed-angle glaucoma and giant cell arthritis as the most dangerous causes.
	2. Red flags in headache include: Chronic progressive headache, early morning headache worse on lying supine, pain disturbing sleep, neurological or visual abnormalities, fever and systemic illness such as immunosuppression or malignancy.

3. The primary headache disorders (tension headache, migraine, cluster headache) present as episodic recurrent headaches, and can be distinguished clinically.

Common Pitfalls	1. Acute closed-angle glaucoma and giant cell arthritis are easy to miss.
	2. CT scans are probably over-used. Not every headache requires a CT scan.
Questions	1. **REFLECT!** Considering the differentials you have learnt in this chapter, what are the key steps in physical examination of a patient presenting with headache?
	2. **EXPLORE!** Learn how a lumbar puncture is performed. What are the contraindications for this procedure? How would you consent a patient for it?
	3. **GO FURTHER!** Cluster headache is one of several trigeminal autonomic cephalgias, which are primary headache disorders. Look up hemicrania continua, paroxysmal hemicrania and short-lasting unilateral neuralgiform headache with conjunctival injection and tearing (SUNCT).

Chapter

23

An Approach to Blackouts: Syncope and Seizure

Clinical Case

Three 18-year-old military recruits present with sudden blackouts.

- *Recruit A loses consciousness mid-way through a timed run. He recovered immediately, and felt well enough that he wanted to continue his run.*

- *Recruit B loses consciousness after standing at attention for 2 hr under the hot sun. His right fingers were observed to 'jerk' several times, and this was associated with urinary incontinence. He managed to get up and fall out of the parade immediately after.*

- *Recruit C loses consciousness while having his meal in the canteen. His right fingers were observed to 'jerk' several times, with no urinary incontinence. He was drowsy after, and had to be carried out on a stretcher.*

For each patient, what is the most likely diagnosis, and what workup would you perform?

Syncope is an acute, transient loss of consciousness with loss of postural tone due to impaired cerebral blood flow. **Seizures** arise from a sudden synchronous discharge of cerebral neurons, which may (or may not!) be associated with a loss of consciousness. Either condition, together with a number of mimics, may present as 'blackouts'. Telling them apart often poses diagnostic difficulty, especially if the event is unwitnessed. Yet this is a critical distinction, for example, identifying a malignant cardiac arrhythmia allows for potentially life-saving intervention; conversely, diagnosing epilepsy carries serious consequences including the loss of driving privileges, limitation of employment and social stigma (Figure 23.1).

Distinguishing Syncope and Seizure

Most patients regain full consciousness by the time they are seen. In a patient who remains drowsy, in addition to considering post-ictal drowsiness, other differentials of altered mental state (Chapter 31) must be considered.

There is no substitute for careful clinical history-taking. Every effort should be made to obtain an eyewitness account, which provides diagnostically useful information. In its absence, however, a presumptive diagnosis can often still be made (Table 23.1).

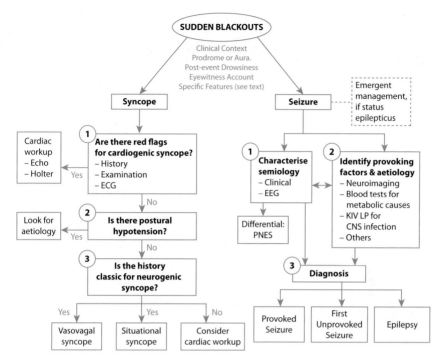

EEG, electroencephalogram; PNES, psychogenic non-epileptic seizure.

Figure 23.1. Approach to transient loss of consciousness (blackouts).

Approach to Syncope

Vasovagal syncope is the most common, and a rather benign, cause of syncope. On the other hand, syncope may be a manifestation of structural heart disease, arrhythmias or postural hypotension. The clinician's challenge is, on one hand to identify any sinister causes of syncope, and on the other, to avoid over-investigation of typical vasovagal syncope. Three questions are useful.

1. Are there red flags for cardiac syncope?
2. Is there postural hypotension?
3. Is the presentation classical for neurogenic syncope?

1. Are There Red Flags for Cardiac Syncope?

A number of cardiac conditions present with syncope (Table 23.2).

Begin with a history, examination and ECG. **Red flags** suggesting cardiac syncope include:

- Syncope on exertion: Suggests insufficient cardiac output under demands of exertion, or provoked arrhythmia.

Table 23.1. Clinical Features to Distinguish Syncope vs. Seizure

	Syncope	Seizure
Context	Prolonged standing, heat, emotion, crowds Postural change Exertion, palpitations, chest pain Known heart disease	Head injury, structural brain disease Infection, metabolic disturbances Sleep deprivation, alcohol, bright lights (triggers) Prior seizures
Pre-event	Usually with a prodrome of light-headedness, fading of vision, pallor, diaphoresis Except cardiac syncope, which is without warning	May have aura[a]: déjà vu feeling, rising epigastric sensation, familiar smell or taste May be sudden, without warning
During event	Sudden loss of tone Hypotension or bradycardia (if observed) Brief motor activity, including clonic jerks	Features more specific for seizure include: – Sustained tonic–clonic or myoclonic movements – Automatisms[a] or blank staring – Lateral tongue biting[a] – Forceful head turn to one side (version)[a]
Post-event	Pallor, diaphoresis, flushing. Rapid, complete recovery to full alertness	Post-ictal drowsiness[a] (especially generalised seizure) May have transient weakness (Todd's paralysis) Nose wiping (in focal seizure)

[a]Features particularly specific to seizures. On the other hand, other features may not differentiate between syncope and seizure, for example, incontinence occurs in both conditions, and unsustained twitches can occur in syncope, potentially leading to misdiagnosis as seizure.

- Syncope when supine: This would be inconsistent with vasovagal syncope or postural hypotension.
- Sudden syncope without warning: A prodrome of light-headedness and blurring of vision is expected in vasovagal syncope. Very sudden syncope without this prodrome, and not associated with postural change, is worrisome for a cardiac cause.
- Chest pain or palpitations at time of syncope.
- Known cardiac disease including pacemakers.
- Family history of sudden cardiac death.
- Abnormal cardiac examination including murmur and fluid overload.
- ECG findings: Look for unexplained sinus bradycardia (< 40 beats/min), sinus pause (> 3 sec), high-grade (Mobitz type II second-degree and third-degree) heart block, wide QRS complex, delta waves, long or short QT, S-T abnormalities and Q waves.

Workup: If there is strong clinical suspicion for cardiac syncope, consider:

- **Echocardiogram** for structural and valvular pathology.
- **Extended ECG monitoring** for paroxysmal arrhythmias. It is reasonable to begin with a 24 hr Holter; however, this may be negative if arrhythmias are less frequent than once in 24 hr. If there is a strong suspicion for arrhythmia in spite

Table 23.2. Cardiac Causes of Syncope

	Condition	Mechanism of syncope	Recognition
Structural heart disease	Critical aortic stenosis Hypertrophic obstructive cardiomyopathy Others: pulmonary stenosis, pulmonary embolism, pulmonary hypertension	Outflow obstruction	Murmur Echocardiogram
	Heart failure	Inadequate cardiac output	Echocardiogram Signs and symptoms
	Aortic dissection	Obstructed carotid perfusion	Chest pain + syncope Widened mediastinum
Arrhythmias	Sinus dysfunction, e.g., sick sinus syndrome High-grade atrioventricular block Ventricular tachycardia Pacemaker malfunction	Arrhythmia leading to sudden fall in cardiac output	ECG
Channelopathies	Long QT syndrome— congenital or acquired (e.g., drugs: antipsychotics, fluoroquinolones)	Paroxysmal arrhythmias, e.g., torsade de pointe	ECG: prolonged QT
	Brugada syndrome	Ventricular tachyarrhythmias	ECG: coved or saddleback ST elevation in V1–V2
	Wolff–Parkinson–White syndrome	Tachyarrhythmias involving accessory pathway	ECG: pre-excitation (delta wave; Figure 5.3)

of negative monitoring, consider other forms of extended ECG monitoring (e.g., trans-telephonic monitoring, etc.).

2. Is There Postural Hypotension?

Giddiness or syncope due to postural hypotension typically presents upon postural change—for example, getting out of bed, standing up from a seated position—and is more common in the elderly. Syncope arises from a failure of blood pressure autoregulation (i.e., peripheral vasoconstriction and compensatory increase in heart rate) in response to postural change, such that postural change leads to transiently inadequate cerebral perfusion.

Measure postural blood pressure supine and after standing for 3 min. Postural hypotension is defined as a sustained reduction in systolic blood pressure ≥ 20 mmHg, or diastolic blood pressure ≥ 10 mmHg.

Aetiologies: If there is postural hypotension, look for a cause. This may be multifactorial.

- **Volume depletion**: Acute dehydration due to vomiting, diarrhoea and hyperglycaemia is usually clinically apparent. Chronic volume depletion due to poor intake is common in the elderly.

- **Drugs**: The sympathetic response may be blunted by pharmacologic agents, including beta-blockers, tricyclic antidepressants.

- **Adrenal insufficiency**: Postural hypotension is a feature of chronic adrenal insufficiency. Consider performing a synacthen test.

- **Autonomic failure**: Neurological disease can affect the baroreceptor—medulla—autonomic ganglia—sympathetic neuron pathway, leading to postural hypotension, neurogenic bladder dysfunction, ejaculation failure and gastrointestinal dysmotility. This is most commonly autonomic neuropathy due to longstanding, poorly controlled diabetes mellitus.

   However, if there are atypical features—absence of longstanding diabetes, autonomic dysfunction out of proportion to peripheral neuropathy, neuropathy out of proportion to renal and retinal microvascular damage, non-length dependent or asymmetric neuropathy or Parkinsonism—think of other causes of autonomic failure.

   - Autonomic failure with peripheral neuropathy (other than diabetes): Metabolic (vitamin B12 deficiency, toxins), paraneoplastic, infective (HIV), inflammatory (Sjogren syndrome, Guillain–Barre syndrome), infiltrative (amyloidosis) and hereditary (hereditary sensory and autonomic neuropathy, etc.).

   - Autonomic failure associated with Parkinsonism, ataxia or dementia: Consider a neurodegenerative disease including multiple system atrophy, Parkinson disease, Dementia with Lewy bodies (see Chapter 30).

   - Isolated autonomic failure: Autoimmune, paraneoplastic and idiopathic causes.

   Consider autonomic function tests; a detailed approach to workup is beyond the scope of this text.

3. Is the Presentation Classical of Neurogenic Syncope?

The typical history of neurogenic syncope is:

- **Vasovagal syncope**: A young, healthy person who loses consciousness *while upright*, when faced with orthostatic stress (prolonged standing, dehydration, hot weather, after physical exertion) or emotional stimuli (e.g., crowded environment, noxious stimuli, e.g., sight of blood, fear of bodily injury). A prodrome (light-headedness, sweating, nausea, a gradual darkening or blurring of vision) is followed by the loss of postural tone. The supine position rapidly restores cerebral blood flow; the patient rapidly and completely regains alertness, although there may be some residual fatigue and pallor.

- **Situational syncope**: Syncope occurs during or immediately after coughing, swallowing, urinating or defecating; again with rapid and complete recovery.

In the presence of such a typical history, and the exclusion of red flags, a positive diagnosis of neurogenic syncope should be made without further investigation. Other times, however, history is atypical for neurogenic syncope, yet there is no suggestion of postural hypotension or cardiac disease, and initial investigation (ECG) is normal. In such patients, vasovagal syncope remains the most likely aetiology, but cardiac workup may be considered if there is a reasonable pre-test probability (e.g., elderly patient with multiple cardiovascular risk factors).

Approach to Seizure

If the episode of loss of consciousness has been firmly established as a seizure, the clinical question depends on the context.

- **First seizure**: The impetus is to search for a provoking cause, which may be life-threatening.

- **Recurrent seizure**: The question is whether a formal diagnosis of epilepsy should be made, and if so, which type of epilepsy, and whether to initiate treatment.

- **Known epileptic with breakthrough seizure**: This is a management issue—addressing any precipitant, adjusting medications to better control seizures.

- **Status epilepticus**: Continuous seizures for ≥ 5 min, or ≥ 2 seizures without full recovery of consciousness in between, requires prompt intervention.

Characterisation of seizure semiology and identification of a precipitant should proceed simultaneously.

1. Characterise the Seizure Semiology

This has historically been a difficult task, as few seizures are witnessed by healthcare professionals or a reliable eyewitness. Today, many patients and family members bring video recordings of their seizures, which is very helpful.

(a) **Clinical characterisation** (based on the 2017 International League Against Epilepsy Classification)

First determine if the seizure began with focal or generalised manifestations.

- **Generalised-onset seizures**:
  - **Motor**: The stereotypical generalised tonic–clonic seizure begins with bilateral tonic stiffening, often with biting of tongue and apnoea, then bilateral clonic limb jerking, followed by post-ictal drowsiness. Other motor manifestations include clonic, tonic, myoclonic and atonic activity (and various combinations).
  - **Non-motor (absence)**: A classic absence seizure can be described as—without warning, the patient stares into space, being unaware of surroundings, and within 10 sec returns to normal as if nothing happened. There is no loss of postural tone and no post-ictal confusion. There are usually recurrent episodes, beginning from childhood, and patients are often thought to be 'daydreaming'.

- **Focal-onset seizures**: As an illustration, consider mesial temporal lobe epilepsy. This begins with an *aura*—a rising epigastric sensation, a Déjà vu feeling or a particular taste or smell. The patient then loses awareness of the surroundings, but may continue to keep eyes open, without loss of postural tone. There may be automatisms (repetitive, stereotyped movements such as lip smacking, unilateral finger fidgeting), dystonic posturing and forceful head turning to one side. There are many different focal-onset seizures; two key characteristics to consider:
  - − **Aware vs. impaired awareness**: In a focal aware seizure (previously 'simple partial seizure'), the patient retains awareness of self and surroundings. In a focal impaired-awareness seizure (previously 'complex partial seizure'), the patient loses awareness at any point during the seizure.
  - − **Motor onset vs. non-motor onset**: Identify the first prominent sign and symptom of seizure. Motor manifestations include unilateral automatisms, clonic, myoclonic or tonic movements. Non-motor manifestations include autonomic, cognitive, emotional and sensory features (such as an aura).
- **Focal to bilateral tonic–clonic**: In these seizures, neuronal activity starts in a particular region of the brain, then propagate to bilateral hemispheres, causing bilateral tonic–clonic movements (known as secondary generalisation in older classifications). The focal onset (e.g., an aura, one limb that begins tonic movement first) may be subtle and easily missed, but it is of significance as it may imply an epileptogenic focus.
- **Unclassified**: At times no further information on onset or manifestations may be available. Such seizures could be described as, for example, 'unknown-onset motor (tonic–clonic) seizure'.

The above classification carries certain implications.

- Semiology may point to aetiology. A focal seizure may suggest a structural intracranial lesion, such a prior stroke (scar epilepsy) or a congenital malformation (e.g., hippocampal sclerosis); the manifestation (motor or non-motor) *localises* to a particular lobe, and the side of involvement (left or right) may *lateralise* to whether left or right brain is responsible. Recurrent episodes of absence seizure, with onset in childhood, is often a genetic *epilepsy syndrome*. On the other hand, generalised tonic–clonic seizures may be due to a number of causes, including idiopathic epilepsy, metabolic, infective and other causes.
- Semiology may be of value in choosing an antiepileptic drug.
- Certain manifestations are inconsistent with organic seizures. For example, to explain bilateral upper limb jerking with full awareness, one would have to invoke a focal seizure involving either motor cortex, which propagates across the corpus callosum to the contralateral motor cortex, sparing everything in between such that consciousness is preserved—a highly unlikely situation! With such presentations, psychogenic non-epileptic seizures (PNES) may need to be considered.

(b) Electroencephalogram (EEG)

In certain circumstances, the EEG has a role in confirming and characterising seizure activity. While a 20- to 30-min EEG recording may not capture any seizure activity, the EEG may be used in several ways:

- **Routine EEG** is helpful in characterising first unprovoked seizures. Even in the interictal period, it may show focal sharp waves (focal epilepsy) or generalised sharp wave complexes (generalised epilepsy). On the other hand, a negative EEG does not rule out seizure, and some findings are nonspecific. Some clinicians omit EEG evaluation if it does not change the treatment plan.

- **Video EEG** monitoring: Can capture EEG at the point of clinical seizures, and correlate EEG features to the clinical manifestation. Used to characterise seizures (especially to distinguish seizure vs. PNES), and also if considering surgery for epilepsy.

- **Role in status epilepticus**: Helpful to confirm resolution of seizure activity, and rule out persistence of non-convulsive status epilepticus (hard to tell clinically once the patient is intubated and paralysed).

2. Identify Provoking Factors and Aetiology

How extensive should the workup be? A first seizure occurs, by definition, in patients who are not expected to have seizures; therefore, an extensive workup should be performed, looking for a treatable cause of provoked seizure, and for any lesion that would predispose to future seizure. On the other hand, the workup for recurrent or breakthrough seizure is generally less extensive, unless there is a strong clinical suspicion of a structural or infective cause.

(a) **First seizure:**

- **Structural**
  - **Intracranial haemorrhage**: Including subarachnoid haemorrhage (SAH), subdural hematoma (SDH), traumatic brain injury. There may be a frank history of trauma or thunderclap headache (ruptured SAH), but SDH can occur without clear-cut trauma.
  - **Stroke**: Especially haemorrhagic stroke, haemorrhagic conversion and cerebral venous thrombosis. There may be signs and symptoms of stroke, for example, weakness, numbness or facial droop.
  - **Epileptogenic mass lesion**: For example, brain abscess, brain tumour or old stroke (scar epilepsy).
  - **Congenital malformation**: For example, hippocampal sclerosis.

Workup
- In the acute setting, obtain urgent CT brain to exclude gross lesions/bleed
- In the stable patient, obtain MRI brain, looking for any epileptogenic mass lesion or congenital malformation

- **Metabolic**
  - **Electrolyte derangement**: Hypo- or hyper-glycaemia, hyponatraemia, hypocalcaemia, hypomagnesaemia and uraemia; these are easily treatable causes.

    – Bedside capillary glucose
    – Basic laboratories: glucose, sodium, calcium, urea, renal and thyroid function

  - **Drugs**: Alcohol or benzodiazepine withdrawal, recreational and other drugs (cocaine, amphetamine) can provoke seizures. Certain prescription medications (e.g., cefepime and ertapenem) may lower seizure threshold.

    – Consider toxicology screen if there is suspicion

  - Other metabolic disorders: For example, thyrotoxicosis, acute intermittent porphyria, inborn errors of metabolism.

- **Infective**
  - In meningitis or encephalitis, seizure may accompany fever, neck stiffness, photophobia and purpuric rash (in meningococcus).
  - Cerebral abscess (see structural lesion earlier).
  - **Others**: Less common aetiologies include cerebral malaria, toxoplasmosis, neurocysticercosis and so forth.

    – Lumbar puncture if there is clinical suspicion (see Chapter 22)
    – Blood cultures
    – Neuroimaging

- **Autoimmune and paraneoplastic encephalitis**: Anti N-methyl-D-aspartate (anti-NMDA) receptor encephalitis is perhaps the best-known autoimmune encephalitis. It presents with emotional and behavioural disturbance, short-term memory loss, drowsiness, seizures and dyskinesia. This is a rapidly expanding field, with many types of encephalitis and new antibodies described in recent years.

  – Specific antibody tests (out of scope of this text)

- **Underlying conditions associated with epilepsy**
  - **Neurocutaneous syndromes**: For example, tuberous sclerosis, Sturge–Weber syndrome. Look for their characteristic cutaneous stigmata.
  - **Neurodegenerative disorders**: Late Alzheimer's disease, among other neurodegenerative disorders, is associated with seizures.
  - **Developmental disorders**: These, including Down's syndrome, may be associated with epilepsy. Developmental delay is a feature of a number of epilepsy syndromes.

(b) **Recurrent or breakthrough seizures**:

- Tests for 'first seizure': Begin with basic electrolytes, considering neuroimaging and lumbar puncture if there is clinical suspicion (known epilepsy does not rule out meningitis!). MRI and EEG should be done for all patients with recurrent seizures, if not already performed.

- Look for precipitants: General medical illnesses (even sepsis, upper respiratory tract infection), sleep deprivation and alcohol may all precipitate seizures.

- Assess compliance to antiepileptic drug therapy. It is useful to send drug levels, as a check on compliance, and to assist titration. Pursue compliance issues.

3. Decide on a Diagnosis

Having characterised the seizure (clinically and on EEG) and obtained information about possible precipitants and structural brain abnormalities, the final step is to synthesise this information to decide on a diagnosis. A *diagnosis* may be:

- **Provoked seizure**: A seizure occurring due to an identifiable precipitant (electrolyte abnormality, drugs, infection, etc.). Further seizures are unlikely if this precipitating factor is removed.

- **Epilepsy**: A condition of *recurrent* seizures, such as:
  - Two unprovoked seizures > 24 hr apart.
  - One unprovoked seizure and high recurrence risk.[1] For example, identifying an epileptogenic mass lesion or malformation, would constitute 'high recurrence risk'.
  - Diagnosis of an epilepsy syndrome: An epilepsy syndrome is a recognised cluster of features including clinical (seizure type, age of onset, comorbidities), imaging and EEG findings. Examples include childhood absence epilepsy, mesial temporal lobe epilepsy and so forth.

- **First unprovoked seizure**: In an *unprovoked* seizure with no feature suggesting high recurrence risk, the diagnosis should be left as 'first unprovoked seizure'. While some of these patients may later develop epilepsy, there is insufficient evidence to diagnose epilepsy now.

---

[1] Defined as probability of further seizures > 60% in 10 years, which is the recurrence risk after two unprovoked seizures.

Using what you have learnt, **pen down your approach** to the Clinical Case at the start of the chapter **BEFORE reading the discussion** below.

Case Discussion

There are crucial differences between the presentations of the three recruits.

Recruit A's blackout is worrisome for cardiogenic syncope. Immediate recovery implies syncope rather than seizure, but the onset of syncope during exertion suggests insufficient cardiac output or arrhythmia provoked by increased cardiac demand. A number of young military recruits have suffered sudden cardiac death from aetiologies such as hypertrophic obstructive cardiomyopathy and congenital long QT syndrome. He should receive echocardiographic and extended ECG monitoring.

Recruit B is likely to have vasovagal syncope. Prolonged standing in hot weather is classic for vasovagal syncope, and he recovered promptly, which is more consistent with syncope than seizure. A few unsustained twitches and even urinary incontinence can occur in syncope. He should be hydrated but otherwise requires no further investigation.

Recruit C has had a seizure. Although his convulsions were brief and he did not have urinary incontinence, simple syncope (unless cardiogenic) has no business occurring while sitting up eating, and he had post-event drowsiness. Eyewitness accounts should be obtained. He should receive workup including electrolytes, EEG, MRI brain and evaluation for provoking factors.

Key Lessons	1. Syncope and seizure can be differentiated based on context, pre-, intra- and post-event features. Aura, lateral tongue biting, semiology characteristic of a seizure (automatisms, version, sustained tonic–clonic movements) and post-ictal drowsiness suggest seizure. Prodromal light-headedness and rapid recovery of alertness suggest syncope.
	2. Most syncope is vasovagal, but look for red flags for cardiogenic syncope, as well as postural hypotension.
	3. In any seizure, look for provoking factors. Consider neuroimaging, blood investigations for metabolic derangements and lumbar puncture (if suspecting infection). Diagnosis hinges on the synthesis of seizure semiology, EEG and MRI findings (i.e., any epileptogenic structural abnormalities).
Common Pitfalls	1. Unsustained twitches can occur in syncope and should not be misdiagnosed as seizure.
	2. Patients with a single unprovoked seizure have a higher risk of seizure recurrence than the general population, but should not be told that they have epilepsy (unless there is a structural abnormality with high recurrence risk, or epilepsy syndrome).

Questions
1. **REFLECT!** Have you, or anyone you know, ever experienced vasovagal syncope? Can you recount the episode?

2. **DISCUSS!** It is not uncommon for elderly patients with multiple medical comorbids to present with sudden loss of consciousness. Suppose a 70-year-old man with ischaemic heart disease, atrial fibrillation, diabetes and hypertension presents with sudden blackouts. What would be some special considerations in this patient, and how would your approach differ, as compared to any of the military recruits we discussed?

3. **EXPLORE!** Why is cardiac syncope worrisome? What are the potential consequences of hypertrophic obstructive cardiomyopathy, long QT and Wolff–Parkinson–White syndrome? What is the implication of syncope occurring in these conditions?

4. **GO FURTHER!** The Internet is rich with countless videos of different types of seizure. Why not have a look at some of them? As you do so, attempt to characterise the seizure semiology (the 2017 international league against epilepsy classification of seizure types may be helpful).

Chapter **An Approach to**
24 Giddiness

Clinical Case

A 38-year-old supermarket cashier presents with giddiness. She was at work when she suddenly felt the room spinning, felt nauseous and had to sit down as she was falling to one side. She also complains of some hemifacial numbness. Although she denies it, her colleagues noticed that her speech was unclear. She had no weakness, facial droop, diplopia, hearing loss or tinnitus. All symptoms completely resolved within 2 hr. She has no past medical history, and has never had giddy spells before. On examination, there are no cranial nerve deficits, no cerebellar signs and power and sensation in all limbs are normal. A CT brain is normal. What is the most likely diagnosis, and what should be done next?

Giddiness is a challenging symptom to approach. A classic description of benign positional postural vertigo, or a clear-cut brainstem stroke is easy to diagnose, but textbook histories are the exception rather than the rule. Furthermore, giddiness is often a non-specific symptom of general medical illness. In navigating this minefield, the clinician's best bet is a careful history and physical examination (Figure 24.1).

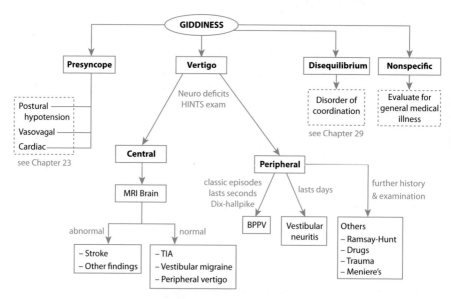

BPPV, benign paroxysmal positional vertigo; HINTS exam, head impulse, nystagmus, test of skew; TIA, transient ischaemic attack.

Figure 24.1. Approach to giddiness.

Types of Giddiness

'Giddiness' means different things to different patients. There are four main types (Table 24.1):

- **Pre-syncope** is a sense of light-headedness, associated with fading of vision, pallor and diaphoresis. There may be a brief loss of consciousness (syncope).
- **Vertigo** is an illusion of motion, for instance, patients may complain that the room is spinning.
- **Disequilibrium** is a sense of imbalance during movement, due to a difficulty in coordination. This occurs only when the patient walks.
- **Non-specific**: Giddiness is often a non-specific symptom of general medical illness.

Table 24.1. Four Main Types of Giddiness

	Pre-syncope	Vertigo	Disequilibrium	Non-specific
Characteristic	Light-headedness Feeling faint Fading of vision	Room spinning	Imbalance during movement	Vague
Giddiness occurs when . . .	Postural change, prolonged standing	May or may not be related to head turning	During movement only	Non-specific
Associated features	Pallor Diaphoresis Postural BP drop	Nausea/vomiting Hearing loss Brainstem signs and symptoms[a] Weakness/ numbness	Ataxic gait Cerebellar signs Parkinsonism	Features of general medical condition
Time course	Transient, short-lived	Brief or prolonged	Resolves when stationary	Prolonged
Aetiology	Impaired cerebral blood flow due to: – Postural hypotension – Vasovagal heart disease	Vestibular pathway dysfunction due to: – Brainstem disease – Ear disease	Disorder of coordination – Cerebellar disease – Proprioceptive loss – Parkinsonism	Anaemia Hypoglycaemia Sepsis Psychosomatic Other illnesses

[a] Including diplopia, dysarthria, dysphagia, facial droop, facial or limb weakness or numbness, ataxia and Horner's syndrome.

In Practice . . .

In many patients, especially the elderly, narrowing to one type of giddiness may not be reliable or even possible. In addition to focusing on the most likely type of giddiness, a practical approach would be to:

- Screen for general medical illnesses by asking about other symptoms, performing a routine physical examination and basic investigations including capillary glucose, haemoglobin, electrolytes and as directed by clinical suspicion.
- Check postural blood pressure (postural hypotension as a cause of pre-syncopal giddiness).
- Do ECG in all patients (arrhythmias as a cause of giddiness).
- Always consider dangerous causes of giddiness especially (a) Posterior circulation stroke or transient ischaemic attack (TIA; see text) and (b) cardiogenic syncope (Chapter 23).

This chapter discusses the approach to vertigo. For patients with pre-syncopal giddiness, see Chapter 23. For patients with disequilibrium, see Chapter 29.

Vertigo: Central vs. Peripheral

If giddiness is vertiginous, the next step is to distinguish between central vs. peripheral vertigo. Peripheral vertigo is often benign, while central vertigo could be a stroke or TIA. The main distinguishing features are given in Table 24.2.

Table 24.2. Distinguishing Peripheral vs. Central Vertigo

	Peripheral vertigo	Central vertigo
Character and time course (see text)	Classic BPPV: recurrent episodes lasting seconds, associated with head movement More prolonged symptoms in other causes of peripheral vertigo	Vertigo lasts hours in stroke, but shorter durations do not rule out TIA. No association with head movement
Nausea and vomiting	Often present, can be marked	Usually absent to mild
Hearing deficits	May have hearing loss or tinnitus	None
Neurologic deficits	**None**	**Any neurological deficit (even if transient)** – Cranial nerve deficits, dysphagia, dysarthria – Weakness or numbness of face or limbs – Diplopia, poor pursuit and inaccurate saccadic eye movements. – Cerebellar signs, ataxic gait – Horner's syndrome
Time course[a]	Seconds, minutes or hours	Minutes or hours (not seconds)
HINTS exam[b]	All three components reassuring	**Any one component worrisome**

BPPV, benign paroxysmal positional vertigo; TIA, transient ischaemic attack.

ᵃA Note on Time Course

Except in classic benign paroxysmal positional vertigo (BPPV) lasting seconds, time course is a poor differentiating feature between central and peripheral vertigo.

- Vertigo lasting seconds: BPPV, also consider postural hypotension (although it is non-vertiginous).
- Vertigo lasting minutes: TIA, in addition to BPPV and postural hypotension.
- Vertigo lasting hours: Stroke, vestibular neuritis and other aetiologies.

ᵇHINTS Exam

The HINTS exam is a rapid bedside examination to identify which patients warrant further evaluation for central vertigo. It should be performed on *patients who are still giddy*:

- **Head impulse**: Before doing this test, check that the patient has no cervical spine instability or neck pain. Asking the patient to look at a midline object, rapidly rotate the head left and right. This tests whether the vestibular ocular impulse is impaired— as occurs in peripheral causes of vertigo.
- **Nystagmus**: Examine extraocular eye movements in the routine way, paying attention to any nystagmus. Nystagmus may also be elicited during other manoeuvres (e.g., Dix–Hallpike, if done).
- **Test of skew**: Asking the patient to focus on a fixed target, alternately cover either eye in rapid succession. Known as cover–uncover testing, this accentuates vertical misalignment of the eye.

Table 24.3. Interpreting the HINTS Exam

	Peripheral vertigo	Central vertigo
Head impulse[a]	Loss of visual fixation followed by corrective saccade back to midline (impaired vestibular-ocular reflex)	No loss of visual fixation or corrective saccade (intact vestibular-ocular reflex)
Characteristics of nystagmus	Unidirectional Horizontal only Jerk or rotational Latency before onset Fatigable Suppressed by visual fixation	Uni- or multidirectional, gaze evoked Can be vertical or horizontal Any pattern including pendular No latency Not fatigable Not suppressed by visual fixation
Test of skew	Uncovered eye does **not** realign (normal vertical alignment)	Uncovered eye quickly moves up/down to realign on the visual target (positive skew deviation)

[a] Patients with peripheral vertigo, who are no longer giddy are likely to have an intact vestibular–ocular reflex (i.e., normal head impulse). This is a misleading finding as it is considered indicative of central vertigo. Therefore, head impulse testing should only be performed on patients who are still giddy.

HINTS is reassuring if all three components are consistent with peripheral vertigo (Table 24.3)—as a sensitive test (as good as MRI), a reassuring HINTS rules out stroke. On the other hand, if any one component suggests central vertigo, a central cause cannot be ruled out and further investigation is warranted.

Central Vertigo

The main concern in central vertigo is posterior circulation stroke. While anterior circulation strokes more commonly present with hemiplegia (with or without sensory, cerebellar and cortical signs), posterior circulation strokes are harder to recognise, often presenting with vertigo, cranial nerve and cerebellar deficits and variable sensory loss (see 'GO FURTHER' on page 238).

Next steps: Unlike anterior circulation strokes, it is difficult to make a clinical diagnosis of posterior circulation stroke without imaging.

- **MRI brain**: This is the preferred modality of imaging in suspected posterior circulation stroke. MRI is far superior because (a) CT visualises the posterior fossa poorly, where many structures are small, and (b) CT is not sensitive to detect acute infarcts.
- **CT brain**: If it is not possible to obtain a timely MRI, CT brain may be performed. Prompt identification of large established infarcts or haemorrhage is important, as these may cause mass effect requiring intervention. On the other hand, a normal CT brain does not rule out brainstem stroke and in most cases, MRI will need to be done later.

Central Vertigo with Abnormal MRI Brain

- **Posterior circulation stroke**: MRI brain is able to identify stroke and distinguish between infarct and haemorrhage. The next questions will then be (a) is the patient a candidate for thrombolysis, and (b) what is the mechanism of the stroke. This is discussed in Chapter 25.
- **Other findings**: MRI may reveal other findings including inflammatory lesions suggestive of multiple sclerosis, malformations and so forth. In the appropriate locations they may explain vertigo; some findings may be incidental.

Central Vertigo with Normal MRI Brain

If the MRI is normal, consider:

- **Posterior circulation TIA**: This is a difficult diagnosis, but important to recognise, as it confers a high risk of subsequent stroke. Be particularly alert to this diagnosis in patients with symptoms or neurologic deficits attributable to brainstem ischaemia (e.g., slurring of speech that got better), patients with strong risk factors (e.g., atrial fibrillation, previous radiotherapy to the neck, hypercoagulable states and cardiovascular risk factors), and if the MR angiogram reveals significant intracranial atherosclerosis. Even with a normal MRI brain, persist with TIA workup (see Chapter 25) if there is high clinical suspicion.

- **Vestibular migraine:** Consider the diagnosis if recurrent episodes of vertigo are associated with migraine headache, photophobia or migraine auras.
- **Causes of peripheral vertigo.** The head impulse can be falsely normal (suggesting a central cause) if giddiness has resolved.

Peripheral Vertigo

The commonest causes of peripheral vertigo are BPPV and vestibular neuritis. These causes can be differentiated with particular attention to time course, provoking factors and bedside examination.

- **BPPV:** Recurrent episodes of vertigo, each *lasting seconds*, provoked by changes in head position (which displaces the calcium debris or otoliths in the semi-circular canal). Vertigo is absent on lying still. A *Dix–Hallpike manoeuvre* on the affected side may reproduce vertigo, together with nystagmus which obeys the rules of peripheral nystagmus—unidirectional, horizontal or rotational, showing latency of onset and fatigability. The Dix–Hallpike manoeuvre is not sensitive, so a negative test does not rule out BPPV.

- **Vestibular neuritis:** Sudden-onset severe vertigo, *lasting for days or longer*, associated with nausea/vomiting and gait instability. There is no relationship to positional change. This is due to viral or post-infectious inflammation of the eighth cranial nerve. If inflammation affects both vestibular and cochlear components of the nerve, there may also be hearing loss or tinnitus.

- **Ramsay Hunt syndrome:** Zoster reactivation in the geniculate ganglion causes vertigo, hearing loss, ear pain ± ipsilateral facial paralysis. Otoscopy reveals vesicles in the auditory canal.

- **Drug vestibulotoxicity:** For example, gentamicin, high-dose furosemide and cisplatin.

- **Labyrinthine trauma:** Trauma may damage of the vestibular nerve, leading to vertigo either immediately or later.

- **Meniere disease:** Recurrent episodes of vertigo, each lasting 20 min to 24 hr, together with ear fullness and fluctuating low-tone sensorineural hearing loss ± tinnitus. Onset is gradual (vs. acute in vestibular neuritis) and disease is progressive. This is a diagnosis of exclusion, thought to be due to excess endolymph in the inner ear.

 Using what you have learnt, **pen down your approach** to the Clinical Case at the start of the chapter **BEFORE reading the discussion** below.

Case Discussion

This is a relatively young lady whose vertigo is associated with features worrisome for brainstem ischaemia (ataxia, facial numbness, dysarthria). A diagnosis of brainstem transient ischaemic attack (TIA) must be considered. Do not be misled by the resolution of symptoms, normal examination and normal CT scan—the neurological deficits of a TIA are transient, and a CT scan is normal by definition (or it would be a stroke). If a HINTS examination were performed, it may have revealed features suggestive of central vertigo, or may be falsely reassuring as her symptoms have resolved.

The next step is an MRI brain and TIA workup (including vertebral artery imaging, monitoring for atrial fibrillation and searching for risk factors for stroke/TIA—see Chapter 25). This lady's MRI showed no acute infarct or haemorrhage, but a CT angiogram subsequently revealed vertebral artery dissection.

Key Lessons	1. Giddiness may be due to pre-syncope, vertigo, disequilibrium or it may be a non-specific symptom of general medical illness. It may not always be possible to distinguish between pre-syncope and vertigo.
	2. Distinguish between central and peripheral vertigo based on the presence of signs or symptoms suggestive of brainstem ischaemia, neurologic deficits and HINTS examination (head impulse, nystagmus and test of skew).
	3. Central vertigo is worrisome for posterior circulation stroke or TIA. Obtain MRI brain.
	4. Common causes of peripheral vertigo include BPPV and vestibular neuritis, which may be distinguished based on time course and provoking factors.
Common Pitfalls	1. A normal CT brain does not exclude posterior circulation stroke or TIA.
	2. Patients with peripheral vertigo can have a 'normal' head impulse (i.e., no corrective saccade) if they are no longer giddy.
Questions	1. **REFLECT!** Have you seen a patient with typical BPPV? How did the patient describe his/her symptoms, and what did the nystagmus look like? (You can also try searching the Internet for videos of nystagmus.)
	2. **DISCUSS!** Compare and contrast BPPV and giddiness due to postural hypotension. How would you tell the two apart?
	3. **EXPLORE!** Do you know how to perform the Dix–Hallpike manoeuvre? A positive Dix–Hallpike should be followed with an Epley manoeuvre, which aims to reposition the otoliths. A successful Epley's can be quite gratifying—you will have a very happy patient the next morning. Why don't you learn both manoeuvres?
	4. **GO FURTHER!** Lateral medullary syndrome is the commonest brainstem stroke syndrome, and is easy to miss as there is no weakness. Read up on its clinical features, and try to explain why these features arise, based on the neuroanatomical structures in the lateral medulla.

Chapter **An Approach to**
25 Weakness

Clinical Case

A 40-year-old lady is admitted for difficulty walking. She first had difficulty climbing upstairs 1 week ago, and was tripping frequently for no apparent reason. In the past 2 days, she has had difficulty walking on level ground. On examination, power in bilateral lower limbs was 4/5 proximally and 3/5 distally. Upper limb power is full. Ankle and knee jerks were difficult to elicit, but upper limb reflexes were normal. Planters were downgoing. There is reduced pinprick sensation over both ankles and feet. She is not able to walk and requires a wheelchair. Examination of the heart, lungs, abdomen, cranial nerves and cerebellar system is normal. How would you approach her complaint?

Weakness is a cardinal presentation of neurologic disease. This may be an acute stroke with a fast-closing window for thrombolysis, a myasthenic crisis with impending respiratory collapse, or a compression neuropathy for which treatment is non-urgent. Clinical history and examination is the key to diagnosis, investigations are usually supportive. The clinician must answer two questions: (1) where is the lesion (neurological localisation), and (2) what is the lesion (aetiology).

This chapter presents a condensed approach to the major causes of weakness, beginning with a general approach, then upper and lower motor neuron weakness. Many beginning clinicians suffer from neurophobia; be encouraged that once understood (rather than memorised), the approach to weakness is quite logical and intuitive to work through. Basic neuroanatomical knowledge and familiarity with the neurologic examination is assumed.

General Approach

Verify True Neurological Weakness

Weakness can mean many things to many people. Verify that there is objective weakness (not always an easy task!). Patients may complain of 'weakness' when they have something else, for example:

- Difficulty walking due to ataxia and poor coordination (cerebellar dysfunction; see Chapter 29), bradykinesia or instability (see Chapter 30).
- Hypoglycaemia is a mimic of neurological weakness and should always be ruled out with a bedside capillary blood glucose. The story is often told of the 'stroke patient' who was cured with IV dextrose!

- Reduced effort tolerance due to cardiac failure, pulmonary disease or anaemia.
- Lethargy due to infection, hypothyroidism, electrolyte imbalance, dehydration.
- Joint or muscle pain.
- Psychiatric illness, for example, conversion disorder: A diagnosis of exclusion only after other investigations are normal.

Having ascertained that there is indeed weakness, proceed to explore the two cardinal questions—(1) where is the lesion, and (2) what is the lesion. General principles are explained here, and specific scenarios given in the subsequent sections.

Where Is the Lesion?

Think of the motor axis. It takes two motor neurons (an 'upper' and a 'lower' motor neuron) for a signal from the brain to be translated into movement. The upper motor neuron's (UMN) cell body is in the motor cortex and its axon descends through the brainstem and spinal cord, to synapse onto the lower motor neuron (LMN) in the anterior horn of the spinal cord. The LMN then exits the spinal cord in a root, then plexus, and through peripheral nerves, to synapse at the neuromuscular junction (NMJ) unto a muscle. Therefore, weakness must be due to pathology somewhere along the neuroaxis: brain–brainstem–spinal cord–anterior horn cell–root–plexus–peripheral nerve–NMJ–muscle. Each location on the neuroaxis presents with unique features.

UMN or LMN lesion: First distinguish between an UMN vs. a LMN pattern of weakness (Table 25.1). A UMN lesion localises the lesion to the brain, brainstem or spinal cord. A LMN pattern localises to anterior horn cells and distally.

Table 25.1. Distinguishing Upper Motor Neuron vs. Lower Motor Neuron Lesions

	UMN: brain, brainstem, spinal cord	LMN: root, plexus, peripheral nerve[2]	LMN: NMJ or muscle
Atrophy	Less marked	Present, may be severe	Variable[3]
Fasciculation	None	May be present	None
Tone	Increased[1]	Decreased	Usually normal[3]
Clonus	≥ 3 Beats[1]	≤ 3 beats	≤ 3 beats
Reflexes	Increased[1]	Decreased	Usually normal[3]
Plantars	Upgoing[1]	Downgoing	Downgoing

Caveats:

[1]An acute UMN lesion (e.g., acute stroke or spinal cord injury) is likely to not demonstrate hyperreflexia or spasticity; these UMN features take time to develop. Plantars may or may not be upgoing acutely.

[2]Anterior horn cell lesions are not included in this classification; they may present with a mix or UMN and LMN signs (see page 249).

[3]Atrophy is usually absent, but severe myopathy may lead to atrophy, hypotonia and diminished reflexes.

What Is the Lesion

Having localised the lesion, the next step is to identify its aetiology. Certain aetiologies are more likely to affect particular locations along the neuroaxis—this is discussed in the subsequent sections. Time course is another other important distinguisher.

- **Hyperacute**—sudden onset in minutes: Usually vascular, for example, cerebrovascular accident and haemorrhage.

- **Subacute**—onset over hours to days: Inflammatory (e.g., Guillain–Barre syndrome, multiple sclerosis [MS]), infective (e.g., bacterial meningitis).

- **Chronic**—slowly progressive over weeks to months or longer: Neoplastic, infective (e.g., TB), degenerative (e.g., Parkinson's disease and cervical myelopathy), or metabolic (e.g., diabetic neuropathy).

- **Episodic**—acute flares with intervening asymptomatic intervals: This is characteristic of disorders like migraine and epilepsy. Rarely, these diseases can present with weakness—that is, hemiplegic migraine and Todd's paralysis post-seizure. The periodic paralyses (thyrotoxic periodic paralysis, hypokalaemic periodic paralysis; page 166) also present episodically.

The next sections discuss UMN weakness, followed by LMN weakness.

UMN Weakness

The distribution of weakness, as well as adjacent involved structures, assists to localise the lesion (Figure 25.1).

- **Brain**: Contralateral limb weakness ± contralateral brainstem signs (e.g., facial droop) ± cortical signs (i.e., deficits due to injury to the cerebral cortex, e.g., aphasia and hemi-neglect).

- **Brainstem**: Contralateral limb weakness ± *ipsilateral* cranial nerve palsies (crossed hemiparesis)—recall that cranial nerves are lower motor neurons that originate from the brainstem; therefore, a *left* pontine stroke may cause a *left* LMN facial palsy and *right* hemiparesis. A large brainstem lesion may lead to drowsiness (disruption of the ascending reticular activating system) and hemodynamic fluctuations (disruption of cardio-regulatory and respiratory centres).

- **Spinal cord**: Classically *bilateral* weakness (the cord is small, so it is hard to only affect half the cord) with a defined *level*. There are UMN signs and sensory loss below the level of the lesion, and LMN signs at the level of the lesion. Bowel or bladder sphincters may be involved, causing urinary retention or incontinence.

The subsequent subsections discuss the approach to UMN weakness based on the distribution of weakness—hemiparesis, para/quadriparesis or weakness in a bizarre distribution (Figure 25.2).

Figure 25.1. Classical distributions of UMN weakness.

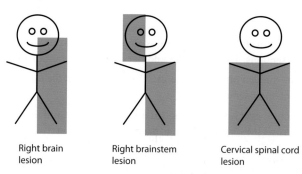

| Right brain lesion | Right brainstem lesion | Cervical spinal cord lesion |

Caveats:

1. A very distal spine lesion (below the termination of the spinal cord at L2), for example, Cauda equina syndrome and Spina bifida, may show LMN signs rather than UMN signs. Conus Medullaris syndrome (affecting the termination of the spinal cord) causes mixed UMN and LMN signs.

2. Cerebellar signs may be present in brainstem lesions, due to their close proximity and common vascular supply, as well as in brain lesions (disruption of the cerebellar–cortical loop, e.g., in the lacunar stroke syndrome of ataxic hemiparesis). Therefore, cerebellar signs may not distinguish between brain and brainstem lesions.

3. Very rarely, a spinal cord lesion may affect only half the cord. The classic example is Brown-Sequard syndrome, first described in farmers who had a violent propensity to transect each other's hemicord with machetes, which presents with ipsilateral UMN weakness (corticospinal tract), ipsilateral loss of vibration sense and proprioception (dorsal columns) and contralateral loss of pain and temperature sensation (spinothalamic tract). This nicely reflects the neuroanatomical fact that the spinothalamic tract decussates one to two vertebral levels above the root supplied, while the corticospinal tract and dorsal columns decussate at the base of the medulla.

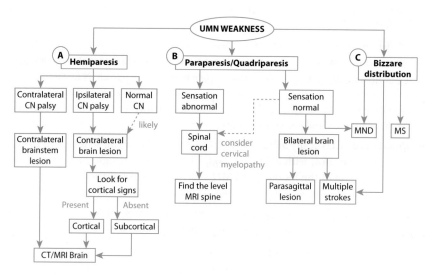

CN, cranial nerve; MND, motor neuron disease; MS, multiple sclerosis.

Figure 25.2. Approach to upper motor neuron (UMN) weakness.

(A) UMN Hemiparesis

Localisation

In UMN hemiparesis, half of the body is weak. This is the result of a CNS lesion in the contralateral brainstem or brain.[1] The lateralisation of cranial nerve abnormalities is significant.

- **Brain lesions**: UMN hemiparesis with *ipsilateral* cranial nerve palsy, for instance, left hemiparesis with left facial droop in a right-sided stroke. Note that this would be an UMN CN VII palsy, involving only the lower half of the face (see Chapter 26).

- **Brainstem lesions**: UMN hemiparesis with *contralateral* cranial nerve palsy at the level of lesion. For example, a *left* pons lesion can result in *right*-sided weakness with *left* LMN facial droop, involving both the lower and upper half of the face (due to involvement of the seventh nerve nucleus, which is an LMN). Similarly, a *left* midbrain lesion can result in *right*-sided weakness and *left* third nerve palsy.

Cortical signs: Brain lesions are further localised as cortical (cerebral hemispheres including the motor cortex), or subcortical (deep structures including internal capsule, thalamus and basal ganglia). Signs of cerebral cortex dysfunction, including gaze deviation, aphasia, hemineglect or cortical blindness, allow a clinical diagnosis of a cortical lesion. Line bisection is a useful test—holding a stethoscope on both ends, ask the patient to divide it in half; a patient with hemineglect will not be able to accurately identify the midpoint.

Brainstem signs: The presence of drowsiness, vertigo, gaze palsies and pupillary abnormalities suggest brainstem involvement, either directly from a brainstem lesion, or due to brainstem compression by a large brain lesion or cerebral oedema.

Aetiology and Workup

Aetiology: The time course is the key.

- Onset in minutes: Usually vascular, for example, cerebral infarct or haemorrhage.
- Onset over hours to days: Inflammatory (e.g., MS), infective (e.g., cranial abscess).
- Progressive over weeks to months: Neoplastic (i.e., brain tumour), infective (e.g., tuberculoma).

Workup begins with cranial imaging.

- CT brain is the imaging modality of choice in suspected acute stroke, is generally easier to obtain, and will reveal gross abnormalities.
- MRI brain provides superior anatomic detail especially in the posterior fossa (i.e., suspecting a brainstem lesion).
- Contrast (either CT or MRI) should be used if infection, inflammation or tumour is suspected. Contrast helps to delineate the lesion.

---

[1] Or rarely, a hemicord lesion (Brown-Sequard syndrome, page 242).

Approach to Suspected Acute Stroke and Transient Ischaemic Attack

Stroke is the commonest cause of UMN hemiparesis and some additional comments are in order. With modern reperfusion therapy (thrombolysis ± thrombectomy), stroke is a time-sensitive diagnosis with a narrow window for life-changing intervention. The important questions to answer are:

1. Is this a stroke?
2. If stroke, is it ischaemic or haemorrhagic?
3. If ischaemic stroke, is the patient a candidate for reperfusion therapy?
4. If stroke/transient ischaemic attack (TIA), what is the mechanism?

1. **Is this a stroke?** Stroke is suspected when a patient presents with sudden-onset one-sided weakness or facial slurring. However, a number of other aetiologies mimic this hyperacute presentation and should be considered.

- TIA: Rapidly improving deficits with a total duration lasting < 1 hr raise the possibility of TIA instead of actual infarction. Nonetheless, TIAs reflect inadequate cerebral blood flow and confer a high risk of early stroke; they require workup much in the same way as acute stroke (for TIA: skip steps 2 and 3, go directly to step 4).

- Other neurologic paroxysms: Hemiplegic migraine (with headache), seizure with Todd's paralysis. These characteristically begin with positive symptoms (e.g., seeing bright lines, hearing noises, paraesthesia, twitching or jerking movements) before negative symptoms (weakness, loss of vision, numbness) present while positive symptoms are not a typical feature of stroke. The distinction can be difficult.

- Hypoglycaemia can mimic hemiplegia, but is easy to rule out with a capillary blood glucose (which must always be done).

- Psychiatric disease including conversion disorder: This is suspected in patients with known psychiatric issues, inconsistent history and examination findings not consistent with a defined arterial territory.

2. **If stroke, is it ischaemic or haemorrhagic?** The next step is to obtain a non-contrast CT brain.

- Normal CT brain: In the presence of typical symptoms (e.g., hemiparesis and/or facial droop) of acute onset, a normal CT brain is perfectly consistent with hyperacute stroke. It must be emphasised that stroke is a clinical diagnosis; the role of imaging is to exclude haemorrhage and differentials, not to diagnose stroke.

- Early signs of cerebral infarction: Subtle signs of infarction, for example, loss of grey–white differentiation or normal gyri and sulci (Figure 25.3a), or large vessel hyperattenuation (e.g., a dense middle cerebral artery [MCA] sign) (Figure 25.3c), are consistent with acute stroke. If there is uncertainty, MRI can be helpful (Figure 25.3d–f).

- Established cerebral infarction: Overt parenchymal hypoattenuation (Figure 25.3b) suggests an established stroke, precluding reperfusion therapy.

- Cerebral haemorrhage: Blood appears bright on CT scan (Figure 25.4). The aetiology and management of haemorrhagic stroke is somewhat different from that of ischaemic stroke.

- Other differentials: For example, intra-cranial tumour, abscess and so forth (which rarely mimic stroke).

3. **If ischaemic stroke, is the patient a candidate for reperfusion therapy (thrombolysis/thrombectomy)?** Reperfusion therapy restores blood flow to the ischaemic penumbra (i.e., neurons that are in danger but not yet dead), but at the risk of cerebral haemorrhage. Therefore, careful selection of patients with a low bleed risk, and hence a favourable risk-benefit ratio, is essential. In the acute assessment of stroke, look for:

- Onset of stroke: Only patients with acute symptom onset are eligible for reperfusion (< 4.5 hr in thrombolysis, up to 24 hr in thrombectomy). It is important to find out when the patient was 'last seen well'; for a patient who wakes up with a stroke, the 'last seen well' time is the time that he/she went to bed (or woke up to go to toilet).

- Severity of stroke: Use objective scoring (National Institutes of Health Stroke Scale [NIHSS]). Patients with very severe deficits may be poor candidates for reperfusion, and patients with mild deficits may not benefit enough from reperfusion to justify its risk.

- Risk factors for bleeding: For example, intracranial haemorrhage, internal bleeding, anticoagulation (novel oral anticoagulant or warfarin with INR > 1.7), severe uncontrollable hypertension, coagulopathy, surgery in 14 days and other factors.

Figure 25.3. Neuroimaging in ischaemic stroke. A 60-year-old man presented with acute left hemiparesis and left UMN facial droop. CT brain 3 hr after symptom onset (a) showed loss of grey–white differentiation and obliteration of normal gyri and sulci in the right fronto-parietal region, indicative of early ischaemic stroke. He did not undergo thrombolysis. Repeat CT brain 5 days later (b) shows an established MCA territory infarct. Another 60-year-old man presented with acute left hemiparesis and left UMN facial droop. CT brain 2 hr after symptom onset (c) showed a dense MCA sign. MRI brain was performed immediately, and confirmed restricted diffusion—bright on diffusion weighted imaging (DWI) (e) and dark on apparent diffusion coefficient (ADC) (f) indicative of acute infarct in the right frontal lobe. MR angiogram visualised an abrupt cut off in the proximal MCA (d), which supplies the territory of infarct.

(a)
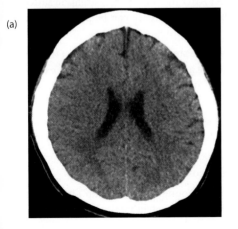

(b)
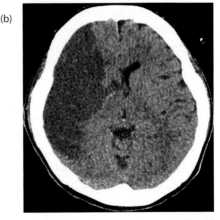

(Cont'd)

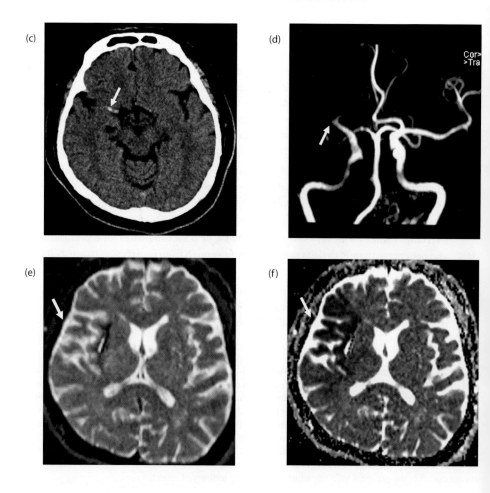

4. **What is the mechanism of this stroke/TIA?** After the acute phase, attention shifts to identifying the mechanism of stroke, such that a recurrence can be prevented. In ischaemic strokes, consider:

- Imaging for arterial disease (e.g., atherosclerotic stenosis, or carotid dissection in younger patients): Both intra-cranial vessels (e.g., CT/MR angiogram) and extra-cranial vessels (e.g., ultrasound carotids or CT angiogram extending downwards to the aortic arch).

- Workup for cardioembolic source: Monitoring for atrial fibrillation, left ventricular thrombus (echocardiography in patients with suspected ischaemic heart disease).

- Workup for risk factors of small vessel disease: For example, screen for hyperlipidaemia (fasting lipids) and diabetes (fasting glucose).

- In young patients, consider other aetiologies ('young stroke workup') including hypercoagulable disorders, paradoxical emboli from a patent foramen ovale, vasculitis and autoimmune disorders.

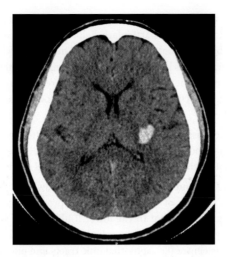

Figure 25.4. Neuroimaging in haemorrhagic stroke. A 50-year-old man with poorly controlled hypertension presented with acute right hemiparesis and right UMN facial droop. CT brain is significant for a haemorrhagic infarct (white) in the left basal ganglia. This is a favourite location for hypertensive bleeds.

(B) UMN Paraplegia/Quadriplegia

In spastic paraparesis, both lower limbs are weak with UMN signs. This is most commonly a spinal cord lesion, as a brain or brainstem lesion has to affect both sides to cause paraplegia or quadriplegia.

UMN Para/Quadriplegia with Abnormal Sensation

If sensation is abnormal, the lesion is almost always at the spinal cord (the terms 'myelitis' and 'myelopathy' refer to spinal cord disease). Bladder and bowel sphincter dysfunction also suggests a spinal cord lesion, and is decidedly less common in lesions of other parts of the neuroaxis. Proceed to find the level of the lesion, and consider an aetiology.

Where is the lesion? Which level of the spinal cord?

- **Examine for brisk *jaw jerk*:** This is an important sign; a brisk jaw jerk implies cranial nerve involvement, suggesting something *more* than just spinal cord disease (e.g., MS, neuromyelitis optica [NMO], motor neuron disease [MND]).
- **Examine for a *motor* level,** *below* which there are UMN signs (due to involvement of descending corticospinal tract fibres), and *at* which there may be LMN signs (due to involvement of anterior horn cells). For example:
  - UMN lower limbs, brisk triceps jerk (C7), absent biceps jerk (C5/6): lesion *at* C5/6.
  - UMN lower limbs, brisk triceps jerk (C7), brisk biceps jerk (C5/6): lesion *above* C5/6—upper cervical cord (normal cranial nerves) or brainstem (cranial nerves involved).

- **Examine for a *sensory* level**: There may be an identifiable dermatome below which sensation is diminished. This is particularly helpful in a thoracic cord lesion, as there are no testable limb reflexes between C7 and L2. This is not always a reliable finding, as there is considerable overlap in sensory dermatomes, and the pattern of sensory loss in chronic myelopathies is often distal (almost resembling peripheral neuropathy). If the sensory level contradicts the motor level, follow the motor level, which is more reliable.

- **Dissociated sensory loss**: Spinal cord disease tends to affect both pain/temperature (spinothalamic tract) and vibration/proprioception (dorsal columns) simultaneously. Rarely, this may not be the case (also see Brown-Sequard syndrome, page 242).

  - Syringomyelia: Pain and temperature loss in a shawl-like distribution over the shoulders, with sparing of fine touch and proprioception. UMN weakness in the upper limbs exceeds that in the lower limbs. This is due to an expanding fluid-filled cavity in the centre of the spinal cord, which affects spinal cord structures closer to the centre (i.e., spinothalamic tracts and upper limb motor tracts).

  - Subacute combined degeneration: UMN paraparesis with isolated proprioception and vibration loss; spinothalamic tracts are spared. This is classically due to vitamin B12 deficiency.

  - Anterior cord syndrome: UMN paraparesis with isolated loss of pain and temperature, with sparing of dorsal columns.

- **Imaging**: Obtain MRI spine to confirm the clinical localisation.

What is the lesion: Identify possible aetiologies in context of the patient:

- **Acute onset, then static (does not get worse)**: Trauma. Usually apparent on history and unfortunately not rare.

- **Subacute onset**:
  - Inflammatory: MS or NMO. In MS, patients may also give a history of prior episodes, demonstrating dissemination in time and space (page 249).
  - Infective: For example, epidural abscess and spinal TB.
  - Neoplastic: For example, metastases and primary bone tumours.

- **Chronic and slowly progressive**:
  - Degenerative: Cervical myelopathy (degenerative in older patients, may be due to rheumatologic disease in younger patients), spinocerebellar degeneration (with cerebellar signs).
  - Metabolic: Subacute combined degeneration from B12 deficiency.
  - Infective: Tabes dorsalis (i.e., neurosyphilis).

- **Static from young**: Congenital causes, for example, hereditary spastic paraparesis.

UMN Para/Quadriplegia with Normal Sensation

Normal sensation makes a spinal cord aetiology less likely. Consider:

- **Bilateral brain disease**:
  - Parasagittal lesion (e.g., meningioma): Classically bilateral lower limb diplegia, as the parasagittal segment of the motor homunculus supplies the lower limbs.
  - Multiple strokes in both cerebral hemispheres.
- **MND**: The combination of UMN and LMN findings (wasting or fasciculation) is classic for MND, however, some variants (primary lateral sclerosis) are purely UMN.
- Hereditary spastic paraparesis.
- Cervical spondylotic myelopathy: Rarely may present with only subtle sensory findings.

(C) UMN Weakness; Bizarre Distribution

This finding cannot be explained with the usual approach. Consider:

- **Multiple strokes** affecting different territories in the brain.
- **Multiple sclerosis (MS)**: Consider MS in a younger patient (often 18–50 years old) with CNS lesions in multiple anatomic locations (dissemination in space), and at different times (dissemination in time). This demyelinating disease can affect any part of the CNS, causing subacute-onset transverse myelitis (bilateral UMN below the spinal cord level), incoordination, optic neuritis (visual deficit with pain on extraocular eye movements and a relative afferent pupillary deficit), gaze palsies or various patterns of sensory impairment. There are *no LMN features*. Contrasted MRI of the brain and spine demonstrates white matter lesions disseminated in space (there some typical sites) and time (e.g., both old and new lesions present at the same time). Lumbar puncture may reveal oligoclonal bands in the cerebrospinal fluid, although this is less commonly done now (see MacDonald diagnostic criteria).
- **Multiple sclerosis (MS) mimics**: MS has a number of mimics, including NMO, lupus and others. A detailed discussion is beyond the scope of this text.
- **Motor neuron disease (MND)**: MND (amyotrophic lateral sclerosis) affects both UMN in the cerebral cortex, as well as anterior horn cells. This results in a classic paradox of mixed LMN (prominent wasting, fasciculation) *and* UMN signs in the same myotome. The best place to look for fasciculation is the tongue at rest in the mouth. *Sensory abnormalities are absent*, unlike MS. Note that MND is a heterogeneous group, some have the classic mix of UMN and LMN, less common variants are purely LMN or purely UMN. Nerve conduction studies (NCS) are normal, but electromyography (EMG) shows a denervation pattern. Imaging may be necessary to rule out differentials.

LMN Weakness

LMN weakness arises from a disorder in the anterior horn cells, nerve root, plexus, peripheral nerve, NMJ or muscle. For clarity of understanding, it is helpful to think of a prototypical disorder for each component of the neuroaxis, and only then consider the exceptions (Table 25.2). An approach is given (Figure 25.5).

Table 25.2. Prototypical Generalisations of the LMN Disorders

Prototypical disorder	Anterior horn cell	Peripheral nerve	Specific nerve, root or plexus	Neuromuscular junction	Muscle
	Spinal muscular atrophy	Diabetic neuropathy	Intervertebral disk prolapse	Myasthenia gravis	Dermatomyositis
Sensation	**Normal**	Impaired	Impaired	**Normal**	**Normal**
Distribution of weakness	Symmetrical proximal	Symmetrical distal	Patchy	Symmetrical proximal	Symmetrical proximal
Reflexes	Diminished	Diminished	Diminished	Normal	Usually normal
Additional characteristics	**Fasciculations** Eye muscles usually spared			**Fatigability**	
Exceptions to the rules	Weakness may be distal and asymmetrical. Reflexes may be brisk in motor neuron diseases	Pure motor neuropathies have normal sensation			There are distal myopathies. Reflexes may be depressed in severe myopathy

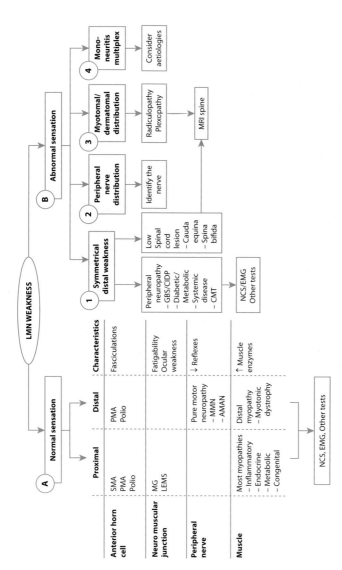

Figure 25.5. Approach to lower motor neuron (LMN) weakness.

AMAN, acute motor axonal neuropathy; CIDP, chronic inflammatory demyelinating polyneuropathy; CMT, Charcot–Marie–tooth; EMG, electromyography; GBS, Guillain–Barre syndrome; LEMS, Lambert–Eaton myasthenic syndrome; MG, myasthenia gravis; MMN, multifocal motor neuropathy; NCS, nerve conduction study; PMA, progressive muscular atrophy; SMA, spinal muscular atrophy.

A note on time course:

- The majority of LMN disorders have an onset in weeks to months.

- Acute LMN weakness (onset in days) suggests Guillain–Barre syndrome or acute nerve compression (e.g., disk prolapse and cauda equina syndrome). Myasthenia gravis (MG) may present with an acute exacerbation of chronic weakness.

- Insidious onset in childhood or early adulthood, very slow progression or with family history: suggestive of hereditary causes, for example, spinal muscular atrophy (SMA) and Charcot–Marie–Tooth.

(A) LMN Weakness + Normal Sensation

Normal sensation makes peripheral neuropathy less likely, with the exception of some pure motor neuropathies. These aetiologies have characteristic clinical features, although NCS and EMG are often required.

Neuromuscular Junction

	Workup
MG: Fluctuating muscle weakness, ptosis, ophthalmoplegia and/or bulbar weakness (dysphagia). *Fatigability* is the key characteristic—muscles are weaker after repetitive movements, ptosis is worse on prolonged upward gaze, and patients complain of increased weakness at the end of the day. Reflexes and sensation are normal. Respiratory failure is a feature of severe MG. This is an autoimmune disorder due to formation of antibodies against the postsynaptic acetylcholine receptor.	– Anti-acetylcholine receptor, anti-MUSK antibody – Repetitive nerve stimulation shows decremental response with repeated stimulation – CT thorax for thymoma
Lambert–Eaton myasthenic syndrome (LEMS): The clinical features are quite distinct from MG. Unlike MG, weakness improves with exercise, is more marked in the lower limbs and ophthalmoplegia is less common. There may be autonomic symptoms, for example, dry eyes or erectile dysfunction. This is a paraneoplastic disorder and up to 50% of cases are associated with small cell lung cancer.	– Anti-voltage gated calcium channel antibody – Repetitive nerve stimulation shows increased amplitude post exercise – Workup for cancer

Muscle

Characteristic features of muscle disease include elevated muscle enzymes (creatinine kinase and aldolase) and a myopathic pattern on EMG.

	Workup
Proximal weakness: The majority of myopathies exhibit proximal weakness.	
Inflammatory—Dermatomyositis and polymyositis: Characteristic skin findings in dermatomyositis include a heliotrope periorbital rash, Gottron's	– Autoantibodies, for example, ANA, anti-Jo-1 and others

papules, mechanics' hands and a photosensitive rash in a shawl-like distribution; such findings are absent in polymyositis. Myalgia may be a feature of both polymyositis and dermatomyositis.[2] These are paraneoplastic disorders.

- **Endocrine**: Proximal myopathy is a feature of Cushing's disease (including iatrogenic steroid myopathy), hypo- or hyperthyroidism. Look for other clinical features of these diseases.

  - Thyroid function
  - As suspected clinically

- **Metabolic**: Alcohol and statins.

- **Inherited**: The muscular dystrophies differ in genetics, severity and age of onset and distribution of weakness. These may be suspected based their onset in childhood or early adulthood and family history. There may be calf pseudohypertrophy.

  - Muscle biopsy
  - Genetic tests

Distal weakness: There are a number of genetic distal myopathies, the most common of which is myotonic dystrophy.

- **Myotonic dystrophy**: This is a trinucleotide repeat expansion disorder, which may present in infancy, childhood or the second to fourth decade. Its hallmark is *myotonia*, that is, slowed relaxation after muscle contraction. A gripped finger is released slowly (grip myotonia), and percussion of the thenar eminence results in thumb abduction with slow relaxation (percussion myotonia). Patients have LMN weakness (mostly distal, proximal in type 2 myotonic dystrophy), muscle pain, a characteristic *hangdog* appearance (due to facial muscle wasting) and frontal balding. Extra-neurological weakness include cardiomyopathy and arrhythmias, endocrine disease and cataracts.

  - May require muscle biopsy
  - Malignancy workup

  - EMG shows myotonia
  - Gene testing
  - Echocardiography

Anterior Horn Cell

The motor findings in these disorders are somewhat heterogeneous:

Workup

- **SMA**: A genetic disorder resulting in the degeneration of anterior horn cells. While most types of SMA have an onset in infancy, there are some late-onset types. Fasciculation, prominent wasting and bulbar weakness is characteristic.

  - Muscle biopsy
  - Genetic test

---

[2] Inclusion body myositis, another inflammatory myopathy, is quite distinct from polymyositis and dermatomyositis. It presents with an insidious onset of asymmetric (vs. symmetric), proximal and distal (vs. proximal) muscle weakness especially affecting finger flexors and quadriceps. Dysphagia may develop but myalgia is minimal. On examination there is atrophy and hyporeflexia. CK is < 10× normal and can be normal.

- **MND**: Some variants (e.g., progressive muscular atrophy) exhibit only progressive LMN signs without UMN dysfunction.

- **Post-polio**: Polio destroys the anterior horn cells (can be proximal or distal), leading to wasting and LMN weakness. This is usually an old childhood infection; wild-type polio has been eradicated in most countries.

    − NCS: normal conduction
    − EMG: neuropathic pattern

Peripheral Nerve

The majority of peripheral nerve disorders present with abnormal sensation. Exceptions that do have normal sensation are:

Workup

- **Multifocal motor neuropathy (MMN)**: Subacute-onset asymmetric patchy upper limb LMN weakness (wasting, fasciculation, normal or depressed reflexes) and *sensory sparing*. This mimics MND.

    − NCS: demyelination with conduction block
    − Anti-GM1 antibodies may be positive

- **Guillain–Barre syndrome variant** (acute motor axonal neuropathy): See Guillain–Barre syndrome below.

    − NCS: axonal neuropathy pattern

- **Charcot–Marie–Tooth**: Sensory examination may be spuriously normal (page 255).

(B) LMN Weakness + Abnormal Sensation

These are disorders of peripheral nerves, roots or plexus. The distribution of weakness is diagnostically important:

1. Symmetrical distal LMN weakness.
2. Weakness/numbness in the supply of a peripheral nerve.
3. Weakness/numbness in a dermatomal/myotomal distribution.
4. Mononeuritis multiplex: Pattern of deficit implies that more than one peripheral nerve is involved.

1. Symmetrical Distal LMN Weakness

Peripheral neuropathy: Symmetrical distal LMN weakness with sensory loss in a 'gloves and stocking' distribution. Sensory changes may be more pronounced than motor weakness. Of these, only Guillain–Barre syndrome presents acutely; the other entities are chronic.

Workup

- **Guillain–Barre syndrome (GBS)**: Symmetrical ascending LMN weakness, areflexia and sensory

    − NCS: demyelinating or axonal pattern

impairment, progressing over a period of 1–2 weeks. There may be a preceding infection (e.g., diarrhoeal illness). The degree of weakness varies from mild, to inability to walk, to respiratory failure requiring intubation; patients must be monitored for signs of respiratory insufficiency (measure forced vital capacity or negative inspiratory force daily). GBS variants include the Miller-Fisher syndrome (MFS), which presents as a triad of ophthalmoplegia, ataxia and areflexia.

- EMG: neuropathic pattern
- CSF: elevated protein with normal white cell (albumino-cytologic dissociation)
- Anti-GQ1b antibody in MFS

- **Chronic inflammatory demyelinating polyneuropathy (CIDP)**: Its features are similar to GBS, but unlike the monophasic course of GBS, CIDP has a slowly progressive or relapsing–remitting course > 8 weeks.

  - NCS: demyelinating
  - CSF: as in GBS

- **Metabolic neuropathies**: Diabetic peripheral neuropathy, B12 deficiency, alcohol, chemotherapy or heavy metal exposure.

  - Fasting glucose/ HbA1c
  - B12

- **Systemic disease**: Chronic HIV infection, hypothyroidism or amyloidosis.

  - HIV screen
  - Thyroid panel

- **Hereditary**: Charcot–Marie–Tooth disease (hereditary motor and sensory neuropathy) presents as a slowly progressive peripheral neuropathy with onset in childhood. There may be pes cavus, bilateral foot drop and wasting of the anterior compartment of the thigh.

Low spinal cord lesion: This should be considered in bilateral lower limb weakness and numbness, with sparing of the upper limbs

- **Cauda equina syndrome** As the spinal cord ends at L2, occlusion of the spinal canal below L2, with compression of exiting nerve roots, results in bilateral lower limb LMN weakness. This presents acutely with back and radicular pain, bilateral lower limb weakness and numbness and bladder dysfunction.

  - MRI spine

  Aetiologies include acute central disk prolapse, compression by metastatic tumour and epidural abscess (see Chapter 51).

- **Spina bifida**: This is a congenital neural tube defect. Examination of the patient's back may find a dimple or tuft of hair.

  - MRI spine

2. Peripheral Nerve Distribution

Identify the peripheral nerve involved by recognising that the pattern of motor and sensory deficit. For example, LMN hand weakness may be due to medial, ulnar and radial nerve pathology (Table 25.3).

Table 25.3. Manifestations of Peripheral Nerve Lesions in the Hand

Lesion	Median nerve	Ulnar nerve	Radial nerve
Weakness	Weak thumb abduction Benediction sign (weak finger flexors)[a] Thenar wasting	Clawed hand Froment sign (weak thumb adduction) Hypothenar wasting	Finger drop Wrist drop[a]
Numbness	Radial 3.5 fingers Thenar eminence[a]	Medial 1.5 fingers Hypothenar eminence[a]	Over first dorsal webspace
Aetiologies	Carpel tunnel syndrome Cubital fossa syndrome	Wrist trauma Cubital valgus	Humeral fracture

[a] Only present in a high lesion (above the wrist).

Distinguish from nerve root: Careful distinction has to be made between a peripheral nerve vs. a nerve root lesion. For example, unilateral isolated LMN foot drop (weak ankle dorsiflexion) can be due to a common peroneal nerve or L5 root lesion. To distinguish them:[3]

- Find a muscle supplied by the L5 root but not by the common peroneal nerve. Hip abduction and ankle inversion fit the bill. These actions are intact in common peroneal nerve lesions, but weak in L5 lesions.

- Consider the pattern of sensory loss: Sensory loss tends to be more extensive in a common peroneal nerve lesion, affecting the lateral shin and whole of the forefoot (this is less reliable than the motor findings).

3. Myotomal/Dermatomal Distribution

This localises to root or plexus. Aetiologies include:

- **Nerve root compression** by a prolapsed intervertebral disk (acute onset with pain), tumour, epidural abscess and so forth (also see Chapter 51).

- **Diabetic amyotrophy**: An microvasculitis affecting the nerve roots, typically in recently diagnosed or well-controlled diabetes. There is an asymmetric focal onset of pain followed by weakness and weight loss. This can involve multiple nerve roots.

- **Neuralgic amyotrophy** (Parsonage–Turner syndrome): Subacute onset of severe pain and patchy weakness in (usually) C5–C6, unilateral or bilateral, ± sensory symptoms and muscle atrophy.

- **Trauma**: For example, root avulsion from traffic accident.

- After radiation therapy.

---

[3] This applies only to LMN foot drop with no other weak muscles and a corresponding pattern of sensory loss. If there is weakness of other muscles, consider a lesion in the lumbosacral plexus, sciatic nerve (loss of ankle jerk, weak leg muscles with sparing of quadriceps and adductors), and polyneuropathies (diabetes, Charcot–Marie–tooth, etc.). If sensation is normal, consider motor neuron disease, myopathy and Charcot–Marie–Tooth. If there are UMN signs, consider spinal cord or cortical disease.

Workup: This usually involves an MRI of the spine (to evaluate for local compressive causes). NCS and EMG may show characteristic findings in diabetic or neuralgic amyotrophy.

4. Mononeuritis Multiplex

Mononeuritis multiple is the involvement of two or more peripheral nerves in separate parts of the body. Aetiologies include:

- Diabetes mellitus.
- Vasculitis: ANCA vasculitis (e.g., granulomatosis with polyangiitis of Wegener, eosinophilic granulomatosis with polyangiitis of Churg Strauss), polyarteritis nodosa, lupus.
- Infective: For example, HIV and leprosy.
- Infiltrative disease: For example, amyloidosis and sarcoidosis.

 Using what you have learnt, **pen down your approach** to the Clinical Case at the start of the chapter **BEFORE reading the discussion** below.

Case Discussion

Where is the lesion? Recognise the key features of this presentation. Firstly, weakness follows an LMN pattern with areflexia and down-going plantars; this makes brain, brainstem or spine disease (except cauda equina) unlikely. Secondly, sensation is impaired—among the LMN causes of weakness, only peripheral nerve, root and plexus lesions affect sensation. Thirdly, the distribution of weakness is symmetrical and distal (tripping over herself also suggests foot drop). Put together, this localises to either a peripheral nerve or low spinal cord lesion.

What is the lesion? Among the causes of peripheral neuropathy, only Guillain–Barre syndrome (GBS) develops in a week; the other aetiologies (e.g., diabetic neuropathy and metabolic causes) are more chronic. Spinal cord disease is a differential. Cauda equina syndrome should be considered particularly if there is back pain or sphincter dysfunction (UMN features are not expected as this occurs below the termination of the spinal cord at L2); do a rectal examination looking for anal tone. Transverse myelitis (e.g., multiple sclerosis) may mimic the time course and LMN findings of GBS, with UMN signs only developing later. Myasthenia gravis presents with a similar time course, but its weakness is fatigable, and sensation and reflexes are normal.

There are various subtypes of GBS, including a demyelinating and an axonal form, as well as a cranial-nerve dominant variant (Miller-Fisher syndrome). Nerve conduction studies and electromyography may reveal useful information of demyelination or axonal conduction defects. Lumbar puncture characteristically shows elevated protein with normal cell count.

Hypoventilation is common in GBS. Check a blood gas for carbon dioxide retention, and monitor forced vital capacity and/or negative inspiratory force. Patients with respiratory failure will require intubation and mechanical ventilation.

Key Lessons	1. Upper motor neuron weakness may be due to lesions in the brain, brainstem or spinal cord. The distribution of weakness (hemiparesis, paraparesis or bizarre), the side of any cranial nerve palsy (ipsilateral or crossed hemiparesis) and the presence of other cortical or brainstem signs help to localise the lesion.
	2. Lower motor neuron weakness may be due to anterior horn cell, root, plexus, peripheral nerve, neuromuscular junction or muscle disease. Important differentiators include the presence or absence of sensory impairment, the distribution of weakness (proximal vs. distal and symmetrical vs. patchy), normal or diminished reflexes and fatigability.
	3. The time course of weakness is helpful in determining its aetiology. Hyperacute presentation suggests a vascular aetiology.
Common Pitfalls	1. Acute stroke is a clinical diagnosis, and CT brain may be normal. Performing CT brain 'to exclude acute stroke' is incorrect.
	2. There is a hierarchy of clinical findings; some are more reliable than others. 'Hard' (i.e., reliable) signs include tone, reflexes, plantars, fasciculation and fatigability. The power examination, and distribution of weakness, is intermediate. Sensation is a soft sign; the pattern of sensory loss can be used to support but not negate hard signs.
Questions	1. **REFLECT!** Cervical myelopathy can resemble a number of other lesions. Have you ever seen a patient with cervical myelopathy? How did he/she present?
	2. **DISCUSS!** Building on the algorithm presented in this chapter, write down how you would approach a patient who presents with foot drop. Discuss in small groups and refine what you have written.
	3. **EXPLORE!** Strokes present in many different ways, depending on the affected part of the brain or brainstem. Read up on the clinical manifestations of the following stroke types—(a) Total or partial anterior circulation infarct, (b) posterior circulation infarct and (c) lacunar infarct.
	4. **GO FURTHER!** Rarely, lesions along the neuroaxis may present as purely sensory loss, with motor weakness either absent or very mild. These include mononeuropathies (e.g., mild Carpal tunnel syndrome), polyneuropathies (e.g., diabetes), spinal cord lesions (syringomyelia), brainstem lesions (classically lateral medullary syndrome) and rarely brain (e.g., isolated sensory cortex lesion). How do these lesions differ in the distribution of sensory loss, and how can they be distinguished?

Chapter

26

An Approach to Cranial Nerve Palsy

Clinical Case

A 45-year-old lady presents with a 1-month history of double vision, which has been getting worse in the last week. Closing one eye makes the double vision go away. Examination reveals partial right-sided ptosis, and impairment of extra ocular eye movements in all directions. Both pupils are equal and reactive to light. Apart from an inability to bury her eyelashes, all other cranial nerves are normal. There is no limb weakness or numbness, and no cerebellar signs. What is the most appropriate next step?

Cranial nerve (CN) palsies present with difficulty seeing (which may mean loss of vision, diplopia or ptosis), difficulty speaking, difficulty hearing or facial droop. A lesion anywhere along the neuroaxis—that is, brain, brainstem, anterior horn cell, peripheral nerve, neuromuscular junction or muscle—may lead to CN palsy. The approach begins with determining whether single or multiple CNs are affected (Figure 26.1).

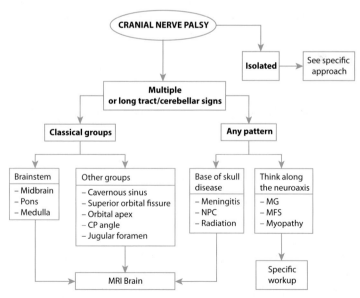

CP angle, cerebellopontine angle; MFS, Miller-Fisher syndrome; MG, myasthenia gravis; NPC, nasopharyngeal carcinoma.

Figure 26.1. General approach to cranial nerve palsy.

This chapter presents the approach to multiple CN palsies, and approaches to diplopia and ptosis (CN III, IV, VI), and facial droop (CN VII). Other chapters discuss an approach to visual loss (see Chapter 27) and hearing loss (see Chapter 28). Isolated CN I, V, XI and XII lesions are rare. Familiarity with how to examine the CNs is assumed.

Multiple CN Palsy

This is more likely a single lesion involving multiple CN, than multiple separate lesions. Attempt to find the most parsimonious localisation that would explain multiple CN involvement.

Classical Groups

Brainstem clubs: The brainstem is a small place with many important structures; lesions tend not to affect CN nuclei alone, but also the other structures coursing through the brainstem. Clues to brainstem disease include long tract signs, cerebellar dysfunction and drowsiness (involvement of the ascending reticular activating system).

- **Midbrain lesion**: CN III and IV palsy, vertical gaze palsies, crossed hemiparesis (e.g., *left* CN III palsy with *right* limb upper motor neuron weakness; see page 241) and cerebellar signs.
- **Pontine lesion**: CN V–VIII palsy, horizontal gaze palsies (e.g., inter-nuclear ophthalmoplegia [INO], page 263), crossed hemiparesis and cerebellar signs.
- **Medullary lesion**: Differences between a medial and lateral lesion arise because some nuclei/tracts are medial, and others are lateral.
  - Lateral medullary lesion: CN IX–X palsy, crossed pain and temperature loss (ipsilateral facial and contralateral body), ipsilateral Horner's syndrome, vertigo and ipsilateral cerebellar signs. *There is no limb weakness.* This is relatively common, due to an infarct of the posterior inferior cerebellar artery.
  - Medial medullary lesion: CN XII palsy (tongue deviation to ipsilateral side), crossed hemiparesis and contralateral loss of vibration and proprioception sense (dorsal columns involved, spinothalamic tracts spared).

Other anatomic localisations:

- **Cavernous sinus**: CN III, IV, VI, V_1 and V_2 ± sympathetic fibres to face. Aetiologies include a large pituitary adenoma.
- **Superior orbital fissure**: CN III, IV, VI ± V_1.
- **Orbital apex**: CN II, III, IV, VI and V_1 ± proptosis.
- **Cerebello-pontine angle**: CN VIII (hearing loss, tinnitus, vertigo), CN VII and V. This is most commonly due to an acoustic neuroma. A large lesion may also encroach on the cerebellum leading to ipsilateral cerebellar signs.
- **Jugular foramen**: CN IX, X, XI ± XII.

Workup: These groups suggest a lesion in a specific anatomical location, and an MRI of the brain (or the specific part of the brain) is generally the next step.

Any Pattern of CN Palsy

These aetiologies can cause any pattern of CN involvement, including isolated CN palsies, and the anatomic groups defined earlier. However, suspicion of these disorders is highest if there are multiple CN palsies that do not conform to the classical groups.

Subacute (days to weeks):

Workup

- **Miller-Fisher syndrome** (a Guillain–Barre syndrome variant): The classic triad is ophthalmoplegia, ataxia and areflexia. Bulbar weakness and respiratory compromise may be severe, requiring respiratory support. The degree of limb weakness and sensory impairment is variable. Interestingly, Miller-Fisher is the only common peripheral neuropathy with prominent involvement of the CNs.
  - Anti-GQ1b antibody
  - Nerve conduction study
  - Consider blood gases and respiratory support

- **Basal meningitis**: For example, due to tuberculosis. Look for any chronic headache, fever, altered mental state or meningism.
  - MRI brain for base of skull enhancement
  - Lumbar puncture

- **Flare of myasthenia gravis** (see the following).

Chronic:

- **Myasthenia gravis**: Fatigability and fluctuating weakness is characteristic. Reflexes and sensation are normal (also see page 252). Again, bulbar weakness and respiratory compromise may be severe.
  - Anti acetylcholinesterase receptor, anti-MUSK antibody
  - Repetitive nerve stimulation
  - CT thorax for thymoma

- **Base of skull disease**: For example, nasopharyngeal carcinoma, other malignancies or previous cranial radiation. These may pick off CNs in a seemingly random fashion.
  - MRI brain

- **Myopathies**: Some myopathies involve the CNs. Look for limb involvement (pages 252–253).

- **Mononeuritis multiplex**: See page 257.

Isolated Diplopia

Diplopia may be due to a lesion in the brainstem nuclei, CNs, neuromuscular junction and orbit (Figure 26.2).

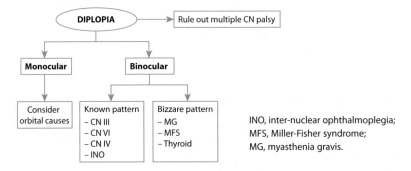

Figure 26.2. Approach to diplopia.

1. Monocular vs. Binocular Diplopia

The first step is to ask the patient if diplopia is present when one eye is closed.

- **Monocular diplopia**: Diplopia present when only one eye is open is suggestive of eye pathology—for example, refractive error, cornea opacity, cataracts, lens dislocation, retinal abnormalities and so forth.

- **Binocular diplopia**: Diplopia present when both eyes are open, absent when one eye is closed, is due to ocular misalignment. Conjugate gaze requires that the extra-ocular muscles of both eyes move in tandem; any lesion of these nerves, neuromuscular junction or muscles will result in binocular diplopia.

2. What Is the Pattern of EOM Palsy

In binocular diplopia, the next step is to characterise the pattern of extra-ocular eye movement (EOM) palsy, and consider if this fits into any known CN pattern.

Known patterns:	Aetiologies and Workup
- **CN III palsy**: Complete CN III palsy causes a 'down and out' (depressed and abducted) eye, ptosis and impairment of all EOM except abduction (CN VI) and depression (CN IV). Partial CN III palsy may present with ptosis, pupillary dilation and various combinations of EOM palsy (sparing abduction and depression).	- See pages 263–264
- **CN VI palsy**: Horizontal diplopia worst on ipsilateral gaze, and impaired abduction.	- Trauma - Microvascular ischaemia

- **CN IV palsy**: Vertical diplopia. There is ipsilateral hyperopia, worse on contralateral gaze (as CN IV is responsible for depression in the adducted position), and on head tilt to the ipsilateral side (as CN IV is unable to intort to keep the eye level). At rest, patients adopt a position that minimises diplopia—head tilt to the contralateral side and chin-down posture.

- **Internuclear opthalmoplegia (INO)**: Adduction failure and nystagmus in the abducting (contra-lateral) eye. This is due to a lesion in the ipsilateral midbrain, more specifically the medial longitudinal fasciculus (MLF).

- **One and a half syndrome**: The combination of a complete horizontal gaze palsy in one eye (which can neither abduct nor adduct—the 'one'), and an INO in the other eye (the 'half'). This is due to a large lesion affecting the parapontine reticular formation (PPRF) and MLF on the side of the 'one'.

Bizarre patterns:

- **Myasthenia gravis**: Any pattern of EOM palsy; all directions may be affected, and the pattern of EOM palsy is variable. Look for fatigability.

- **Miller-Fisher syndrome** (a Guillain–Barre syndrome variant): Again, any pattern of EOM palsy, classically with ataxia and areflexia and a variable degree of limb weakness or numbness.

- **Thyroid ophthalmopathy**: EOM restriction due to infiltration, rather than EOM muscle weakness. There may be proptosis and other thyroid eye signs (see Chapter 36).

- Intracranial mass lesions (false localising VI): do MRI brain
- Minor head trauma
- Idiopathic
- Congenital
- Microvascular ischaemia

- MRI brain for brainstem lesion

- MRI brain for brainstem lesion

- See workup on page 261

- See workup on page 261

- Thyroid function tests

Approach to Isolated CN III Palsy

Additional notes on isolated CN III palsy are in order (Figure 26.3).

- The most feared cause of CN III palsy is compression by an enlarging intracranial aneurysm, most commonly of the posterior communicating artery. As the parasympathetic fibres responsible for pupillary constriction are on the outside of CN III, while the motor fibres are in the inside, external compression of the nerve can cause a dilated pupil ('surgical CN III'). Therefore, any CN III palsy with a dilated pupil is concerning for an intracranial aneurysm, and MRI/MRA should be performed.

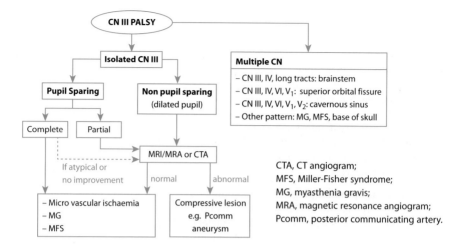

Figure 26.3. Approach to CN III palsy.

- Microvascular ischaemia ('medical CN III') is the most common cause of CN III palsy, and usually presents acutely and improves over weeks. If the pupils are spared in spite of complete CN III palsy (i.e., totally unable to open eyes), an aneurysm is very unlikely and MRI can be omitted.[1] MRI is still indicated in an incomplete CN III palsy, if there are atypical features, or if the patient fails to improve with time. Microvascular ischaemia is usually blamed on one or more vascular risk factors like diabetes, hyperlipidaemia, hypertension, and smoking. Work up for these conditions.

- Aetiologies like myasthenia gravis and Miller-Fisher syndrome remain in the differential diagnosis and can cause isolated CN III palsy.

Isolated Ptosis

The eyelids are kept open by the levator palpebrae superioris, a skeletal muscle supplied by CN III, as well as by smooth muscles supplied by sympathetic fibres. Therefore, lesions affecting the sympathetic chain, and lesions affecting the supply of CN III (midbrain–course of CN III–neuromuscular junction–muscle) may cause ptosis. Patients with ptosis often attempt to compensate, leading to frontalis overactivity.

Important differentiating features in the approach to ptosis include:

- **Unilateral vs. bilateral**: Horner's syndrome and CN III palsy are unilateral (except nuclear CN III palsy, page 265).

- **The presence of ophthalmoplegia**, which would be consistent with CN III palsy or MG.

---

[1] There is some debate on this; some clinicians opt to image all CN III palsies, even if complete and pupil-sparing.

- **Pupil size**: Miosis is typical of Horner's syndrome; dilated pupils suggest CN III palsy.
- **Fatigability**: Suggests myasthenia gravis.
- **Other CN palsy**: This may be subtle, for example, inability to bury eyelashes suggesting a mild CN VII palsy. Local causes, Horner's syndrome, and isolated CN III palsies should not cause other CN to be involved.

First consider whether ptosis is unilateral or bilateral. Then look for other features that might suggest a specific aetiology of ptosis (Figure 26.4). These are discussed in turn.

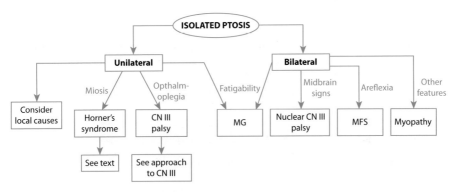

MFS, Miller-Fisher syndrome; MG, myasthenia gravis.

Figure 26.4. Approach to ptosis.

Horner's Syndrome

Horner's syndrome is the triad of ptosis, miosis and anhidrosis, due to disruption of sympathetic innervation to the head and neck. The lesion may be located anywhere along the course of sympathetic supply (brainstem–T1/2 nerve root–lung apex–common and internal carotid artery–cavernous sinus).

	Major aetiologies and Workup
• **Brainstem**: Most commonly the lateral medullary syndrome from posterior inferior cerebellar artery occlusion; other features include vertigo, crossed sensory loss and cerebellar signs.	– MRI brain
• **Spinal cord disease**: For example, syringomyelia, cervical cord trauma (see Chapter 25) may lead to Horner's syndrome, in addition to other long tract signs.	– See pages 247–248
• **Lung apex**: Classically a 'Pancoast tumour' in the lung apex. There may be constitutional symptoms of malignancy, weak and wasted hands (T1 nerve root involvement) and cervical lymphadenopathy.	– Chest X-ray or CT thorax

- **Ascending sympathetic fibres**: For example, carotid arterial dissection (neck pain and Horner's
syndrome), cavernous sinus lesions.

– CT angiogram of neck
for carotid dissection

CN III Lesions

There are two distinct types of CN III lesions:

- **CN III palsy (fascicular)**: The 'usual' CN III palsy with ptosis, impaired extra-
ocular movements (sparing abduction and depression), causing a 'down and out' eye,
± pupillary dilation (page 263).

- **Nuclear CN III palsy**: In addition to the other signs of CN III palsy (as above), a
lesion of the CN III nucleus in the midbrain results in bilateral partial ptosis (the
levator palpebrae superioris is controlled by a single central subnucleus) and bilateral superior rectus weakness (each superior rectus subnucleus supplies bilateral
superior recti muscles). There may also be other long tract signs.

Other Causes of Ptosis

- **Myasthenia gravis**: Unilateral or bilateral ptosis, any pattern of EOM palsy, but
with characteristic fatigability (page 261).

- **Miller-Fisher syndrome** (Guillain–Barre syndrome variant): Bilateral ptosis, any
pattern of EOM palsy, areflexia and ataxia (page 261).

- **Myopathies**: Some myopathies cause ptosis; these include myotonic dystrophy,
mitochondrial myopathy, for example, chronic progressive external ophthalmoplegia, and others. There may be other limb features (see Chapter 25).

- **Local causes**: Consider after ruling out neurological causes.
  - **Senile (aponeurotic) ptosis**: Due to dehiscence of the levator aponeurosis,
    usually in elderly patients, but also from contact lens trauma in younger patients.
  - **Congenital ptosis**: Non-progressive ptosis since birth.

Isolated Facial Droop

UMN CN VII Palsy

This affects the contralateral lower face with sparing of the frontalis and orbicularis
occuli. There would be limb weakness on the same side as the CN VII palsy (see
pages 241–243).

LMN CN VII Palsy

This affects the entire ipsilateral face. Think along the course of the VII nerve
(pons–cerebello-pontine angle–petrous part of temporal bone [internal acoustic
meatus]–parotid), as well as neuromuscular junction and muscle.

Isolated unilateral facial droop:

- **Bells' palsy**: The commonest cause of LMN CN VII palsy, this presents with a sub-acute onset of unilateral complete facial droop. It is an idiopathic, usually self-limiting disorder. Imaging is not required for diagnosis unless features are atypical or the patient fails to improve (but be sure to exclude any other CN or long tract involvement).

- **Ramsay Hunt syndrome**: Herpes zoster affecting CN VII and causing ipsilateral conductive hearing loss. Otoscopy may find vesicles.

- **Mastoid disorders**: For example, mastoiditis and mastoid fractures.

- **Parotid disorders**: For example, parotid tumour, facial nerve injury as a complication of parotid surgery. Look for a parotid mass or previous scars.

Bilateral facial droop (facial diplegia):

- Myasthenia gravis (page 261).

- Myotonic dystrophy (the classic 'hangdog appearance').

- Miller-Fisher syndrome.

- Other causes: Mononeuritis multiplex, sarcoidosis and so forth.

Complex facial droop: Facial droop with other CN or long tract signs:

- **Pons**: LMN CN VII palsy with crossed hemiparesis (see Chapter 25).

- **Cerebellopontine angle lesions**: LMN CN VII palsy with CN VIII palsy.

 Using what you have learnt, **pen down your approach** to the Clinical Case at the start of the chapter **BEFORE reading the discussion** below.

Case Discussion

Binocular diplopia with ptosis resembles a CN III lesion. Before a conclusion of isolated CN III palsy can be made, other diagnoses including brainstem disease, a base of skull (meningeal) process, neuromuscular junction and peripheral nerve aetiologies have to be considered. This involves an examination of the limbs for long tract signs (brainstem disease), areflexia (Miller-Fisher syndrome) and looking for drowsiness, neck stiffness or cervical lymph nodes (nasopharyngeal carcinoma), which could suggest a base of skull disease. Careful examination to rule out multiple cranial nerve involvement should be performed.

This lady has a number of features that would be inconsistent with an isolated CN III palsy. This includes impaired extraocular eye movements in all directions, and inability to bury the eyelashes (suggesting CN VII palsy). Furthermore, CN III palsy due to microvascular ischaemia tends to present acutely; her diplopia developed over 1 month. The next step is to examine for fatigability, the hallmark of myasthenia gravis, which is the most likely diagnosis. Miller-Fisher syndrome is a differential, in which case the limbs may show features of peripheral neuropathy. Further workup for myasthenia includes anti-acetylcholine receptor and anti-MUSK antibodies, repetitive nerve stimulation testing and CT thorax for thymoma.

Key Lessons	1. Cranial nerve palsies may occur in defined 'groups' with specific anatomical localisations. Base of skull disease, myasthenia gravis and Miller-Fisher syndrome may result in any pattern of CN palsy.
	2. Diplopia may be monocular (local orbit causes) or binocular. In binocular diplopia, rule out multiple CN palsy, and observe if the EOM palsy fits into a CN III, VI, IV, or INO pattern. A dilated pupil in CN III palsy is concerning for extrinsic compression by an intracranial aneurysm. Myasthenia gravis, Miller-Fisher syndrome, and thyroid eye disease can cause any pattern of EOM palsy.
	3. Common causes of isolated ptosis include CN III palsy, Horner's syndrome, and myasthenia gravis. Important differentiating features include the presence of ophthalmoplegia, pupil size, and fatiguability.
Common Pitfalls	1. Failure to consider brainstem, base of skull, neuromuscular junction and peripheral nerve diseases in the differential diagnosis for any cranial nerve palsy.
	2. The lateral medullary syndrome is easy to miss as there is no motor weakness.
Questions	1. **REFLECT!** Myasthenia gravis may present in a number of ways. Have you seen a patient with myasthenia gravis? How did the patient describe his/her symptoms, and how was the diagnosis made?
	2. **DISCUSS!** 'The best way to examine the cranial nerves is to examine in order from CN II to CN XII'. Do you agree?
	3. **EXPLORE!** Draw out the brainstem circuitry responsible for controlling conjugate gaze movements. Can you make sense of (a) inter-nuclear ophthalmoplegia, (b) one and a half syndrome, (c) nystagmus in vestibular disorders, (d) gaze deviation in frontal lobe stroke?

An Approach to Red Eye and Loss of Vision

Clinical Case

A middle-aged marketing executive presents with a 2-day history of redness and a 'sticky' discharge in her right eye. She was reluctant to see a doctor but finally presented because the eye was getting increasingly uncomfortable. As she walks into the clinic, you notice that she tries to keep her right eye closed. What are the key differentials, and what would you look for on examination?

Ocular pathology may present with red eyes, visual loss or both. Some of these conditions rapidly lead to permanent visual loss if unaddressed, others appear alarming but are actually relatively harmless, and yet others are insidious thieves of sight that do not announce themselves until late. The initial approach must aim to identify which patients require emergent specialist intervention, and which can be managed in primary care.

Red Eye

1. Identify Red Flags and Dangerous Causes

Begin by evaluating the patient's symptoms, assessing visual acuity and directly inspection the eye with a pen-torch (fundoscopy adds little in this setting). Look for these **red flags**:

- Any pain in excess of mild discomfort. This may be eye pain, painful eye movements, headache (referred pain) or a generally unwell patient.

- Any complaint or objective evidence of visual loss.

- Severe photophobia, i.e. patient cannot keep eye open—this suggests a corneal process. Slight grittiness in the eye is acceptable.

- Risk factors: History of ocular trauma, recent ophthalmologic procedure or immunocompromise.

- Worrisome examination findings: Hypopyon, hyphaema, corneal opacity or haziness, ciliary flush (a violaceous ring around the cornea), chemosis.

Identify the **dangerous causes** of red eye (Table 27.1).

Table 27.1. Dangerous Causes of Red Eye

Aetiology	Symptoms and history	Initial examination	Further investigation
Acute angle-closure glaucoma	Headache or eye pain Nausea/vomiting Patient generally unwell	Fixed mid-dilated pupil Ciliary flush Corneal haziness	Measure intra-ocular pressure Slit lamp: shallow anterior chamber Consider differentials of headache
Endophthalmitis	Recent ophthalmologic procedure or bacteraemia Eye pain, visual loss	Hypopyon: A layer of pus forming a meniscus in the anterior chamber Hazy cornea	Slit lamp: cells and flare Culture of aqueous media or vitrectomy
Trauma or spontaneous hyphaema	Photophobia, visual loss History of eye trauma	Hyphaema: A layer of blood forming a meniscus in the anterior chamber	Specialist examination for other eye injury
Bacterial keratitis	Inability to keep eye open History of improper contact lens use	Corneal opacity Thick mucopurulent discharge	Corneal scraping for gram stain and culture
Herpetic keratitis	Eye pain	May have a faint opacity Watery discharge	Fluorescein staining: branched dendritic ulcer
Anterior uveitis (iritis)	Photophobia History of autoimmune disease— spondyloarthropathy, immunodeficiency (CMV retinitis), etc.	Ciliary flush Unreactive, irregular pupil	Slit lamp: cells and flare Workup for aetiology if not apparent
Scleritis	Severe eye pain History of autoimmune disease, e.g., rheumatoid arthritis	Diffuse redness and vascular engorgement May have a nodular elevation of the sclera	Slit lamp: dilated deep episcleral vascular plexus Workup for aetiology
Orbital cellulitis	Diplopia, painful eye movements Visual loss Fever, toxicity History of sinusitis	Swollen, erythematous eyelids Chemosis, proptosis, limitation of ocular motility May have signs of optic neuropathy	Septic workup CT orbits (urgent)

CMV, cytomegalovirus.

2. Non-Serious Aetiologies

In the absence of any red flag or suggestion of dangerous pathology, consider the following aetiologies, which can generally be managed in a primary care setting.

Bilateral red eyes:

- **Infective conjunctivitis**: An acute history of bilateral red eyes with only mild discomfort, in an otherwise well patient with full visual acuity. There may be a discharge—purulent in bacterial conjunctivitis, watery in viral conjunctivitis and the eye may be 'stuck shut' with crusting in the morning. Very often one eye is affected first, before spreading to the other eye. There may be a positive contact history—it is quite contagious.

- **Allergic conjunctivitis**: Pruritic, watering eyes, often associated with an atopic setup (rhinitis, asthma, eczema). Unlike infective conjunctivitis, there is usually minimal discharge, pruritus is more severe, and both eyes turn red at the same time.

- **Dry eyes** (keratoconjunctivitis sicca): Mild erythema and discomfort, worse on visual strain (e.g., reading). If this is severe, consider a secondary cause of dry eyes, for example, Sjogren's syndrome.

Unilateral red eyes:

- **Conjunctivitis**: Infective conjunctivitis can be unilateral.

- **Sub-conjunctival haemorrhage**: A well patient with the sudden appearance of well-demarcated haemorrhage on the eye, which may be spontaneous or associated with coughing, sneezing or straining (which increases intraocular pressure). There is no discharge. This appears frightening but is actually harmless.

- **Episcleritis**: Mild irritation and sectorial (or diffuse) vascular congestion. This is usually self-limiting.

- **Preseptal cellulitis**: An erythematous and swollen eyelid, usually reflecting ascending spread of infection from sinusitis. Distinguish from orbital cellulitis in which there are also red flags of chemosis, visual loss, ophthalmoplegia and toxicity.

Acute Visual Loss

Acute visual loss is almost always a serious pathology and should not be dismissed. Identify the clinical picture (Figure 27.1):

- **Persistent visual loss with red eye**: Think of serious anterior segment pathology, for example, acute closed-angle glaucoma (see Section 'Red Eye').

- **Persistent painful visual loss**: Consider anterior segment pathologies (see Section 'Red Eye'), as well as optic neuritis and arteritic ischaemic optic neuropathy.

- **Persistent painless visual loss**: Examine for a relative afferent pupillary defect (RAPD)—its presence suggests a significant optic nerve or large retinal pathology (note: cataracts and refractive error do not cause RAPD). Examine the posterior segment using direct fundoscopy, and refer for indirect ophthalmoscopy and slit lamp examination.

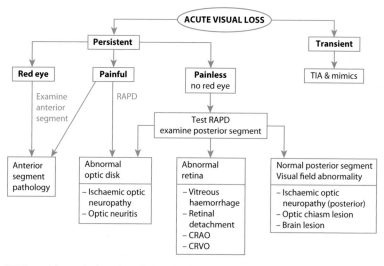

CRAO, complete retinal artery occlusion; CRVO, complete retinal vein occlusion; RAPD, relative afferent pupillary defect; TIA, transient ischaemic attack.

For anterior segment pathology, see approach to red eye in this chapter.

Figure 27.1. Approach to acute visual loss.

- **Transient visual loss (amaurosis fugax):** Consider transient ischaemic attack (TIA) and its mimics (page 244).

Persistent Painless Visual Loss: Abnormal Optic Disk

- **Ischaemic optic neuropathy (anterior):** Decreased colour vision, RAPD and an *inferior altitudinal field defect*. The optic disk is swollen if the anterior segment of the optic nerve is affected. Examine the other cranial nerves to rule out a superior orbital fissure or cavernous sinus syndrome (see Chapter 26). There are two types of ischaemic optic neuropathy:
  - Arteritic: Due to vasculitis, for example, giant cell arteritis (ask about headache, jaw claudication, scalp tenderness and do ESR).
  - Non-arteritic: Due to microvascular disease (e.g., diabetes, hypertension, etc.).
- **Optic neuritis:** Monocular visual loss with decreased colour vision, RAPD and optic disk swelling. There may be pain on eye movement. Aetiologies include auto-immune disease such as multiple sclerosis, as well as infective and post-infective causes—there may be other neurological symptoms or signs, which point to the underlying aetiology.

Persistent Painless Visual Loss: Abnormal Retina

The retinal causes of painless visual loss are directly identified on posterior segment examination via fundoscopy (Table 27.2).

Table 27.2. Retinal Causes of Painless Visual Loss

Aetiology	History	Initial examination	Workup
Vitreous haemorrhage	Sudden blurring of vision Floaters	Diminished red reflex Blood in the vitreous	Look for secondary causes—e.g., diabetic neovascularisation, trauma, retinal tear
Retinal detachment	Floaters Photopsia (flashes of light) May have partial visual field defect	Visible retinal tear and elevation May have RAPD or visual field loss	Look for secondary causes, e.g., diabetes
Retinal artery occlusion	Sudden profound visual loss	Pale fundus with cherry red spot at fovea RAPD Visual field loss in branch retinal artery occlusion	Consider temporal arteritis (evaluate symptoms, do ESR) Look for embolic source
Retinal vein occlusion	Subacute visual loss, may be mild to marked	'Blood and thunder' fundus: flame haemorrhages, cotton wool spots, dilated veins Swollen optic disk May have RAPD (in ischaemic causes)	Workup for pro-thrombotic diathesis, vasculitis and microvascular disease

RAPD, relative afferent pupillary defect; ESR, erythrocyte sedimentation rate.

Persistent Painless Visual Loss: Normal Posterior Segment

With a normal posterior segment examination, the likely pathology is in the posterior optic nerve or brain. The distribution of visual field loss is the key.

- **Bitemporal hemianopia:** An optic chiasm lesion, for example, pituitary adenoma.

- **Homonymous hemianopia:** A lesion in the contralateral optic tract, optic radiation or occipital lobe. A parietal lobe lesion tends to cause contralateral inferior quadrantanopia, while a temporal lobe lesion tends to cause contralateral superior quadrantanopia. Occipital lobe lesions affect both inferior and superior quadrants, and may have macular sparing.

- **Inferior altitudinal field defect:** Often ischaemic optic neuropathy (optic disk is normal if only the posterior segment is affected). See ischaemic optic neuropathy (page 272).

Workup: The hemianopias should be worked up with an MRI of the brain and/or pituitary fossa.

Transient Painless Visual Loss

Amaurosis fugax is a sudden presentation of transient painless visual loss. Some differentials in this scenario are:

- **Transient ischaemic attack (TIA)**: This is the main fear; as visual loss may indicate disruption of blood supply to the ophthalmic artery. The classic history is negative visual phenomena (a 'black curtain descending') lasting 5 to 10 min. Workup urgently as for any other TIA (page 244), and entertain a diagnosis of temporal arteritis.

- **Migraine with aura**: Visual loss may precede, occur with, or occur independently from headache. Distinction from a TIA can be tricky—some clues: (1) migraine aura can present with positive visual phenomena (e.g., white out of vision) instead of negative phenomena, (2) migraine aura usually lasts longer (e.g., 30 min) than TIA (not absolute, some TIAs can last quite long), (3) there may be a history of recurrent episodes, (4) patients usually have a lower cardiovascular risk profile—in a vasculopath with multiple comorbidities, be cautious about attributing an episode of visual loss to migraine aura.

- **Seizures with aura**: Blindness is rare; other auras are far more common.

- **Hypoglycaemia**: Bilateral visual loss with other sympathetic symptoms (tachycardia, palpitation, diaphoresis), relieved with a glucose snack/drink.

Chronic Visual Loss

A few diseases are responsible for the bulk of gradual-onset, painless progressive visual loss. They may be symmetrical or asymmetrical.

- **Refractive errors**: For example, presbyopia. Improvement of visual acuity with pinhole suggests refractive error amenable to optical correction.

- **Cataract**: Presents as general blurring of vision, increased glare and 'starbursts' around lights and increase in myopia (due to change in refractive index of the lens). Look for secondary causes of cataract (e.g., DM, steroids) and other pathology that would limit visual acuity should surgery be performed.

- **Glaucoma**: Unlike acute angle-closure glaucoma, chronic closed-angle or open-angle glaucoma causes insidiously progressive visual loss, loss of peripheral visual field ('tunnel vision') and halos around lights. Fundoscopy reveals increased cup-to-disk ratio (> 0.6), or even optic atrophy if severe. Measure intraocular pressure, which is invariably high (> 21 mmHg).

- **Age-related macular degeneration (AMD)**: Presents as poor central vision (loss or distortion). Fundoscopy shows macular drusen, atrophy, macular neovascularisation (dry AMD) or exudates and haemorrhage (wet AMD). Patients may also find the lines in Amsler grids wavy or irregular.

- **Diabetic retinopathy**: Fundoscopy reveals haemorrhages, exudates, macular oedema and neovascularisation. This is initially asymptomatic, but may progress to visual loss. Patients usually have a long history of poorly controlled diabetes. If visual loss is acute, or there is sudden worsening, consider vitreous haemorrhage or traction retinal detachment which are associated with diabetic retinopathy.

- **Corneal blindness**: For example, trachoma, keratitis causing corneal opacification visible on careful anterior segment inspection.

- **Drug toxicity**: For example, due to hydroxychloroquine, ethambutol.

Using what you have learnt, **pen down your approach** to the Clinical Case at the start of the chapter **BEFORE reading the discussion** below.

Case Discussion

The history is of a unilateral red eye with discharge. The most common cause is conjunctivitis, but unusually, there is a disproportionate degree of discomfort, and she seems to be unable to keep her eye open. These are red flags. The main differential is bacterial keratitis.

She should be carefully examined for corneal opacities, visual loss or hypopyon (rare). Ask if she wears contact lens, and if so, whether there is any history of improper use (e.g., re-using disposables, inadequate cleaning of hard lenses, etc.), which further heightens the suspicion of keratitis. She should be advised to discontinue contact lens wear immediately, and be referred for ophthalmological care; slit lamp examination with fluorescein staining will confirm the diagnosis.

Key Lessons	1. Initial evaluation of a red eye should focus on identification of red flags, which may suggest dangerous pathology such as acute closed-angle glaucoma, hypopyon, hyphaema, keratitis, iritis, scleritis or orbital cellulitis.
	2. In acute visual loss, consider the dangerous causes of red eye, examine for a relative afferent pupillary defect, and perform fundoscopy for retinal and optic disk abnormalities. If both retina and optic disk are normal, consider optic nerve or brain pathologies.
	3. Patients with transient visual loss (amaurosis fugax) should be urgently worked up for a transient ischaemic attack.
Common Pitfalls	1. Eye pain, severe photophobia, visual loss, corneal opacities or ciliary flush are not features of conjunctivitis. More dangerous aetiologies of red eye must be considered.
	2. Refer patients with amaurosis fugax urgently to neurology, not ophthalmology. Incorrect referral causes delays.
Questions	1. **EXPLORE!** Look up pictures of (a) the different causes of red eye, and (b) fundoscopic pictures of the various aetiologies of visual loss. Describe the findings, and learn to recognise these pathologies.
	2. **REFLECT!** Have you ever encountered a patient with red eyes, in whom the diagnosis was not conjunctivitis or subconjunctival haemorrhage? What made you/your team recognise that this was not simply conjunctivitis?

Chapter

28

An Approach to Hearing Loss

Clinical Case

A 70-year-old gentleman presents with a complaint of bilateral hearing loss. He struggles to understand speech, especially in a noisy environment. He first noticed this problem 3 years ago, but it has been getting worse over time. He is otherwise well, with no ear pain, discharge or other symptoms. His past medical history includes diabetes, hypertension and hyperlipidaemia. How would you approach this patient?

Hearing loss is a common problem at any age. It may be sudden and frightening, or insidiously progressive, causing significant functional impairment over time. The diagnostic evaluation aims to identify treatable causes of hearing loss, so that they may be addressed. Congenital aetiologies of hearing impairment will not be covered here (Figure 28.1).

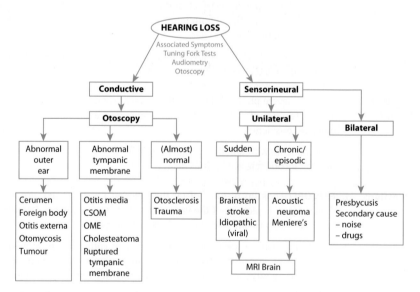

CSOM, chronic suppurative otitis media;
OME, otitis media with effusion.

Figure 28.1. Approach to hearing loss.

Conductive vs. Sensorineural

Normal hearing requires both sound conduction from the external environment to the inner ear, as well as intact sensorineural pathways from the inner ear to the brain. Therefore, hearing loss may be divided into:

- **Conductive**: Any defect limiting sound conduction from the auricle and external ear canal, through the middle ear, into the inner ear.

- **Sensorineural**: A lesion in the inner ear, auditory nerve or brainstem.

- **Mixed**: Both conductive and sensorineural.

The first step in approaching hearing loss is determining if it is conductive or sensorineural. This narrows down the possible aetiologies.

Clinical Differentiators

A clinical distinction can be made based on associated symptoms, tuning fork tests and otoscopy (Table 28.1). Two tuning fork tests are employed.

- **Weber's test**: Place a 512 Hz tuning fork on the forehead between the eyes; it is normally equally loud in both ears.

- **Rinne's test**: Place a 512 Hz tuning fork on the mastoid bone behind the ear (testing bone conduction). Once the sound is no longer audible, hold the tuning fork near the external auditory canal and ask the patient if the sound is still audible (air conduction). Air conduction is normally better than bone conduction.

Table 28.1. Distinguishing Conductive vs. Sensorineural Hearing Loss

	Conductive hearing loss	Sensorineural hearing loss
Associated symptoms	Ear pain, discharge Ear fullness	Vertigo Cranial nerve abnormality
Weber's test	Louder in bad ear (may be normal in bilateral hearing loss)	Louder in good ear (may be normal in bilateral hearing loss)
Rinne's test	Bone conduction better than air conduction	Air conduction better than bone conduction
Otoscopy	Abnormal	Normal

Audiometry

Formal audiometry should be performed in most patients without an obvious cause of hearing loss (e.g., ear wax). Pure tone testing quantifies air and bone conduction across a range of sound frequencies. This determines the severity of hearing loss, identifies any air/bone gap (bone conduction better than air conduction, suggesting conductive loss) and it may give clues on possible aetiologies (some aetiologies affect certain frequencies more than others). Apart from pure tone testing, other components of audiological assessment are helpful in determining function and whether the tympanic membrane is normal.

Conductive Hearing Loss

Most causes of conductive hearing loss can be identified on otoscopic examination. A systematic approach to otoscopy is important—focusing first on the outer ear, then visualising all quadrants of the tympanic membrane.

Abnormal Outer Ear

- **Cerumen impaction (ear wax)**: Ear fullness and hearing loss (usually mild). Dense cerumen is obvious on otoscopy. If severe and recurrent, consider keratosis obturans. Hearing should be re-examined after the ear is syringed, as there can be another abnormality lurking behind the ear wax.
- **Foreign body**: This would also be obvious on otoscopy.
- **Infection**: Outer ear infections present with hearing loss, otalgia, ear discharge and pruritus. Look out for any tympanic membrane perforation, suggesting concomitant otitis media.
  - **Otitis externa** (bacterial infection): Otoscopy reveals oedema, erythema and debris in the external ear canal.
  - **Otomycosis** (fungal infection): Otoscopy finds fungal spores and hyphae in the external ear canal.
- **Tumour**: For example, squamous cell carcinoma, basal cell carcinoma. This resembles otitis externa and is often only suspected after treatment failure.

Abnormal Tympanic Membrane

- **Acute otitis media**: This is an acute bacterial infection. Fluid accumulation in the middle ear results in hearing loss, painful ear fullness ± fever. The tympanic membrane appears bulging, red and inflamed.
- **Chronic suppurative otitis media**: This is a chronic middle ear infection. Patients complain of persistent ear discharge and conductive hearing loss. Examination reveals tympanic membrane perforation with discharge from the middle ear; discharge may be purulent when there is active infection.
- **Otitis media with effusion** (secretory otitis media): Chronic Eustachian tube dysfunction or obstruction results in negative middle ear pressure, leading to fluid build-up. Patients report hearing loss. On otoscopy, the tympanic membrane appears grey, dull and there may be visible bubbles. Nasopharyngeal cancer may involve the Eustachian tube opening and cause otitis media with effusion; always examine the nasopharynx especially in patients of southern Chinese ancestry.
- **Cholesteatoma**: This is a benign epithelial ingrowth into the middle ear, which invariably becomes infected. It presents as a chronically draining ear with poor

response to antibiotics. Otoscopy shows tympanic membrane attic retraction, perforation and sometimes a pearly mass behind (may not always be visible). Left alone, a cholesteatoma may erode adjacent structures, causing sensorineural hearing loss, facial palsy, vertigo, intracranial sepsis and sagittal sinus thrombosis.

- **Ruptured tympanic membrane**: May be due to foreign body, barotrauma or head injury (as well as chronic suppurative otitis media). These causes are identifiable from the history.

(Almost) Normal Otoscopy

- **Otosclerosis**: This is a process of bony overgrowth, leading to progressive fixation of the stapes. It presents with gradual-onset, progressive hearing loss, which may be unilateral or bilateral. There may also be a component of sensorineural hearing loss. Tympanic membrane is normal or may show a Schwartz sign (Flamingo Pink Sign).
- **Trauma**: Can disrupt the ossicular chain, leading to conductive hearing loss.

Further Investigations

The aetiology of conductive hearing loss is usually diagnosed clinically. Investigations may include:

- **CT temporal bone** in unexplained or atypical conductive hearing loss, which may confirm otosclerosis, ossicular disruption or other middle ear disease.
- **Tympanometry** to measure middle ear impedance. This may identify abnormal tympanic membrane motility (e.g., perforated tympanic membrane, middle ear effusion), or negative middle ear pressure (in Eustachian tube dysfunction).

Sensorineural Hearing Loss

The causes of sensorineural hearing loss can be divided into (a) unilateral and sudden onset, (b) unilateral, episodic or chronic and (c) bilateral.

(a) Sudden Unilateral Sensorineural Hearing Loss

- **Idiopathic, often viral**: The aetiology of most cases of sudden sensorineural hearing loss is uncertain. Many cases may be due to viral cochleitis. There may be tinnitus. If the vestibular component of the eighth nerve is also affected, patients may also have vertigo (see Chapter 24).
- **Brainstem neurological lesions**: A brainstem stroke[1] or other inflammatory lesion (e.g., multiple sclerosis) can cause sensorineural hearing loss. In most cases other cranial nerves ± long tracts would be affected (see Chapter 26).

---

[1] Particularly a lesion of the anterior inferior cerebellar artery.

- **Trauma:** In addition to conductive hearing loss, trauma may lead to temporal bone fracture, causing sensorineural hearing loss.

- **Other disease:** Other lesions like haemorrhage into an acoustic neuroma may present with sudden hearing loss.

Approach: Patients with sudden unilateral sensorineural hearing loss should undergo MRI brain to exclude a neurological lesion, before diagnosing idiopathic sudden sensorineural hearing loss.

(b) Episodic/Chronic Unilateral Sensorineural Hearing Loss

- **Meniere disease:** Episodic aural fullness, hearing loss or tinnitus, and vertigo with nausea or vomiting. Each episode lasts 20 min–24 hr. Sensorineural hearing loss is initially unilateral, low-frequency and present only during attacks, but may progress to become permanent or bilateral.

- **Acoustic neuroma:** This is a benign tumour, arising in the cerebellopontine angle from the eighth cranial nerve. It presents with slowly progressive unilateral sensorineural hearing loss ± vertigo. When large enough, it may also cause lower motor neuron seventh, fifth and sixth nerve palsies.

- **Post-infective:** Hearing may not fully recover after meningitis or cochleitis.

Approach: These patients should also undergo contrasted MRI internal acoustic meatus to look for an acoustic neuroma.

(c) Bilateral Sensorineural Hearing Loss

- **Presbycusis:** An elderly person with slowly progressive (years), symmetrical, bilateral sensorineural hearing loss, most affecting higher frequencies. This is a degenerative disease. Patients often complain most of difficulty hearing speech in a crowded environment.

- **Damage from noise exposure:** Elicit an occupational or recreational exposure to loud noise.

- **Drug ototoxicity:** May occur due to aminoglycosides, high-dose furosemide, chemotherapy (cisplatin, 5-FU), erythromycin or tetracycline antibiotics.

Approach: First determine that hearing loss is truly symmetrical; if not, MRI brain should be performed as per (b). Look for secondary causes of hearing loss, before concluding that it is due to presbycusis.

Using what you have learnt, **pen down your approach** to the Clinical Case at the start of the chapter **BEFORE reading the discussion** below.

Case Discussion

In an elderly man with slowly progressive bilateral hearing loss, the likely diagnosis is presbycusis. However, other causes of hearing loss must be excluded before diagnosing presbycusis. Perform otoscopy and audiometry. Ensure that there is no conductive hearing loss, such as cerumen impaction—this is common and easily remediable (but finding impacted cerumen does not exclude another diagnosis). Check that sensorineural hearing loss is symmetrical—any asymmetry should prompt MRI brain looking for pathology such as an acoustic neuroma. Look for secondary causes of hearing loss such as occupational noise exposure and ototoxic drugs.

Key Lessons	1. Hearing loss may be conductive or sensorineural. These can be distinguished based on associated symptoms, tuning fork tests, otoscopy and audiometry.
	2. Most causes of conductive hearing loss can be identified on otoscopy—either an abnormal outer ear, or an abnormal tympanic membrane.
	3. The commonest cause of bilateral sensorineural hearing loss is presbycusis, and that of sudden unilateral sensorineural hearing loss is idiopathic/viral. Any unilateral sensorineural hearing loss usually requires an MRI brain, as it may be due to a focal neurological lesion (e.g., acoustic neuroma and brainstem stroke).
Common Pitfalls	1. Asymmetrical hearing loss is not consistent with presbycusis. Acoustic neuroma must be ruled out.
	2. Cerumen impaction may not be the only cause of hearing loss. Re-test hearing and repeat otoscopy after ear syringing; there may be a second pathology.
Questions	1. **EXPLORE!** Look up otoscopic images of the various aetiologies of conductive hearing loss. Try to recognise them.
	2. **REFLECT!** What are some of the challenges in performing and interpreting the tuning fork tests, and how may they be overcome?
	3. **GO FURTHER!** What are some complications of ear infections (e.g., otitis media), and how would you look out for them?

Chapter

29

An Approach to Ataxia

Clinical Case

A 75-year-old gentleman has had frequent falls in the past year. He also has longstanding diabetes, a lacunar infarct 10 years ago with good recovery, and a 2-year history of urinary problems, because of which he has started to wear diapers. His wife reports that he become mentally 'slow' and has lost interest in his usual activities. On examination, he falls forward when getting up from a chair, and has an unsteady gait consisting of small steps with difficulty turning. Tone, power, reflexes, pin prick and proprioception sense are normal in all limbs. What will be your next diagnostic step?

Walking seems easy but is neurologically complex, requiring the coordination of pyramidal (motor), extrapyramidal, sensory, vestibular and cerebellar circuits. Some patients have difficulty walking, not because of weakness, but because of **ataxia**—a problem with balance or coordinating movements.

Clinical Approach

Distinguish ataxia from difficulty walking because of

- Weakness or spasticity (see Chapter 25).
- Giddiness and vestibular dysfunction (see Chapter 24).
- Bradykinesia and postural instability as seen in extrapyramidal disorders (see Chapter 30).
- Non-neurological causes, for example, poor vision (see Chapter 27), joint pain (see Chapter 48), poor effort tolerance or cognitive decline (see Chapter 31).

Then determine if ataxia is due to cerebellar dysfunction, sensory (proprioceptive) dysfunction or cortical disorders (Figure 29.1).

Cerebellar Ataxia

Ataxia is one of many signs of cerebellar disease. A lesion affecting the midline cerebellar structures causes **truncal ataxia** (e.g., falling to one side when standing straight) and cerebellar eye signs such as horizontal gaze-evoked (multidirectional) nystagmus and jerky pursuit (saccadic intrusion). A lesion affecting the cerebellar hemispheres causes ipsilateral **limb ataxia,** with past-pointing, dysdiadochokinesia and intention tremor. There may be scanning speech, that is, speech which varies in rate and volume.

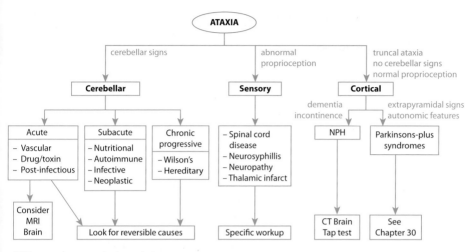

Figure 29.1. Approach to ataxia.

NPH, normal pressure hydrocephalus.

As usual, the answer to 'what is the lesion' requires consideration of time course and distribution. A lesion affecting only *half* the cerebellum (i.e., unilateral dysmetria) is more likely a focal lesion (e.g., a stroke, tumour or multiple sclerosis plaque) rather than a diffuse process (e.g., metabolic and drugs).

Acute Cerebellar Ataxia

- **Vascular**: Infarct or haemorrhage in two locations present with ataxia: (a) ataxic hemiparesis syndrome from a lacunar stroke, in which ataxia is accompanied by hemiplegia ± ipsilateral upper motor neuron facial nerve palsy, and (b) a posterior circulation stroke with ataxia, vertigo, other cranial nerve deficits and long tract signs. Ataxia in this situation is usually unilateral.

- **Drugs and toxins**: Antiepileptic drugs (phenytoin, carbamazepine, lamotrigine), chemotherapy and acute alcohol toxicity (which classically affects trunk more than limbs).

- **Post-infectious cerebellitis**: After viral infection in young adults or children.

Workup: Look through the medication list. Consider MRI brain for stroke, especially if ataxia is hyperacute (within minutes) (also see page 244).

Subacute Cerebellar Ataxia

- **Nutritional**: Alcohol abuse, thiamine deficiency (Wernicke encephalopathy—ataxia, ophthalmoplegia and altered mental state), vitamin E deficiency.

- **Autoimmune disease**: Many entities may present with ataxia. Of note, the triad of ataxia, ophthalmoplegia and areflexia suggests Miller-Fisher syndrome (page 261).

Cerebellar ataxia is common in multiple sclerosis, and may even be its first manifestation (i.e., a clinically isolated syndrome). Other autoimmune disease including acute disseminated encephalomyelitis (ADEM), glutamic acid decarboxylase (GAD) antibody associated ataxia, celiac disease and systemic autoimmune diseases (e.g., lupus, Sjogren's syndrome, Hashimoto thyroiditis) may present with ataxia.

- **Infective**: Creutzfeldt–Jakob disease presents with rapidly progressive dementia (weeks), ataxia and myoclonus. Cerebellar ataxia is also a feature of progressive multifocal leucoencephalopathy (due to JC virus reactivation) and Whipple's disease.

- **Mass lesions**: Cerebellar tumour or abscess.

- **Paraneoplastic**: Paraneoplastic cerebellar degeneration is a rare manifestation of systemic cancer; onconeuronal antibodies may be positive.

- Hypothyroidism.

Workup: The goal of workup is to identify reversible causes of ataxia. Screen for thyroid function, vitamin E ± anti-thyroid and onconeuronal antibodies. Further tests depend on clinical suspicion and may include MRI brain, lumbar puncture and other autoantibodies for systemic autoimmune disease.

Chronic Progressive Cerebellar Ataxia

- **Wilson's disease**: Copper accumulation causing a variety of neurologic manifestations (ataxia, movement disorders, psychiatric symptoms), liver disease (hepatitis to cirrhosis) and Kayser–Fleischer rings. Consider a screen of serum ceruloplasmin and 24 hr urinary copper. While uncommon, Wilson's disease is treatable and should not be missed.

- **Hereditary ataxias**: The list of hereditary ataxias include spinocerebellar ataxia, Friedreich ataxia, episodic ataxias, mitochondrial diseases, ataxia telangiectasia and others. There may be other neurologic manifestations and a positive family history. The details of these diseases are out of the scope of this text.

Sensory Ataxia

Loss of proprioceptive feedback impairs coordination of movements, which is especially bad in the dark (this is the basis of the Romberg's test—visual input compensates for sensory ataxia, so cutting out visual input exacerbates ataxia). Suspect sensory ataxia if proprioception is abnormal, if proprioception is abnormal or Roberg's is positive. Consider the sensory axis from peripheral nerves—dorsal columns—thalamus—sensory cortex:

	Workup
- **Spinal cord disease (myelopathy)** affecting the posterior columns: For example, cervical myelopathy, subacute combined degeneration from vitamin B12 or copper deficiency.	– MRI spine – Serum B12 and copper

- **Tabes dorsalis**: Always consider neurosyphilis.

  − Serum VDRL

- **Polyneuropathy**: For example, Miller-Fisher syndrome, sensory neuronopathy (e.g., in diabetes), paraneoplastic neuropathy, chronic immune sensory polyradiculopathy (details omitted).

  − Nerve conduction studies
  − Other tests based on clinical suspicion

- **Thalamic infarct**: Rarely, a thalamic infarct (the location of the third order sensory neuron) may cause sensory ataxia. This would be of acute onset.

  − MRI brain if suspected

Cortical Causes

In a patient with truncal ataxia with little cerebellar signs, and normal proprioception, two diagnoses must be considered:

- **Normal pressure hydrocephalus**: This is a classic triad of dementia, gait ataxia and urinary incontinence. Patients demonstrate a magnetic gait and turning in numbers. CT brain reveals dilated ventricles out of proportion to cortical atrophy/sulcal enlargement. Large-volume lumbar puncture results in marked improvement in gait (a 'tap test'). This is an important diagnosis as it is eminently treatable.

- **Parkinson's-plus disorders**: Ataxia is a prominent feature in multiple system atrophy (MSP) and progressive supranuclear palsy (PSP; see Chapter 30).

 Using what you have learnt, **pen down your approach** to the Clinical Case at the start of the chapter **BEFORE reading the discussion** below.

Case Discussion

This elderly gentleman appears to have frequent falls because of incoordination. The triad of gait difficulty, urinary problems and cognitive decline suggests normal pressure hydrocephalus.

Differentials include cerebellar ataxia and a Parkinsonian syndrome. Examine carefully for cerebellar signs (e.g., nystagmus and past pointing) and cranial nerve palsies, which may suggest cerebellar ataxia—he could have had another stroke, this time in the posterior circulation, although that would be likely to present more acutely. Examine for autonomic dysfunction (e.g., postural hypotension) and Parkinsonian features, which could suggest multiple system atrophy (MSA) or progressive supranuclear palsy (PSP).

The next step depends on the findings of this examination. If suspecting normal pressure hydrocephalus, the next step is a CT brain. However, MRI is superior if cerebellar lesions (e.g., infarct) or MSA/PSP are suspected.

Key Lessons	1. The causes of cerebellar ataxia can be divided into acute (especially vascular and drugs/toxins), subacute (nutritional, autoimmune, infective or neoplastic) and chronic progressive (mainly hereditary) causes.
	2. Ataxia may be due not only to cerebellar dysfunction, but also proprioceptive loss, normal pressure hydrocephalus and Parkinson-plus disorders.
Common Pitfalls	1. The Romberg's test is not specific for posterior column dysfunction. It is a test of latent disequilibrium; dysfunction in either position sense or vestibular coordination is sufficient to give a positive test.
Questions	1. **REFLECT!** Have you ever seen a patient with cerebellar ataxia, or abnormal past-pointing on the neurological examination? What was his/her ataxia due to, and what differentials did you consider?
	2. **EXPLORE!** How would you examine a patient's gait? What abnormalities might you find in (a) UMN weakness, (b) LMN weakness, (c) foot drop, (d) Parkinson's disease, (e) cerebellar disease and (f) hip or knee pain?

An Approach to
30 Abnormal Movement

Clinical Case

A 56-year-old premorbidly well gentleman complains of difficulty using his right hand, which has been getting steadily worse over the past year. It shakes when he eats or writes; the left hand is only mildly affected. He also reports numerous falls, especially when rising from a chair, and recent urinary incontinence. On examination, blood pressure is 120/80 mmHg supine, and 90/50 mmHg standing. There is a low-amplitude rest tremor, more prominent on the right, as well as decreased facial expression and soft speech. Extraocular movements are intact although pursuit movements are jerky. Repetitive finger tapping is slow. Finger–nose testing reveals dysmetria. What is the likely diagnosis?

Abnormal movements encompass a decrease in voluntary movements (hypokinetic disorder), or an increase in involuntary movements (hyperkinetic disorder). The presence of abnormal movements is obvious, but arriving at a diagnosis requires a working knowledge of the common conditions, and a suspicion for when something might be more than the usual.

Hypokinetic Disorders

Parkinsonism is the main presentation of the hypokinetic movement disorders. The approach to these disorders can be summarised as:

1. Identify parkinsonian features.
2. Is it idiopathic Parkinson's disease (PD) or a Parkinson's-plus syndrome?
3. Are there causes of secondary parkinsonism?

1. Identify Parkinsonian Features

The four cardinal features of parkinsonism (the 'TRAP') are a pill-rolling rest *tremor*, **rigidity** (distinguish from spasticity; Table 30.1), *akinesia* or **bradykinesia** and **postural instability**. Other features include hypophonia, hypomimia and non-motor symptoms including sleep disturbances, fatigue, aches and pains.

The most common cause of parkinsonism is idiopathic PD. However, parkinsonism is also seen in Parkinson's-plus syndromes and secondary parkinsonism.

Table 30.1. Hypertonic Limbs—Rigidity vs. Spasticity

	Characteristic	Cause
Cogwheel rigidity	Tremors superimposed on rigidity: muscle gives way in little jerks	Parkinsonism
Leadpipe rigidity	Stiffness remains uniform throughout range of movement and does not vary with speed of movement (velocity-independent)	Parkinsonism
Clasp-knife spasticity	Joint suddenly gives way as applied force increases—hypertonia present only at start of movement. Spasticity is only elicited at high-speed (i.e., velocity dependent)	Upper motor neuron lesion, e.g., stroke
Percussion myotonia	Tapping the muscle causes contraction, which only slowly relaxes	Myotonic dystrophy

2. Is It Idiopathic PD or a Parkinson's-Plus Syndrome?

Idiopathic PD is a clinical diagnosis; investigations are not required if features are consistent with idiopathic PD, and there are no atypical features. However, atypical features, as well as young age of onset, prompts consideration of the Parkinson's-plus syndromes. The Parkinson's-plus syndromes may initially resemble idiopathic PD (even in response to levodopa), only to evolve atypically later; therefore, the diagnosis of PD should be continually reassessed. Table 30.2 highlights the differences between idiopathic PD and the Parkinson's-plus syndromes.

3. Are There Causes of Secondary Parkinsonism?

Look for secondary causes of parkinsonism. This includes:

Workup

- **Drug-induced parkinsonism**: Parkinsonian side effects from dopaminergic agents (antipsychotic drugs, metoclopramide) may take up to a year to resolve. There is usually little rest tremor.

  − Clinical history
  − Trial off medications

- **Vascular parkinsonism**: For example, multiple basal ganglia infarcts. Symptoms begin and progress in a stepwise manner (i.e., with each new stroke), and the lower limbs are disproportionately affected. These patients are vasculopaths with prior strokes (clinical or asymptomatic).

  − CT/MRI brain: multiple chronic infarcts and/or haemorrhages

- **Wilson's disease**: A hereditary copper storage disease, usually a young patient with various neurologic manifestations (ataxia, parkinsonism, chorea, psychiatric symptoms), liver disease (hepatitis, cirrhosis) and Kayser–Fleischer rings.

  − Screen: serum ceruloplasmin, 24 hr urinary copper

- **CNS infections** including encephalitis, neurosyphilis, HIV or Creutzfeldt–Jakob disease.

  − MRI brain
  − Lumbar puncture in the appropriate context

Table 30.2. Idiopathic Parkinson's Disease vs. Parkinson's-Plus Syndromes

	Idiopathic Parkinson's disease (PD)	Progressive supranuclear palsy (PSP)	Multiple system atrophy (MSA)	Corticobasal degeneration (CBD)	Lewy body dementia (LBD)
Symmetry	Unilateral onset, *asymmetry persists*	More symmetrical	More symmetrical	*Asymmetrical*	More symmetrical
Levodopa response	*Excellent and sustained*; clinical course 10+ years	Poor or non-sustained	Poor or non-sustained	Poor or non-sustained	Poor or non-sustained
Postural and autonomic features	Absent or mild at first presentation	*Early postural instability, falls.* Parkinsonism is mainly axial	*Early autonomic dysfunction, postural hypotension*	Absent or mild	Absent or mild
Other neurological dysfunction	Normal pyramidal and cerebellar systems	*Abnormal vertical gaze*	*Bilateral cerebellar and/or pyramidal signs*	*Unilateral pyramidal,* parkinsonian, and dystonic signs	*REM sleep behaviour disorder*
Cognitive and psychiatric features	Late. Dementia can develop after many years	Early cognitive impairment	Late	Early dementia	Visual hallucinations, fluctuating consciousness; *Sensitivity to antipsychotics*

REM, rapid eye movement.

Hyperkinetic Disorders

The hyperkinetic movement disorders include tremor, choreoathetosis, dystonias and tics.

Tremor

A tremor is a rhythmic oscillation of a body part produced by alternating or synchronous contractions of agonist and antagonist muscles. Its aetiology can be differentiated by identifying (1) when the tremor is worst, (2) whether the tremor is symmetrical (asymmetry occurs in parkinsonism and cerebellar disease).

- **Rest tremors**: Occur even when the limb is completely supported, resting on a surface.
  - An *asymmetric* rest tremor is seen in parkinsonism, together with other features of rigidity, akinesia/bradykinesia and postural instability. This tremor can momentarily stop when the limb is voluntarily moved, and restart after ('re-emergent tremor').
  - Overflow from essential tremor (see the following).
- **Postural tremor**: These tremors occur with hands outstretched against gravity.
  - **Asterixis**: As seen in decompensated cirrhosis or uraemia. These conditions should be obvious from the clinical context.
  - **Enhanced physiologic tremor**: Due to enhanced sympathetic activity as in hyperthyroidism, adrenergic drugs (e.g., salbutamol, nicotine, antidepressants), anxiety, hypoglycaemia and smoking/alcohol withdrawal. Exclude these causes before diagnosing essential tremor.
  - **Essential tremor**: A bilateral, symmetrical tremor affecting the upper limbs and head. There should be an otherwise normal neurological examination (minor cogwheeling is acceptable). There is usually a long history without progressive symptoms, symptom relief with alcohol and good response to beta blockers. There may be a positive family history.
  - **Primary writing tremor**: This tremor occurs only during writing.
- **Intention tremor**: Worst at the extremes of voluntary motion, an intention tremor signifies cerebellar disease (see Chapter 29). It may be symmetrical or asymmetrical, depending on the aetiology of cerebellar disease.

Chorea and Athetosis

Chorea refers to brief, unpredictable movements affecting any body part but especially the distal limbs. Classic signs include a darting tongue, dish-spooning arms and effeminate gait. When mild, patients may look fidgety and incorporate the chorea into other purposeful movements. **Athetosis** is characterised by slower, writhing movements.

(a) **Genetic causes**—these are usually symmetrical and develop insidiously. Depending on the disease, onset may be in childhood or adulthood. There may be a family history.

- **Huntington's disease**: An autosomal dominant trinucleotide repeats disease. In addition to chorea, there is cognitive decline and behavioural changes.

- **Wilson's disease**: See page 288.

- There are many other genetic syndromes that cause chorea. Look for associated neurological features (especially ataxia, dementia and peripheral neuropathy) as these are associated with specific aetiologies.

(b) **Acquired causes**—these may be acute or sub-acute.

	Workup
• **Focal basal ganglia lesion**: A unilateral lesion may cause *asymmetric* chorea. Aetiologies include infarction, haemorrhage, tumour.	– MRI brain
• **Metabolic**: Hyperglycaemia, hyperthyroidism, hypocalcaemia, hypoglycaemia.	– Screen glucose, thyroid and electrolytes
• **Drugs**: Chronic use of dopaminergic agonists (antipsychotics, metoclopramide, prochlorperazine) causes *tardive dyskinesia*, most commonly an elderly patient with protruding tongue movements, lip smacking or chewing movements.	– Review drug history
• **Infective and inflammatory**: Sydenham's chorea (acute rheumatic fever in childhood), lupus, encephalitis and other autoimmune choreas.	– Autoimmune workup if indicated
• **Oestrogen**: Pregnancy and oral contraceptive pills.	– Pregnancy test

Other Hyperkinetic Disorders

These disorders will not be covered in detail.

- **Dystonia**: Abnormal, involuntary posturing affecting various body parts (e.g., torticollis, blepharospasm, limb dystonia, facial dystonia). This can be caused by various genetic and metabolic disorders, including Wilson's disease and ischaemic or infective damage to the basal ganglia. Acute dystonia is a known adverse effect of dopaminergic agonists (antipsychotics and metoclopramide).

- **Tics**: Involuntary, stereotyped movements, which may be both motor and vocal. The main cause is Tourette syndrome.

Using what you have learnt, **pen down your approach** to the Clinical Case at the start of the chapter **BEFORE reading the discussion** below.

Case Discussion

The combination of parkinsonism (rest tremor, bradykinesia, hypomimia, hypophonia), cerebellar dysfunction (falls, dysmetria, jerky pursuit) and autonomic dysfunction (postural hypotension, urinary incontinence) is most consistent with multiple system atrophy. While cerebellar and autonomic dysfunction can occur in idiopathic Parkinson's disease, they tend to occur late, certainly not within one year. Progressive supranuclear palsy (PSP) is a differential, given early postural instability, but cerebellar dysfunction and normal vertical gaze make PSP less likely. The gradual, instead of step-wise, onset of symptoms goes against vascular parkinsonism.

Key Lessons	1. The cardinal features of parkinsonism are tremor, rigidity, akinesia/brady-kinesia and postural instability (the 'TRAP').
	2. Idiopathic Parkinson's disease is asymmetrical, progresses gradually and responds excellently to levodopa. If there are atypical features (early cognitive, cerebellar and autonomic symptoms, vertical gaze palsy, or prominent hallucinations), consider Parkinson's-plus syndromes. Also look for secondary causes.
	3. The types of tremor include rest tremor (parkinsonism), intention tremor (cerebellar disease) and postural tremor (essential tremor, asterixis and enhanced sympathetic activity, as in hyperthyroidism).
Common Pitfalls	1. Wilson's disease should be considered in any young patient with a new onset of abnormal movements, especially if liver enzymes are abnormal. It is rare but treatable.
Questions	1. **EXPLORE!** Look up videos of (a) parkinsonian tremor, (b) essential tremor, (c) choreiform movements, (d) tardive dyskinesia, (e) dystonia and (f) tics. After watching the videos, try to describe the movements in your own words.
	2. **DISCUSS!** What might be the presenting complaint of a patient with early Parkinson's disease (without florid 'TRAP' features)?

Chapter

31

An Approach to Altered Mental State and Cognitive Decline

Clinical Case

A 76-year-old lady is brought in by her family for abnormal behaviour. She was premorbidly well with no chronic medical conditions. In the last year, she has become very suspicious of her family members and especially the domestic helper. She frequently misplaces objects and accuses others of stealing them. She has also stopped buying lottery tickets, and no longer cooks. Her family is bringing her in now because her behaviour has deteriorated further in the past few days—she woke up the entire house at night, and called the police to report that the domestic helper was trying to poison her. She did have cough and fever last week, but has since recovered with medication from the GP. What investigations would you do, and what is the most likely diagnosis?

A number of descriptors (altered mental state, delirium, confusion, drowsiness, coma) are commonly used to describe disordered mental function of varying severity, from slight confusion to unarousable unresponsiveness. The number of non-specific terms used reflects the heterogeneity of diseases that present with decreased alertness and/or loss of higher cognitive function. Altered mental state may be a consequence of intra-cranial lesions, such as stroke, seizure, or dementia. It may also the result of systemic illness (e.g., sepsis and metabolic derangements) manifesting in the organ of least reserve—which, in the elderly, is often the brain. This wide range of possibilities, coupled with the patient's inability to give a history, presents a unique clinical difficulty.

Identifying Altered Mental State

The presence of altered mental function is usually not in doubt. A number of scoring systems exist to quantify the severity of mental dysfunction. The **Glasgow Coma Scale** (GCS; Table 31.1) characterises severity of drowsiness in poorly responsive patients, but will not identify subtle confusion in communicative patients. The **abbreviated mental test** (AMT)[1] is a quick screen in conversant patients. The **Mini-Mental State examination** (MMSE)[1] is a more difficult and comprehensive assessment, usually used when

---

[1] There are country- and language-specific differences in the questions used in the AMT or MMSE. For example, patients in the UK may be asked to name the present monarch; this is modified to the name of the sitting prime minister in other countries. Many countries have validated a version of the AMT and MMSE for use in their population.

Table 31.1. Glasgow Coma Scale (GCS)

	Eyes	Verbal	Motor
1 Point	No eye opening	No sounds	No movement
2 Points	Open eyes to pain	Incomprehensible sounds	Extension to pain (decerebrate)
3 Points	Open eyes to speech	Inappropriate words	Flexion to pain (decorticate)
4 Points	Open eyes spontaneously	Confused speech	Withdrawal to pain stimuli
5 Points	—	Orientated	Localises pain
6 Points	—	—	Obey commands

The minimum GCS is 3, the maximum is 15. Pain can be elicited by supraorbital or nail bed pressure, or sternal rub. Intubation or tracheostomy invalidates the verbal component.

dementia is being considered. None of these scoring systems provides any information on the aetiology of altered mental state, and do not distinguish dementia from delirium.

Aetiological Diagnosis

Identifying an aetiology begins by distinguishing acute from chronic altered mental state (Figure 31.1). Patients with chronic dementia who develop a change in mental state should be approached as for acute altered mental state, as it may imply a new, potentially reversible cause.

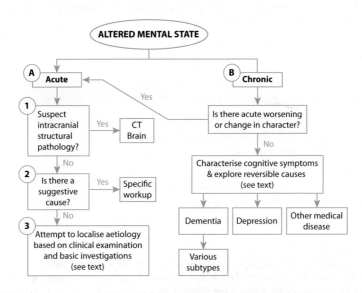

Figure 31.1. Approach to altered mental state.

Acute Altered Mental State

Acute altered mental state presents as two overlapping clinical pictures:

- **Delirium**: An acute-onset, fluctuating disturbance in mental state. Patients are inattentive and have disordered thinking or altered consciousness (hyperactive, e.g., agitation, or hypoactive, e.g., drowsiness).
- **Drowsiness**: Ranges from slight drowsiness to total coma (unarousable unresponsiveness).

The algorithm in Figure 31.1 is expounded upon below:

1. Is Structural Intracranial Pathology Suspected?

Not every intracranial lesion causes drowsiness. To do so, it must affect either the ascending reticular activating system in the brainstem, or bilateral cerebral hemispheres. Certain factors are worrisome for such a lesion:

- **Focal neurological deficit** (during or preceding coma): For example, cranial nerve palsy, unequal or unreactive pupils, dysfunctional brainstem reflexes.
- **Signs of raised intracranial pressure**: For example, dilated or sluggish pupils, Cushing's reflex (hypertension and bradycardia), vomiting, or papilloedema. (Note: bilateral miosis or mydriasis may be due to toxins and not a neurological abnormality).
- **Headache or nuchal rigidity**: Worrisome for intracranial bleed or meningitis.
- **History of head trauma**: Even a minor fall, months ago, may be sufficient to result in subdural haemorrhage in the elderly. Worrisome examination findings include Battle's sign (mastoid fracture), Raccoon's eyes (orbital fracture) and haemorrhage from ears or nostrils (base of skull fracture).
- **Very sudden onset over minutes**: Suspicious for an acute vascular event.
- **Severe drowsiness**.

Concern for structural intracranial pathology prompts emergent CT imaging of the brain. If brainstem pathology is suspected, MRI brain better delineates the posterior fossa.

2. Is There a Suggestive Cause?

Attempt to elicit signs or symptoms to direct further investigation. While patients may not be able to give a history, make every effort to obtain a collaborative history from family members or contacts. The ambulance notes are often helpful (In what condition was the patient found? Who called the ambulance and why?). This may provide information on:

- **Localising symptoms**: For example, fever and cough before onset of drowsiness suggests pneumonia with septic encephalopathy or hypercapnic respiratory failure.
- **Precipitants**: For example, a fall which may cause intracranial haemorrhage.

- **Predisposing factors**: For example, known cirrhosis raises suspicion of hepatic encephalopathy.

- **Recognise aphasia** (expressive or receptive): This may mimic altered mental state, but it should be identifiable upon careful interaction with the patient. While aphasia may be a part of dementia, aphasia alone without the other hallmarks of impaired cognitive function suggests a cortical lesion. Evaluate for a stroke in a compatible anatomical territory (left frontal or temporal).

- **Psychiatric illness** (e.g., psychosis and catatonic depression) may mimic delirium. Nonetheless the imperative is to exclude organic causes before ascribing the mental dysfunction to psychiatric illness.

The presence of any suggestive cause directs further workup.

3. Approach to Non-Specific Altered Mental State

These patients would benefit from having the proverbial net cast wide. Consider a broad range of precipitants for altered mental state ('Vitamin C'):

Workup

- *V*ascular:
  - Cerebrovascular accident
  - Acute myocardial infarction
  - Hypertensive encephalopathy.

    — Take blood pressure
    — ECG
    — Consider CT brain if no other cause of drowsiness identified

- *I*nfective: For example, pneumonia, urinary infection, intracranial infections.

    — Septic workup, look for source

- *T*oxins:
  - **Substances**: Alcohol intoxication, recreational drug use or withdrawal, or poisoning. Look for toxidromes and symptom clusters, for example, Wernicke encephalopathy (ataxia, confusion, ophthalmoplegia)—a confused patient with bizarre nystagmus should receive immediate thiamine!

    — Clinical history
    — Toxicology screen
    — May attempt trial of naloxone and flumazenil

  - **Drugs**: Anticholinergics, narcotics, sedatives, antihypertensives, anticonvulsants, many more.

    — Drug history including complementary medicine

- *A*utoimmune: Autoimmune encephalitis, systemic vasculitis or autoimmune conditions with CNS manifestations.

    — Specific autoimmune workup if indicated

- *M*ajor organ and *M*etabolic:
  - Glucose: Hypoglycaemia, diabetic ketoacidosis, hyperglycaemic hyperosmolar state (see Chapter 37).

    — Begin with a blood gas, electrolytes and liver panel

- Electrolyte imbalance especially hyponatraemia (see Chapter 17).

- Cardiac: Ischaemia/infarction, heart failure.

- Pulmonary: Hypoxia, hypercapnia.

- Liver: Hepatic encephalopathy.

- Renal: Uraemia, dehydration.

- Endocrine: Thyroid storm, myxoedema coma, adrenal insufficiency.

- Environmental: Heat injury is a thermoregulatory disorder occurring in individuals who exert in the heat (e.g., athletes, soldiers, construction workers). Its milder form, heat exhaustion, presents with non-specific neurological symptoms (headache, nausea, vomiting, dizziness, lightheadedness). Its most severe form, heat stroke, manifests with drowsiness, confusion or seizures, and subsequently leads to end-organ damage. A high index of suspicion is necessary. Conversely, hypothermia may also cause altered mental state.

- *Ictal* (**Epilepsy**): Absence or non-convulsive seizures, post-ictal state.

- *Nutritional*: For example, deficiency of vitamin B12, folate or thiamine.

- **Comfort factors**

  - Urinary or faecal retention.

  - Severe pain: For example, undiagnosed fractures.

(right column annotations)

- Subsequent investigations based on clinical suspicion

- Heat injury: rectal temperature > 37.7°C (note that tympanic or oral temperature is unreliable).

- Consider electro-encephalogram

- Clinical examination
- X-rays

Chronic Cognitive Decline

The presenting complaint may be memory loss, cognitive dysfunction or behavioural symptoms. Patients with acute worsening should be evaluated as for acute altered mental state. For a patient at a stable baseline:

1. What are the patient's symptoms?
2. Are there reversible causes?
3. Which type of dementia?
4. How is the patient coping?

1. What Are the Patient's Symptoms?

(a) **Evaluate cognitive function**—elicit history from patient and family; consider the domains[2] of:

- Amnesia: Short and long-term memory loss, losing things, confabulation or catastrophic reactions.

- Aphasia: Difficulty finding words, expressing self or any other communication issues.

- Apraxia: Difficulty with common actions, for example, buttoning, dressing, feeding, using a television remote and so forth.

- Agnosia: Getting lost in familiar places, difficulty recognising familiar people or objects.

- Executive function: Difficulty handling money or making plans, poor decision-making, increasingly disorganised.

(b) **Evaluate functional impact**—consider social or occupational functioning, loss of independence in community, home and self-care.

(c) **Formal assessment**—clinic assessment includes MMSE and clock drawing tests. Consider formal neuropsychological testing if the diagnosis is uncertain, atypical or cognitive decline is suspected in spite of 'normal' MMSE (as may occur in highly educated individuals, in whom MMSE is insensitive).

2. Are There Reversible Causes?

Search hard for any reversible component. Consider the mnemonic 'DEMENTIA':

	Workup
• *Depression or Delusion*: Psychiatric disease may mimic dementia.	− Clinical screening
− Depression (pseudodementia): Look for poor mood, loss of interest, feelings of guilt, poor energy, appetite and sleep. Observe for blunted affect (Table 31.2).	

---

[2] These are the DSM IV domains, which has since been superseded by DSM V; DSM V defines dementia (now re-named major neurocognitive disorder) as cognitive decline in a broader range of domains (learning and memory, language, executive function, complex attention, perceptual-motor and social cognition), interfering with independence in daily activities. The change was made to de-emphasise memory dysfunction as a central criterion, as some patients with non-Alzheimer's dementia have relatively intact memory, and did not meet DSM IV criteria for dementia. For educational purposes, however, the DSM IV domains remain valuable, as they better characterise the prototypical dementia patient.

- Delusion: Atypical presentations of schizophrenia with prominent negative symptoms (disorganised, withdrawn behaviour) may mimic the behavioural and psychological symptoms (BPSD) in advanced dementia.

- **Ethanol**: Chronic alcoholism leading to Korsakoff dementia.

- **Metabolic**: Hypercalcaemia, B12/folate or thiamine deficiency.
  - B12/folate and calcium levels

- **Endocrine**: Hypothyroidism may mimic dementia.
  - Thyroid function tests

- **Neurologic**: For example, subdural haematoma, brain tumour, normal pressure hydrocephalus (triad of cognitive impairment, gait disturbance and urinary incontinence).
  - Routine CT brain in dementia workup

- **Toxic**: Chronic heavy metal poisoning, medication (e.g., diazepam).

- **Infective**: For example, neurosyphilis and HIV.
  - Screen VDRL and HIV

- **Autoimmune**: For example, paraneoplastic, Hashimoto encephalopathy.

3. Which Type of Dementia?

Dementia is diagnosed in a patient who has acquired cognitive impairment in ≥1 domain, which interferes with independent function,[3] and is not better accounted for by delirium (Table 31.2) or another mental disorder.

There are different types of dementia:

- **Alzheimer's dementia**: This is the most common type of dementia. It is of insidious onset and slowly progressive over many years. Amnesia is prominent. CT brain reveals generalised brain atrophy.

- **Vascular dementia**: Presents with an irregular, stepwise decline in cognitive function, on a background of cerebrovascular disease and vascular risk factors. Neuroimaging reveals multiple chronic infarcts.

- **Lewy body dementia**: Patients exhibit fluctuating cognition and alertness, early visual hallucinations and prominent parkinsonism, which is exacerbated by antipsychotic drugs.

- **Frontal–temporal dementia**: A younger patient (in the 50s age group) with personality change (e.g., disinhibition, apathy), aphasia and frontal lobe atrophy on imaging. Memory may be relatively preserved.

---

[3] Some patients have mild cognitive deficits, which do not significantly interfere with function. These patients may be described to have **mild cognitive impairment**, an intermediate state between normal aging and dementia proper.

- **Parkinson's disease dementia**: Dementia occurs late, when Parkinson's disease is well established.

- **Creutzfeldt–Jakob disease**: *Rapidly progressive* (weeks) dementia with *focal neurological abnormalities* (ataxia, myoclonus, upper motor neuron or extrapyramidal features). MRI may initially be normal but subsequently shows basal ganglia hyperintensities. There are characteristic cerebrospinal fluid and electroencephalographic changes.

Table 31.2. Differentiating Confusional States in the Elderly

	Delirium	Dementia	Depression
Onset and Course	Acute onset (days) and fluctuating course	Insidious onset (months–years) and progressive course	Variable onset; if acute, a stressor may be identifiable
Orientation	Disorientated	Clear until late stages	Usually unimpaired
Attention	Inattention, unable to talk	Attentive, often cooperative	Inattentive, not interested to talk
Memory	Poor memory	Consistent pattern of amnesia, affecting short-term memory more than long-term memory	Variable pattern of amnesia, equally affecting recent and remote events; may give 'don't know' answers
Insight	Incoherent and illogical	May deny memory problems (attempt to minimise disability), confabulate or exhibit catastrophic reactions	May or may not realise that he/she has low mood. May instead be more concerned about memory loss (attempt to emphasise disability)
Hallucinations	Simple visual hallucinations and illusions are common	Uncommon (except Lewy body dementia—visual hallucinations)	May have mood-congruent hallucinations (e.g., derogatory voices)
Delusions	May have transient and fragmented delusions	Delusions of theft common (e.g., maid steals items)	May have mood-congruent delusions (e.g., nihilistic, poverty)
Sleep	Disturbed sleep-wake cycle	Sleep-wake reversal; sun-downing	Early morning awakening is characteristic

4. How Is the Patient Coping?

It is important to assess function and care issues. Consider:

- **Activities of daily living**: Self-care, home-care, continence (bladder and bowel) and function in the community.

- **Behavioural and psychological symptoms (BPSD)**: For example, agitation, depression, anxiety, sleep-wake reversal, delusions of theft and so forth.

- **Caregiver issues**: Care needs, caregiver coping.
- **Danger**: Fire risk (leave stove unattended), risk of unwise decisions or exploitation.
- **End-of-life planning**.
- **Feeding**: Interest in food declines as a natural progression of dementia.

 Using what you have learnt, **pen down your approach** to the Clinical Case at the start of the chapter **BEFORE reading the discussion** below.

Case Discussion

This 76-year-old lady has two cognitive issues. Firstly, she has a 1-year history of amnesia, confabulation and impaired executive function. This is suspicious for dementia. Super-imposed on top of this, she appears to have an acute deterioration in mental function— possibly due to an acute infection, or due to the medications that she was given (e.g., antihistamines, which cause confusion in the elderly). This is not surprising as patients with chronic cognitive decline are predisposed to acute episodes of delirium.

She should undergo a basic delirium work up, including a neurological assessment, chest X-ray, electrolytes, full blood count, inflammatory markers and urine microscopy. Obtaining a CT brain, thyroid, B12 and folate levels will also be helpful in view of the suspicion of dementia, and this can be done now. In the current instance, it would be inappropriate to diagnose dementia, as acute delirium precludes assessment of her cognitive baseline. When she is well, reassess her cognitive state, exclude pseudodementia (depression) and other reversible causes, and identify the type of dementia she has.

Key Lessons	1. A huge range of systemic illnesses can cause acute-onset altered mental state. However, focal neurological deficits, signs of raised intracranial pressure, nuchal rigidity, trauma and severe drowsiness should prompt imaging for structural intracranial pathology.
	2. In an elderly patient with chronic cognitive decline, consider delirium, depression and other reversible causes before making a diagnosis of dementia. There are different types of dementia, each with a unique clinical syndrome.
Common Pitfalls	1. Hypercapnia quite reliably causes drowsiness. It can be missed as routine blood tests are normal, and oxygen saturations can be normal when on supplemental oxygen. A blood gas is helpful.
	2. Do not diagnose dementia when a patient is acutely ill.
Questions	1. **REFLECT!** Have you ever encountered a patient with pseudodementia? What features pointed to depression rather than dementia? It would be tragic to misdiagnose depression as dementia, as the former is treatable.

2. **DISCUSS!** Too many CT scans are performed for acute confusion. Do you agree?

3. **EXPLORE!** What should one look for on a CT brain done as part of dementia workup?

4. **GO FURTHER!** Some patients with memory impairment are diagnosed with mild cognitive impairment (MCI). What distinguishes MCI from dementia, and what are the implications of MCI?

Blood

Chapter
32

An Approach to Anaemia

Clinical Case

A 60-year-old lady is admitted for community-acquired pneumonia. Her past medical history includes poorly controlled diabetes, and rheumatoid arthritis on methotrexate (recently started). She had been well and active until 3 days ago, when she developed fever and cough. Her admission laboratories showed:

Haemoglobin	*8.7 g/dL (baseline 12.0 g/dL, 1 year ago)*
White cells	*17 × 10⁹/L*
Platelets	*350 × 10⁹/L*
Reticulocytes	*1.5%*
MCV	*82 fL*
Iron saturation	*8%*
B12	*Normal*
Folate	*Normal*
Creatinine	*121 umol/L (eGFR 42 mL/min, close to baseline)*

Why is she anaemic, and what workup should she receive?

The clinical presentation of anaemia depends on its severity, and whether its onset is abrupt or gradual.

- Mild to moderate chronic anaemia is often asymptomatic, and only incidentally diagnosed on blood tests.

- Severe chronic anaemia may be symptomatic, with lethargy, giddiness, dyspnoea and tachycardia. Physical findings include conjunctival and cutaneous pallor, a bounding heartbeat and a systolic flow murmur. Inadequate myocardial oxygen delivery can precipitate cardiac ischaemia.

- In acute blood loss, features of hypovolaemia dominate, such as postural hypotension, hypovolaemic shock and end organ hypoperfusion (cardiac ischaemia, delirium, acute kidney injury, etc.).

Normal FBC Values:

Hb	13–17 g/dL (male)
	12–16 g/dL (female)
WBC	3.4–9.6 × 10⁹/L
Plt	150–400 × 10⁹/L
MCV	80–95 fL
Retics[a]	0.5%–2%
RDW[b]	10.5%–16%

[a]Reticulocyte count.
[b]Red cell distribution width.
Normal ranges vary based on lab.

FBC, full blood count;
Hb, haemoglobin;
MCV, mean corpuscular volume;
WBC, white blood cells.

- Brisk acute intravascular haemolysis presents with jaundice, acute back pain, hae-moglobinuria and kidney injury.
- Chronic extravascular haemolytic anaemia may be well compensated, may manifest with symptoms of severe chronic anaemia, or with jaundice and signs of extramed-ullary haematopoiesis (see text).

Initial Approach

Begin by distinguishing broad classes of anaemia (Figure 32.1).

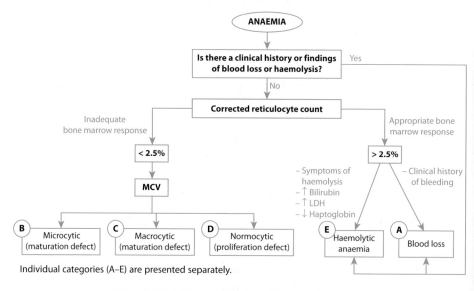

Individual categories (A–E) are presented separately.

Figure 32.1. Distinguishing broad classes of anaemia.

First, identify any clinical history of acute blood loss (e.g., trauma, massive gastro-intestinal bleed) or acute haemolysis (page 312). In the absence of such a history, initial tests include a full blood count, reticulocyte count, blood film, iron studies (ferritin, iron, total iron binding capacity (TIBC), B12 and folate levels. If there is any suspicion of haemolysis, do haemolytic markers (bilirubin, lactate dehydrogenase [LDH] and haptoglobin).

Reticulocytes are red blood cells that have recently been released from the bone marrow; their numbers reflect bone marrow production activity. The marrow is expected to respond to established anaemia of at least moderate severity (Hb < 10 g/dL) by increasing red cell production rate by 2 to 3× or more. Anaemia increases the per-centage of reticulocytes while the absolute number remains unchanged; a corrected reticulocyte count can be calculated as:

Corrected reticulocyte count (%)

$$= \text{Reticulocytes (\%)} \times \frac{\text{Patient's haemoglobin (g/dL)}}{\text{Expected haemoglobin for age and sex (g/dL)}}$$

A corrected reticulocyte count (also known as reticulocyte index) of >2.5% implies adequate bone marrow response, suggesting that the patient's anaemia is due to either blood loss or haemolytic destruction. These aetiologies can be distinguished on clinical history and from haemolytic markers. Recent repletion of iron, B12 or folate may also result in reticulocytosis, but this would be known in the clinical history.

Conversely, a corrected reticulocyte count of <2.5% suggests inadequate bone marrow response. In this situation, the next step will be to look at the mean corpuscular volume (MCV). Macrocytic (MCV > 95 fL) and microcytic (MCV < 80 fL) anaemia reflect red cell maturation defects. Normocytic anaemia (MCV 80–95 fL) suggests a decrease in red cell proliferation.

Subsequent sections discuss the individual categories of anaemia. Anaemia is often multifactorial—known thalassaemia does not preclude iron deficiency from colorectal malignancy!

A. Blood Loss

It is important to understand the different presentations of blood loss.

Following an acute haemorrhagic event, the first presentation is with symptoms and signs of hypovolaemia. As whole blood (both red cells and plasma) is lost, a haemoglobin level drawn at this point may be normal—do not be misled! It is only after fluid resuscitation (whether by physicians or by the body's own fluid conservation mechanisms) that haemoglobin levels fall, as a fixed amount of red cells is diluted by an increased plasma volume. If the bone marrow is normal, increased erythropoiesis kicks in, leading to a rise in reticulocyte count within 10 days.

The increase in erythropoiesis cannot go on indefinitely. In chronic blood loss, haematopoietic factors in the bone marrow become depleted, leading to a fall in erythropoiesis and therefore a fall in reticulocyte count. Iron is usually the first haematopoietic factor to be depleted. Therefore, the commonest presentation of chronic blood loss is asymptomatic iron-deficient anaemia—reticulocytes < 2.5% and low MCV. This is further discussed in page 308.

Clinical Approach

A sudden drop in haemoglobin with negative haemolytic markers (remember that reticulocytes may be normal for the first 10 days) suggests acute blood loss. The aetiology may be apparent from the clinical history, for example, trauma, gastrointestinal bleeding, vaginal bleeding or peri-procedural blood loss. Clinical examination may reveal fresh blood or melena in the rectal examination, or bleeding from an operative wound or vascular access line. Occult bleeding, most notably intra-abdominal haemorrhage, requires a high index of suspicion and CT imaging for diagnosis.

In chronic anaemia with either (a) elevated reticulocytes > 2.5% and negative haemolytic markers, or (b) chronic iron deficiency anaemia, search for symptoms of gastrointestinal or vaginal bleeding (see Chapters 11 and 52). If there are no symptoms, consider endoscopic evaluation of the gastrointestinal tract, which is the commonest source of occult chronic blood loss.

B. Production Defect: Microcytic

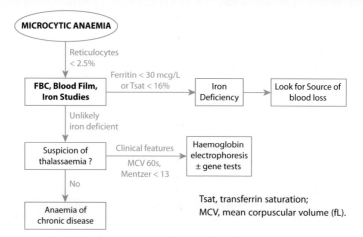

Figure 32.2. Approach to microcytic anaemia.

In microcytic anaemia, red cells are normal but there is insufficient haemoglobin to fill each cell, hence each red cell is small. Common aetiologies are (Figure 32.2):

- **Iron-deficiency anaemia**.

- **Thalassaemia**: Adults who present with microcytic anaemia usually have milder phenotypes (α thalassaemia trait, β thalassaemia minor). Severe phenotypes (β thalassaemia major, HbH disease) present in childhood with microcytic anaemia, splenomegaly and haemolysis.

- **Anaemia of chronic disease**: This may be normocytic or microcytic.

- **Sideroblastic anaemia**: A defect in incorporation of iron into heme, due to lead poisoning, drugs, congenital enzyme deficiencies and myelodysplastic syndrome. These are rare.

Approach

- **The FBC** gives an idea of whether thalassaemia is likely. In thalassaemia, red cells are very small (MCV in 60s) and uniform (low red cell distribution width [RDW]); blood film may also show target cells. In contrast, the red cells in iron deficiency are not as small (MCV 70s, although MCV 60s can occur in very severe iron deficiency) and less uniform (higher RDW). A Mentzer index (MCV divided by RBC count) < 13 is suggestive of thalassaemia (but neither sensitive nor specific).

- **Iron studies**: Iron studies should be obtained in all patients with microcytic anaemia. Ferritin reflects iron stores, and very low levels (e.g., < 30 mcg/L) are specific for iron deficiency; inflammation raises ferritin approximately threefold so in an inflammatory state, up to 100 mcg/L may indicate iron deficiency. Transferrin saturation (iron divided by total iron binding capacity) reflects the amount of iron binding to (i.e., 'saturating') iron binding proteins, levels < 16% suggest iron deficiency. Higher cut-offs are used in pregnancy and other conditions (e.g., renal impairment) where the threshold for iron supplementation is low.

- **Further testing in iron deficiency**: If iron deficiency is identified, search for an aetiology. The commonest cause is chronic occult gastrointestinal blood loss, which depletes iron stores. Ask for any history of blood loss (e.g., menorrhagia), and perform endoscopy for gastrointestinal causes of blood loss or malabsorption.
- **Suspected thalassaemia**: Pursue confirmatory tests:
  - β-thalassaemia: Haemoglobin electrophoresis[1] finds HbF ($\alpha_2\gamma_2$) and HbA2 ($\alpha_2\delta_2$); these are alternative haemoglobin types, which do not incorporate the defective β chain.
  - α-thalassaemia: Haemoglobin electrophoresis may reveal low levels of HbH (inclusion bodies of β_4, the normal globin chain, which is over-produced relative to the defective α chain), but may be normal, in which case diagnosis would require sequencing of the alpha-globin gene.

C. Production Defect: Macrocytic

In macrocytic anaemia, there is sufficient haemoglobin, but not enough red cells to fill with haemoglobin; this reflects defective red cell synthesis. Exclude reticulocytosis, which can raise the MCV as reticulocytes are larger than mature red cells (Figure 32.3).

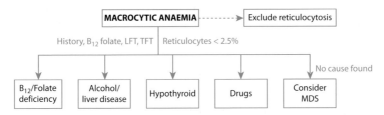

LFT, liver function test; MDS, myelodysplastic syndrome; TFT, thyroid function test.

Figure 32.3. Approach to macrocytic anaemia.

The aetiology of macrocytic anaemia can usually be identified on history and simple tests:

- **Megaloblastic anaemia—B12/folate deficiency**: This anaemia is named after red cells with large immature nuclei and multi-lobed neutrophils seen on the blood film. Macrocytosis may be severe (MCV > 115 fL), and other cell lines may be involved (may cause pancytopenia). Aetiologies of B12/folate deficiency include gastrointestinal malabsorption (e.g., in pernicious

Investigations

- B12 and folate levels
- If low—anti-intrinsic factor antibodies for pernicious anaemia

---

[1] Haemoglobin electrophoresis has been replaced by high performance liquid chromatography methods in some laboratories.

anaemia, gastrectomy, ileal resection, inflammatory bowel disease) and dietary insufficiency in vegans.

- **Alcohol and liver disease**: Heavy chronic alcohol use and non-alcoholic liver disease.

  – Liver function tests

- **Hypothyroidism**: The mechanism of macrocytosis is not well described.

  – Thyroid function tests

- **Drugs**: Especially hydroxyurea, cotrimoxazole, anti-retrovirals for HIV and chemotherapy drugs.

- **Myelodysplastic syndrome** should be considered if there is no other cause for macrocytosis found (see Chapter 34).

D. Production Defect: Normocytic

Normocytic anaemia, with low or inappropriately normal reticulocytes, reflects a bone marrow proliferation defect. First identify which cell lines are affected (Figure 32.4):

- **Hyper-proliferation** of one cell line (raised cell count), with suppression of other cell lines. This occurs in a bone marrow proliferative disorder, for example, leukaemia. See Chapter 34.

- **Isolated anaemia**: Proliferation defect affects only red cells, white cell and platelet counts are normal.

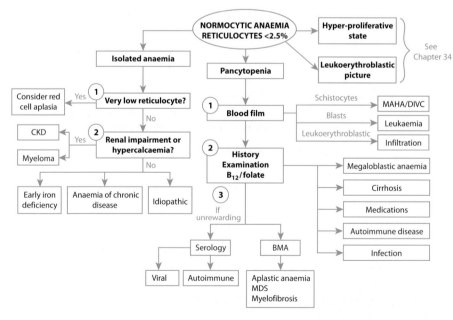

BMA, bone marrow aspirate; CKD, chronic kidney disease; DIVC, disseminated intravascular coagulation; MAHA, microangiopathic haemolytic anaemia.

Figure 32.4. Approach to normocytic anaemia.

- **Pancytopenia or bicytopenia**: Proliferation defect affecting multiple cell lines. The approach to bicytopenia is, in most cases, similar to that to pancytopenia.

- **Leukoerythroblastic picture**: Blood film showing immature RBCs and WBCs (nucleated RBC, myelocyte, metamyelocytes), and teardrop-shaped erythrocytes. This reflects bone marrow replacement, commonly by malignancy or myelofibrosis (Chapter 34).

Isolated Anaemia

Initial investigations include reticulocytes, serum creatinine, calcium and iron studies.

1. Profound anaemia with very low reticulocytes suggests **red cell aplasia**, a disorder due to immunologic attack on red cell precursors. Workup usually includes a bone marrow aspirate. Causes include:

   - Idiopathic.

   - Associated with myelodysplastic syndrome or myeloproliferative disease.

   - Autoimmune disorders: Lupus, rheumatoid arthritis.

   - Infection: Parvovirus B19, milder episodes with other viral illnesses (e.g., hepatitis, HIV, Epstein–Barr virus [EBV], cytomegalovirus [CMV]).

   - Congenital (Diamond–Blackfan anaemia).

   - Thymoma.

2. In the presence of renal impairment, consider:

   - **Chronic kidney disease (CKD)**: Grades 4–5 CKD (eGFR < 30) are associated with erythropoietin deficiency (which is produced by the kidneys) and normocytic anaemia. Rule out concomitant iron deficiency, which must be treated before starting erythropoiesis stimulating agents.

   - **Multiple myeloma**: The cardinal features are hyper*c*alcaemia, *r*enal impairment, *a*naemia and lytic lesions in *b*one (the 'CRAB' symptoms), not all of which may be present at initial presentation. Patients may be symptomatic from anaemia, hypercalcaemia or bone lesions, or be entirely asymptomatic. If myeloma is suspected, do serum calcium, serum and urine protein electrophoresis, plus serum free light chain as an initial screen.

3. After the above have been excluded, consider:

   - **Early iron deficiency**: This may be normocytic initially before microcytosis sets in.

   - **Anaemia of chronic disease**: Chronic infection, inflammation or malignancy may be associated with anaemia. This is common, but it is a diagnosis of exclusion.

   - **Myelodysplasia**: This may present as isolated anaemia. Presence of significant morphologic dysplasia (≥ 10% of red cells, white cells or platelets) should prompt suspicion of myelodysplasia.

   - **Idiopathic**: There are a number of patients who have unexplained anaemia.

Pancytopenia (or Bicytopenia)

The mechanisms of pancytopenia can be divided into bone marrow infiltration, aplasia or blood cell destruction. A stepwise approach:

1. Be sure to consider the following potential emergencies, on clinical history and blood film.

   - **Microangiopathic haemolytic anaemia (MAHA)** and disseminated intravascular coagulation (DIVC): Suggested by findings of haemolysis (elevated bilirubin and LDH, haptoglobin consumption, schistocytes and fragmented red cells on blood film), in a sick patient (page 322).

   - **Leukaemia**: Occasionally there are circulating blasts on the FBC, without overall elevation of the white cell count (see Chapter 34).

   - **Marrow infiltration**: Will show a leukoerythroblastic blood film (see Chapter 34).

2. Next, attempt to identify the following aetiologies based on clinical history, examination, B12 and folate levels.

   - **Megaloblastic anaemia**: Severe B12 or folate deficiency can present not only with macrocytic anaemia, but also with pancytopenia. MCV is elevated, and large immature nuclei and multi-lobed neutrophils are seen on blood film.

   - **Medications**: Cytotoxic drugs predictably cause pancytopenia. Other drugs may cause pancytopenia as an idiosyncratic side effect, these include antibiotics (linezolid, cotrimoxazole, others), antiepileptics, anti-thyroid medication and immunosuppressants.

   - **Cirrhosis with hypersplenism**: Pancytopenia occurs in cirrhotics due to splenic sequestration (see Chapter 10).

   - **Autoimmune disease**: Patients with autoimmune disease (e.g., lupus, rheumatoid arthritis, sarcoidosis) often have cytopenias, which may be due to the disease itself, B12/folate deficiency or as a side effect of drugs (e.g., methotrexate).

   - **Infection**: Marrow suppression may occur in malaria and some viral infections (e.g., HIV, hepatitis, EBV).

3. If (2) is unrewarding, consider:

   - **Serological screen** for autoimmune disease (antinuclear antibody [ANA], dsDNA) and viral illness (HIV, hepatitis, EBV, CMV).

   - **Bone marrow aspirate**: For aplastic anaemia, ineffective erythropoiesis in myelodysplastic syndromes, or marrow replacement in myelofibrosis.

E. Haemolytic Anaemia

Haemolytic anaemia is a syndrome of increased red cell destruction outside the bone marrow, resulting in a shortened red cell lifespan. Haemolysis may occur within blood vessels (intravascular), within the spleen (extravascular) or both.

Apart from general features of anaemia, patients may have signs and symptoms arising directly from haemolysis. Bilirubin breakdown results in *jaundice, dark urine* and bilirubin gallstones. Acute intravascular haemolysis results in the release of free haemoglobin, causing back pain, haemoglobinuria and renal impairment. Chronic extravascular haemolysis preferentially occurs in the spleen, resulting in splenomegaly and to a lesser extent, hepatomegaly. Severe congenital haemolytic anaemia (particularly thalassaemia) leads to extramedullary haematopoiesis, and the classic 'thalassaemic facies' with frontal bossing, maxillary prominence and dental malocclusion. There may be a family history in congenital causes. However, the absence of any symptoms does not exclude the possibility of haemolytic anaemia.

Biochemical evidence of haemolysis includes elevated unconjugated bilirubin, elevated LDH (released from lysed red cells) and low haptoglobin (this binds to free haemoglobin and so is consumed; it is also an acute phase reactant so levels in inflammatory states may be misleadingly normal). The bone marrow is normal and compensates for haemolysis by increasing erythropoiesis, leading to reticulocytosis. However, in all types of haemolytic anaemia, an intercurrent illness (e.g., infection) may depress erythropoiesis, leading to decompensation and more severe anaemia.

A classification of the haemolytic anaemias is first presented, followed by a suggested approach to distinguish major causes, and then a discussion of certain aetiologies.

Pathophysiologic Classification

The causes of haemolytic anaemia may be mechanistically classified into broad groups:

Inherited

- Red cell membrane or cytoskeletal defects
  - Hereditary spherocytosis
  - Hereditary elliptocytosis
- Red cell enzyme defects
  - Glucose 6-phosphate dehydrogenase (G6PD) deficiency
  - Others
- Haemoglobinopathies
  - Thalassaemia
  - Sickle cell anaemia
  - Others, for example, HbE

Acquired

- Autoimmune haemolytic anaemia (AIHA)
  - Warm AIHA
  - Cold AIHA
- Alloimmune haemolytic anaemia
  - Haemolytic transfusion reaction
  - Haemolytic disease of the new-born
- Paroxysmal nocturnal haemoglobinuria
- Microangiopathic haemolytic anaemia (MAHA)
  - Disseminated intravascular coagulation
  - Thrombotic thrombocytopenic purpura–Haemolytic uraemic syndrome (TTP–HUS)
- Mechanical red cell fragmentation
  - Cardiac: prosthetic valves
  - March haemoglobinuria
- Infections: Malaria, others

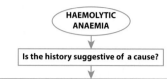

History	Suggested diagnosis	Further testing
– Haemolysis during or after blood transfusion	→ Haemolytic transfusion reaction	→ Check for ABO mismatch → Repeat GXM + direct Coombs' test Contact blood bank
– Episodic haemolysis triggered by oxidative stress	→ G6PD deficiency	→ G6PD enzyme activity
– Septic patient	→ Malaria → TTP-HUS, DIVC	→ Thick & thin blood films → PT/PTT, Platelets, Fibrinogen, D-dimers
– Haemolysis from childhood, family history	→ Congenital causes	→ Peripheral blood film Haemoglobin electrophoresis Other specific tests
– Classic thalassaemic facies	→ Thalassemia	→ Haemoglobin electrophoresis
– Haemoglobinuria, unusual site thrombosis	→ Paroxysmal nocturnal haemoglobinuria	→ Flow cytometry
– Prosthetic valve with regurgitation	→ Mechanical haemolysis	

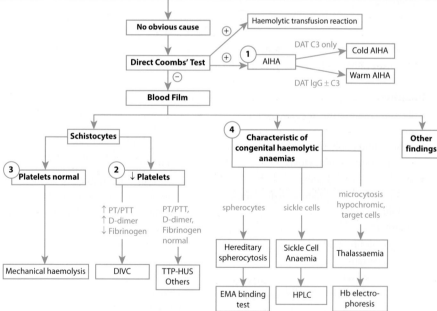

AIHA, autoimmune haemolytic anaemia; DAT, direct antiglobulin test (Coombs' test); DIVC, disseminated intravascular coagulation; EMA, eosin-5'-maleimide; HPLC, high performance liquid chromatography; TTP–HUS, thrombotic thrombocytopenic purpura–haemolytic uraemic syndrome.

Figure 32.5. Approach to haemolytic anaemia.

A Clinical Approach

Begin with a clinical history, which may suggest a particular cause (Figure 32.5). If so, specific confirmatory testing should be pursued. Two other basic tests are particularly helpful.

- **Direct antiglobulin test** (direct Coombs' test): This detects anti-RBC antibodies by reacting washed RBCs with anti-human antibodies. A positive test suggests autoimmune haemolytic anaemia (AIHA) or transfusion-related haemolysis.

- **Peripheral blood film**: Look for schistocytes, that is, fragmented red cells (in MAHA), spherocytes (in hereditary spherocytosis and AIHA), sickle cells (sickle cell anaemia), microcytic hypochromic red cells and target cells resembling iron-deficiency anaemia (thalassaemia), Heinz bodies and bite cells (glucose 6-phosphate dehydrogenase [G6PD] deficiency or oxidative haemolysis).

If there is clinical suspicion of haemolysis and the patient will receive a blood transfusion, consider sending the Coombs' test and blood film prior to transfusion, as they can be inaccurate after transfusion.

1. Autoimmune Haemolytic Anaemia

A positive direct Coombs' test is followed by testing with anti-IgG and anti-C3d.

This identifies two forms of autoimmune haemolytic anaemia (AIHA):

- Cold-related haemolysis (Anti-C3d positive)
  - **Cold agglutinin disease (Cold AIHA):** Anaemia and symptoms on cold exposure, including skin changes (livedo reticularis, acrocyanosis of extremities), which disappear on warming, or discomfort on swallowing cold liquids. There are IgM antibodies, which fix complement to RBC membrane antigens at cold temperatures, leading to intravascular haemolysis. Peripheral blood film shows agglutination of red cells with a falsely raised MCV.

  - **Paroxysmal cold haemoglobinuria:** Intravascular haemolysis and haemoglobinuria (dark urine, flank pain, jaundice) on exposure to cold. There is a specific IgG antibody (the Donath–Landsteiner antibody) that binds RBC in the cold, and causes haemolysis on rewarming.

Aetiologies: Workup for:

- Infection: especially mycoplasma and EBV
- Malignancy, especially chronic lymphocytic lymphoma (CLL)—consider protein electrophoresis, flow cytometry and bone marrow aspirate

- Post-infective: classically syphilis, more commonly viral illness
- Autoimmune disease
- CLL and lymphoma

- **Warm AIHA** (Anti-IgG positive): Caused by IgG antibodies (± complement) that bind to RBC antigens at 37°C, marking RBCs for phagocytic destruction by splenic macrophages (i.e., extravascular haemolysis). Peripheral blood film may show spherocytes. Immune thrombocytopenia may accompany AIHA (Evans syndrome). Haemoglobin can drop quite rapidly in warm AIHA.

  − Autoimmune disease: e.g., SLE
  − Infections: viral infections, HIV
  − Malignancy, for example, lymphoma, CLL
  − 50% are idiopathic

- **Either pattern—Drug-induced autoimmune haemolysis**: A number of drugs may precipitate autoimmune haemolysis, most notably cephalosporins, penicillins and NSAIDs.

2. Microangiopathic Haemolytic Anaemia

The MAHA result from mechanical shearing of red cells as they pass through intravascular microthrombi. Hallmarks are features of haemolysis (jaundice, raised LDH, low haptoglobin), evidence of red cell fragmentation (schistocytes on blood film), and thrombocytopenia. The MAHA syndromes include:

- Thrombotic thrombocytopenic purpura–haemolytic uraemic syndrome (TTP–HUS).
- Disseminated intravascular coagulation (DIVC).
- Pre-eclampsia and haemolysis, elevated liver enzymes and low platelets (HELLP) syndrome: These are serious complications of pregnancy, with hypertension, proteinuria, transaminitis, thrombocytopenia and MAHA.
- Other thrombotic microangiopathy syndromes.

TTP–HUS and DIVC are discussed in greater detail on page 322.

3. Non-MAHA Causes of Mechanical Red Cell Fragmentation

Apart from MAHA, the other mechanical causes of red cell fragmentation show a normal platelet count. Evidence of mechanical haemolysis (schistocytes) is still seen. These aetiologies include:

- Malignant hypertension.
- Haemodynamic turbulence around prosthetic intravascular material, most commonly seen in leaky prosthetic valves. Also seen in stenotic native valves, ventricular assist devices or AV malformations.
- March haemoglobinuria: Direct trauma to red cells in peripheral blood vessels, classically seen in soldiers after a long march, marathon runners or drumming enthusiasts.

4. Congenital Causes

The congenital haemolytic anaemias may be due to defects in red cell membrane or cytoskeleton, enzymes or haemoglobin (listed on page 313). They may be identified based by a classic history (as in glucose 6-phosphate dehydrogenase [G6PD]), by blood film findings, or on more specific screening tests. The commonest congenital haemolytic anaemias are:

Diagnostic investigations:

- **Hereditary spherocytosis**: A disorder of erythrocyte membrane due to defective spectrin. Extravascular haemolysis in the spleen leads to splenomegaly. Spherocytes are seen on blood film (also seen in AIHA)

  − Eosin-5'-maleimide (EMA) binding test (has replaced osmotic fragility test)

- **Thalassaemia**: Discussed on page 308. Haemolysis is typically less marked than anaemia and extramedullary haematopoiesis.

  − Haemoglobin electrophoresis

- **Sickle cell disease**: HbS, a beta globin chain variant, leads to sickling of red cells, which can be visualised on blood film. Apart from haemolytic anaemia, patients suffer vaso-occlusive phenomena including painful vaso-occlusive crises, acute chest syndrome, stroke, renal infarction, myocardial infarction and venous thromboembolism.

  − High performance liquid chromatography to identify HbS
  − Sickling test/Sickle solubility test

- **Glucose 6-phosphate dehydrogenase (G6PD) deficiency**: This presents in males (X-linked disease) with episodes of acute intravascular haemolysis precipitated by oxidative stress, when exposed to (a) fava beans, (b) infections and (c) drugs, particularly co-trimoxazole, primaquine, dapsone and rasburicase. Acute episodes can be severe, but with complete recovery and no symptoms between attacks.

  − Measure G6PD enzyme levels (may be falsely normal after a haemolytic episode—may need to recheck)

5. Others

Diagnostic investigations:

- **Haemolytic transfusion reaction**: *Acute* haemolytic transfusion reactions, due to ABO incompatibility, present with immediate hypotension, fever, features of intravascular haemolysis (flank pain, haemoglobinuria, renal injury) and coagulopathy (features of DIVC)—this is an emergency. *Delayed* transfusion reactions arise from an antibody response to minor red cell

  − Clerical check of whether the correct blood product has been transfused
  − Repeat group and cross-match (GXM) and antibody identification

antigens, and usually occurs 5 to 10 days after transfusion. Direct Coombs' test is positive.

- **Paroxysmal nocturnal haemoglobinuria**: Unexplained Coombs' negative *haemolytic anaemia*, and/or other *cytopenias*, and/or venous *thrombosis* in atypical locations (e.g., portal vein, mesenteric vein). There may be episodes of jaundice and pink/red urine from haemoglobinuria, which classically occur at night. This is due to an acquired PIG-A gene mutation in a haematopoietic stem cell, creating a population of *clonal RBCs*, which lack a cell membrane protein (CD55, CD59). This results in increased susceptibility of RBCs to complement lysis.

  – Flow cytometry: detects deficiency of CD55, CD59
  – Ham's test used to be done in the past
  – Look for associated bone marrow failure syndromes, for example, aplastic anaemia, myelodysplastic syndrome

- **Infections—especially Malaria**: Always consider in a patient who presents with sepsis and anaemia after travel to a malaria-endemic location.

  – Thick and thin blood films

 Using what you have learnt, **pen down your approach** to the Clinical Case at the start of the chapter **BEFORE reading the discussion** below.

Case Discussion

This lady has developed moderate anaemia in one year. Other cell lines are unaffected. Given no history of acute blood loss or haemolysis, and a corrected reticulocyte count of 1.5% × (8.7/12) = 1.1% (low), her anaemia is likely due to decreased red cell production. Low iron saturations (8%) provide evidence of iron deficiency which should cause microcytic anaemia. Unexpectedly, her MCV is normocytic, suggesting that she has a concomitant microcytic (iron-deficiency) and macrocytic anaemia. The latter is most probably due to methotrexate, which inhibits dihydrofolate reductase, leading to a functional folate deficiency even if measured folate levels are normal. She has chronic kidney disease but this is unlikely to cause moderate anaemia until eGFR < 30 mL/min. Finally, there may also be a component of anaemia of chronic disease, due to her chronic inflammatory state.

In the first instance, she should be evaluated for a cause of iron deficiency—in particular, endoscopic evaluation for a gastrointestinal malignancy should be considered.

Key Lessons	1. The causes of anaemia can be divided into blood loss, haemolysis, or decreased production (microcytic, microcytic or normocytic), based on corrected reticulocyte counts and MCV.
	2. Common causes of microcytic anaemia with low reticulocytes are iron deficiency, thalassaemia and chronic disease.

3. Common causes of macrocytic anaemia with low reticulocytes are B12/folate deficiency, alcohol or drug use and hypothyroidism.

4. The approach to normocytic anaemia with low reticulocytes begins by identifying which cell lines are affected. Anaemia alone is seen in renal disease, myeloma, red cell aplasia and chronic disease. Pancytopenia is seen in microangiopathic haemolysis, malignancy including myelodysplastic syndromes, severe B12/folate deficiency, medications, infections, cirrhosis, autoimmune disease or aplastic anaemia.

5. Evidence of haemolysis includes jaundice, elevated bilirubin and LDH and reduced haptoglobin. History, blood film and a direct Coombs' test divides the causes of haemolysis into: autoimmune haemolysis, transfusion reactions, microangiopathic haemolysis, infective and congenital causes.

Common Pitfalls

1. Patients often have multiple concomitant causes of anaemia; MCV can be spuriously normal.

2. Blood transfusion may obfuscate the results of anaemia workup (except ferritin, which is not affected by transfusion). Except in an emergency, attempt to collect all specimens required for anaemia workup before transfusing blood.

Questions

1. **REFLECT!** Have you ever met a patient with G6PD deficiency? Was he (usually not she) symptomatic? What are the common medications that he should not take?

2. **DISCUSS!** There are many patients with anaemia. How do you decide if a patient (a) can be investigated and treated in the community, (b) should be referred for endoscopy or (c) should be referred to a haematologist?

3. **EXPLORE!** When should you correct a patient's anaemia with blood transfusion?

4. **GO FURTHER!** Look for pictures of the following blood films: iron deficiency, thalassaemia, megaloblastic anaemia, acute leukaemia, leukoerythroblastic picture, schistocytes, bite cells, sickle cells and spherocytes.

Chapter **An Approach to**

33 **Abnormal Bleeding**

Clinical Case

A 30-year-old lady presents with a 1-month history of petechial rashes, epistaxis and gum bleeding. She works as a teacher and has no medical history. Apart from an oral contraceptive, she does not take any drugs. Examination is unremarkable except for non-palpable dark macules on bilateral lower limbs. There is no splenomegaly. A full blood count shows: haemoglobin 12.8 g/dL, WBC 7.0 × 10⁹/L, platelet 28 × 10⁹/L. PT and aPTT are normal. What is the most likely diagnosis? What are the disorders to exclude?

This chapter discusses the systemic causes of abnormal bleeding. Where bleeding presents in a single organ, consider local anatomical abnormalities causing bleeding—see the approaches to gastrointestinal bleed (see Chapter 11), menorrhagia (see Chapter 52), haemoptysis (see Chapter 8) and haemorrhagic stroke (see Chapter 25).

Normal haemostasis requires (1) vasoconstriction, (2) platelet plug formation and (3) coagulation cascade activation. Hence, the causes of a bleeding diathesis may be pathophysiologically classified in Table 33.1.

Table 33.1. Pathophysiologic Classification of a Bleeding Diathesis

	Coagulation defect	Platelet defect	Vascular defect

Inherited	Haemophilia
	Von Willebrand
	  disease
		(rare)	Connective tissue
			  disease
			HHT

Acquired	Over-anticoagulation
	DIVC
	Liver disease
	Vitamin K deficiency
	Massive transfusion
	Drugs
		Decreased production:
		  bone marrow dysfunction
		  (malignancy, aplasia, myelodysplasia),
		  megaloblastic anaemia
		
		Increased destruction:
		  primary (ITP),
		  secondary (SLE, TTP–HUS, DIVC, dengue, HIV),
		  drugs
		
		Abnormal function:
		  myelofibrosis, uraemia, drugs
			Vasculitis
			Meningococcaemia

DIVC, disseminated intravascular coagulation; HHT, hereditary haemorrhagic telangiectasia; ITP, immune thrombocytopenia; SLE, systemic lupus erythematosus; TTP–HUS, thrombotic thrombocytopenic purpura–haemolytic uraemic syndrome.

A Clinical Approach

The traditional classification is conceptually helpful. Clinically, however, it is far more efficient to streamline the likely aetiology based on the clinical picture (Figure 33.1).

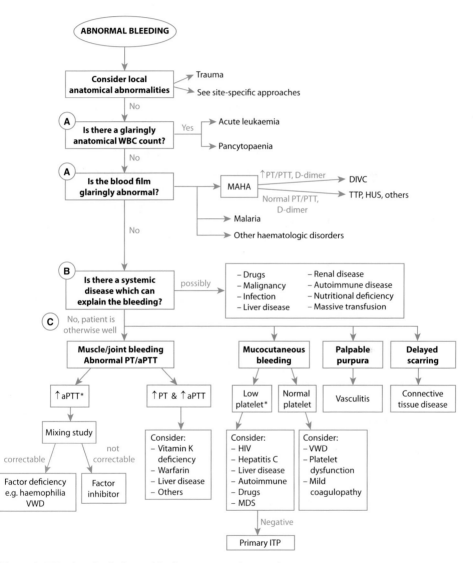

*Elevated aPTT or low platelet but no bleeding: see caveat (page 326).

DIVC, disseminated intravascular coagulation; HUS, haemolytic uraemic syndrome; ITP, immune thrombocytopenia; MAHA, microangiopathic haemolytic anaemia; MDS, myelodysplastic syndrome; TTP, thrombotic thrombocytopenic purpura; VWD, Von Willebrand disease.

Figure 33.1. Clinical approach to a bleeding diathesis.

A. Glaringly Abnormal WBC/Blood Film

Having considered local anatomical abnormalities, look at the full blood count and the peripheral blood film. These may reveal glaring abnormalities—in these disorders bleeding is merely a proverbial tip of the iceberg!

- **Acute leukaemia**: Blasts > 20%, usually (but not always) with a grossly elevated white cell count (page 332).
- **Pancytopenia**: Reduced red cells, white cells and platelets (see page 312).
- **Microangiopathic haemolytic anaemia (MAHA)**: Schistocytes, fragmented red cells and thrombocytopenia (discussed later).
- **Fulminant malaria**: At high parasite densities, a good haematology technician may spot plasmodia in a blood film. At lower parasite densities, however, you will probably have to order thick and thin blood films for diagnosis.
- **Suggestion of other haematological disease**: Leukoerythroblastic picture (immature red and white cells, teardrop cells—page 335), myelofibrosis (giant platelets, fragmented megakaryocytes) or myelodysplasia (significant morphologic dysplasia).

These disorders demand immediate attention and workup. On a less urgent note, the blood film may also detect other abnormalities suggesting specific diseases, for example, B12/folate deficiency (megaloblasts, hypersegmented neutrophils), uraemia (echinocytes)—these are also helpful when considering systemic causes.

Microangiopathic Haemolytic Anaemia

The MAHA deserve further discussion. These result from mechanical shearing of red cells as they pass through intravascular microthrombi. MAHA usually presents as an ill patient with thrombocytopenia (which may cause bleeding), haemolysis (jaundice, raised LDH, low haptoglobin) and red cell fragmentation (schistocytes). The MAHAs include:

- **Disseminated intravascular coagulation** (DIVC): Pathological activation of the coagulation cascade causes widespread thrombosis, consuming platelets and clotting factors, which then causes paradoxical bleeding. Antecedent triggers include severe sepsis, malignancy, trauma and severe pre-eclampsia; patients are usually very sick with multi-organ dysfunction. Biochemical testing reveals coagulopathy, and fibrinogen consumption leading to low fibrinogen and elevated fibrin degradation products (e.g., D dimer). Diagnosis of DIVC mandates evaluation for a cause—a source of sepsis, an acute leukaemia (especially acute promyelocytic leukaemia) and so forth.
- **Thrombotic thrombocytopenic purpur**a (TTP): Decreased ADAMTS13 activity causes accumulation of very large Von Willebrand Factor multimers, which bind platelets at the endothelium, leading to microvascular haemolysis. The decrease in ADAMTS13 activity may be acquired, due to an autoantibody inhibitor, or hereditary, due to an inherited mutation. The pentad of TTP includes MAHA, thrombocytopenia, fever, neurological dysfunction (confusion, headache, seizures)

and renal injury; unlike DIVC, the coagulation cascade is not activated and PT/aPTT is normal. TTP should be suspected in the presence of MAHA and thrombocytopenia with normal PT/PTT; fever, neurological and renal dysfunction are late signs, and delaying treatment is associated with poor outcomes.

- **Haemolytic uraemic syndrome (HUS)**: Shiga toxin released by pathogenic *Escherichia coli* triggers a multisystem disease. This is typically a child who first suffers bloody diarrhoea, and 5 to 10 days later, develops MAHA, thrombocytopenia and acute kidney injury (more severe than TTP); there may also be neurologic dysfunction (milder than TTP) and colitis.

- **Pregnancy-related MAHA**: Pre-eclampsia (hypertension and proteinuria), HELLP syndrome (*h*aemolysis, *e*levated *l*iver enzymes and *l*ow *p*latelets) are serious pregnancy-related disorders.

- There are other thrombotic microangiopathy syndromes; MAHA may also be triggered by drugs, hereditary deficiencies of complement or coagulant pathway proteins and severe B12 deficiency. The nomenclature and classification of these disorders is rapidly evolving, as their pathophysiology becomes better understood.

B. Bleeding Due to Systemic Disease

A number of systemic diseases can lead to bleeding. These may be known diagnoses, suspected on history and examination, or identified on basic laboratory investigations (e.g., renal function, liver panel, etc.)

	Workup
• **Drug**: A complete drug list should be scrutinised. Identify drugs which may cause coagulopathy (anticoagulants in excess) or bone marrow suppression (chemotherapy, antithyroid agents, methotrexate, etc.). Some drugs cause idiosyncratic platelet destruction—for example, antibiotics (linezolid, cotrimoxazole, beta lactams) and anticonvulsants.	– Clinical suspicion – PT/INR for over-warfarinization
• **Malignancy** may lead to bleeding in many ways: (a) marrow suppression or infiltration, (b) DIVC, (c) tumour-related immune thrombocytopenia and other autoimmune mechanisms, (d) treatment-related complications.	– Clinical suspicion based on constitutional symptoms, focal symptoms and so forth
• **Certain acute infections**: For example, malaria, meningococcaemia and dengue fever are particularly known for bleeding. Other forms of severe sepsis may cause DIVC, or thrombocytopenia from myelosuppression.	– Workup based on clinical suspicion, e.g., dengue serology
• **Liver disease**: Defective clotting factor synthesis in acute liver failure results in coagulopathy. Hypersplenism in cirrhosis results in thrombocytopenia (even pancytopenia).	– Liver function test

- **Renal disease**: Uraemia causes platelet dysfunction despite a normal platelet count.
  − Serum creatinine

- **Autoimmune disease**: There may be autoimmune platelet destruction (e.g., in lupus, rheumatoid arthritis), or palpable purpura as a presentation of vasculitis.
  − Specific workup, serology

- **Nutritional deficiency**: Fat malabsorption (see Chapter 13) may result in vitamin K deficiency, and inadequate synthesis of clotting factors.
  − aPTT/PT

- **Massive blood transfusion**: Results in depletion of clotting factors. This is why massive transfusion protocols always include fresh frozen plasma, to provide clotting factors.
  − Clinical history

Caveat: The very presence of any of these diseases does not necessarily imply that it is the cause of bleeding; it may well be an innocent bystander. For instance, aspirin may exacerbate bleeding due to another cause, but it alone does not typically cause bleeding.

C. An Otherwise Well Patient

These are patients who do not have a systemic disease that can explain bleeding, or whose systemic disease is deemed unlikely to be the cause of bleeding. They are usually well and asymptomatic apart from bleeding. Before proceeding with further workup, repeat the platelet count and PT/aPTT. Ensure that there are no platelet clumps on the blood film; this may artificially lower the platelet count (pseudothrombocytopenia). Consider four main presentations (Figure 33.1).

- **Coagulopathies**: These typically present with intramuscular haematomas and haemarthrosis, which may arise from minor trauma and fail to stop. PT and/or aPTT is deranged.

- **Platelet disorders**: Mucocutaneous bleeding (petechiae, purpura, gum bleeding) and menorrhagia is typical. The platelet disorder may be quantitative (thrombocytopenia) or qualitative (normal platelet count).

- **Vasculitis**: Palpable purpura is suggestive of a vasculitic disorder (page 389).

- **Connective tissue disease**: Delayed scarring is suggestive of a connective tissue disease (in contrast, patients with platelet disorders tend to bleed immediately after vascular trauma). In younger patients, consider Ehler–Danlos syndrome and hereditary haemorrhagic telangiectasia (HHT). In older patients, consider skin atrophy due to senile purpura, topical steroids or Cushing's disease. This will not be covered in further detail.

Coagulopathies

Identify if aPTT is prolonged, PT is prolonged or both are prolonged. Common causes are presented:

(a) **Prolonged aPTT**: The next step is to perform a mixing study (adding normal serum, which contains clotting factors, to patient serum):

- **Correctable on mixing**: Suggests factor deficiency, for example, haemophilia A (factor 8 deficiency) or B (factor 9 deficiency) (rarely factor 11 deficiency). These are X-linked recessive diseases, which present in males. Confirm the diagnosis by testing factor activity (8 and 9 initially, if normal then consider 11). Severe Von Willebrand disease (VWD) manifests with intra-articular bleeding, mimicking haemophilia, other cases demonstrate prolonged aPTT but have a mucocutaneous pattern of bleeding.

- **Not correctable**: Suggests a factor inhibitor causing acquired haemophilia (cannot be overcome by adding normal serum). These may be idiopathic, or associated with rheumatoid arthritis, lupus, malignancy or drug reactions.

(b) **Prolonged PT ± aPTT**:

- Warfarin use or other cause of vitamin K deficiency.
- Early liver disease.
- Mild coagulopathy.
- Rarer causes, for example, abnormalities of fibrinogen, rarer inherited factor deficiency (factor 7 deficiency presents with isolated prolonged PT; factor 2, 5 or 10 deficiency present with prolonged PT/aPTT).

Platelet Disorders

(a) **Mucocutaneous bleeding with thrombocytopenia**: A patient with no other cause of thrombocytopenia (drugs, overt infection, liver disease), no coagulopathy and an otherwise normal white cell count and blood film is most likely to have immune thrombocytopenia (ITP, also known as idiopathic thrombocytopenic purpura). This may be:

- **Secondary ITP**: Screen for HIV, hepatitis C. Consider autoimmune workup if there are suggestive clinical features.

- **Primary ITP**: This is a relatively common disease. Patients are well apart from mucocutaneous bleeding. It is a diagnosis of exclusion not requiring bone marrow aspirate. However, it is common practice to perform bone marrow aspirate if the case is atypical, if the patient is over 50 (to exclude myelodysplastic syndrome), or if the patient does not respond to first-line treatment.

(b) **Mucocutaneous bleeding without thrombocytopenia**

- **Von Willebrand disease (VWD)**: VWD is often asymptomatic, or may present with mucocutaneous bleeding or menorrhagia. Rarely, bleeding is severe and may mimic haemophilia. Platelet levels are usually normal, aPTT may be normal or prolonged. Unlike haemophilia, this may occur in males and females. If suspecting VWD, perform an initial screen—VWF antigen, ristocetin cofactor activity and factor 8.

- **Platelet dysfunction**: Rare causes, including Bernard–Soulier syndrome, Wiskott–Aldrich syndrome and so forth. Platelet function testing should be performed if suspected.

- Mild coagulopathies may show a normal aPTT/PT.

Caveat: Thrombocytopenia or Coagulopathy with Paradoxical Thrombosis

These disorders should be considered in the work up of a patient with incidentally detected thrombocytopenia or prolonged aPTT, but no bleeding manifestations. They paradoxically present with thrombosis rather than bleeding.

- **Antiphospholipid syndrome**: The lupus anticoagulant results in a prolonged aPTT that is not correctable on mixing with normal serum. This is a laboratory artefact—the antiphospholipid syndrome is associated with thrombosis (venous thrombosis, stroke and transient ischaemic attack, recurrent pregnancy loss, etc.) instead of bleeding. It may be a primary disorder, or associated with lupus.

- **Heparin-induced thrombocytopenia**: Typically, thrombocytopenia develops 5 to 10 days after starting heparin, with platelets falling more than 30% to 50% but with a nadir $> 20 \times 10^9$. Patients may develop arterial or venous thrombosis. The 4Ts score provides a clinical probability estimate. If the 4Ts score is of intermediate or high probability, send anti-PF4 antibodies and begin empiric treatment.

- **Paroxysmal nocturnal haemoglobinuria**: Haemolytic anaemia, other cytopenias, atypical venous thrombosis (page 318).

   Using what you have learnt, **pen down your approach** to the Clinical Case at the start of the chapter **BEFORE reading the discussion** below.

Case Discussion

This is a young lady who is well apart from thrombocytopenia and mucocutaneous bleeding. The history is suggestive of immune thrombocytopenia (idiopathic thrombocytopenic purpura), but this is a diagnosis of exclusion; more serious causes of bleeding should first be excluded.

Examine a blood film to ensure that there are no schistocytes (MAHA, although this is clinically unlikely with a 1-month history) or dysplastic cells. Take a careful history to exclude drugs that may cause thrombocytopenia (e.g., antibiotics for urinary tract infection, herbal supplements, etc.). Ask for any symptoms that would suggest autoimmune disease (e.g., joint pain, malaria, rash, etc.). It is important that her shin macules are non-palpable, as palpable purpura would suggest a vasculitis. Perform HIV, hepatitis C and liver function testing. If the above are all negative, a diagnosis of primary immune thrombocytopenia can be made.

Key Lessons	1. Four questions are helpful in the initial approach to abnormal bleeding: (a) are there site-specific anatomical abnormalities? (b) Is the WBC count normal? (c) Is the blood film normal? (d) Are there systemic diseases that can explain bleeding?
	2. Glaring causes of bleeding to rule out are: acute leukaemia, pancytopenia, microangiopathic haemolytic anaemia and fulminant malaria.
	3. In an otherwise well patient, consider four main presentations: (a) muscle/joint bleeding from coagulopathy, inherited (haemophilia) or acquired (e.g., warfarin); (b) mucocutaneous bleeding with thrombocytopenia (as in immune thrombocytopenia), or with normal platelet counts (as in Von Willebrand disease); (c) palpable purpura in vasculitis; and (d) delayed scarring in connective tissue disorders.
Common Pitfalls	1. Not all patients who bleed while on aspirin or warfarin do so because of the drug. Evaluate for other causes of bleeding, before blaming the antiplatelet or anticoagulant. Failure to do so may miss potentially serious disorders.
	2. Some acute leukaemias (most notably acute promyelocytic leukaemia) present with bleeding, and should be a differential in patients who present with acute bleeding.
Questions	1. **REFLECT!** Have you ever encountered a patient with MAHA? What did he/she present with, and was MAHA suspected immediately? If not, what was the initial diagnosis, and what prompted suspicion of MAHA?
	2. **DISCUSS!** A patient first presents with a bleeding diathesis. On the physical examination, what will you look out for?
	3. **EXPLORE!** When would platelet transfusion be indicated to correct thrombocytopenia?
	4. **GO FURTHER!** Platelet clumping causes pseudothrombocytopenia. How would you overcome this laboratory error?

Chapter
34

An Approach to
High Cell Counts

Clinical Case

A 50-year-old lady presents with a 3-month history of fatigue. A full blood count (FBC) reveals: haemoglobin 9.2 g/dL, leukocytes 35 × 10⁹/L (70% neutrophils) and platelets 680 × 10⁹/L. Examination is remarkable for mild pallor and splenomegaly of four finger breaths. What is the most likely diagnosis, and what investigations will you pursue?

This chapter presents a basic introduction to the non-haematological and haematological causes of high cell counts, focusing on common diseases while omitting rare ones. **Polycythaemia** refers to a raised haemoglobin, red blood cell (RBC) count and haematocrit above age and gender appropriate reference values. **Thrombocytosis** is a platelet count above 450×10^9/L. **Leucocytosis** is a white blood cell (WBC) count above 11×10^9/L.

Polycythaemia

The causes of polycythaemia may be divided conceptually into:

- **Primary polycythaemia** (polycythaemia vera [PV]): A bone marrow disorder which results in clonal overproduction of red cells, which in turn suppresses erythropoietin levels.

- **Secondary polycythaemia**: An elevated erythropoietin level drives red cell overproduction. This elevated erythropoietin level may be an appropriate response to hypoxia, inappropriately produced by a tumour or due to exogenous injection of erythropoietin.

- **Spurious causes**.

A suggested clinical approach is given in Figure 34.1.

1. Spurious Polycythaemia

Haemoconcentration may lead to a spurious rise in red cell counts. Such situations include:

- **Dehydration**: The clinical history should be fairly obvious. Look for decreased skin turgor, dry mucous membranes, and a postural fall in blood pressure.

- **Dengue**: Haemoconcentration indicates plasma leakage, which is one of the warning signs in dengue.

- **Iatrogenic**: Over-transfusion or blood doping in competitive sportsmen.

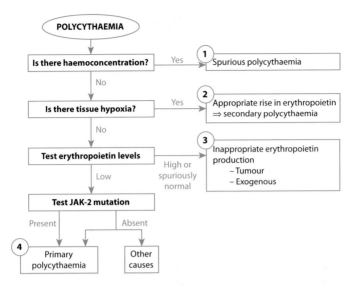

Figure 34.1. Approach to polycythaemia.

2. Secondary Polycythaemia: Tissue Hypoxia

Tissue hypoxia may be assumed with an appropriate clinical history, or demonstrated by blood gas testing. Hypoxia is a physiological trigger of raised erythropoietin and polycythaemia. Causes include:

- **Smoking**: Cigarettes release carbon monoxide, which binds haemoglobin to form carboxyhaemoglobin. This reduces the oxygen carrying capacity of blood. Blood gas measures oxygen dissolved in plasma, and remains normal.

- **Chronic lung disease**: For example, chronic obstructive pulmonary disease, interstitial lung disease and obstructive sleep apnoea. An arterial blood gas would demonstrate resting hypoxaemia.

- **Cyanotic heart disease** with right to left shunt, for example, congenital cyanotic heart disease, left to right shunt with Eisenmenger's syndrome.

- High altitude.

3. Secondary Polycythaemia: Inappropriate Erythropoietin Production

Inappropriate production of erythropoietin, in the absence of hypoxia, may be due to:

- **Erythropoietin-producing tumour**: Search for a renal (renal cell carcinoma, polycystic kidney), adrenal (tumour), hepatic (hepatocellular carcinoma) or uterine (fibroid) cause. Workup may include CT abdomen and liver function tests.

- **Exogenous**: Erythropoietin injections in sportsmen, as a means of cheating.

- **High affinity haemoglobin**: Rare; only detectable on measuring haemoglobin O_2 affinity.

4. Primary Polycythaemia

PV should only be diagnosed after exclusion of secondary causes. The classical history is a flushed patient complaining of *aquagenic pruritus*—itch after a hot bath. There may be hepatosplenomegaly and mild elevations in platelet and white cell counts. Erythropoietin levels are suppressed. JAK-2 is mutated in 90% of cases.[1]

PV may lead to complications, including:

- Hyperviscosity symptoms: Mainly neurological, for example, headache, vertigo, visual disturbances.
- Thrombosis: Arterial (e.g., stroke) or venous (e.g., deep vein thrombosis [DVT], Budd–Chiari syndrome).
- Bleeding.
- Transformation to leukaemia or secondary myelofibrosis (MF) (watch for marked splenomegaly, thrombocytopenia).

Thrombocytosis

Thrombocytosis is most commonly a reaction to inflammation. It may also be a clonal disorder, or hereditary (rare: will not be discussed). A clonal disorder is more likely if there is splenomegaly, giant platelets on blood film and complications of thrombocytosis (see the following). A clinical approach:

1. Is there a pro-inflammatory state or other cause of reactive thrombocytosis?
2. If indeed primary thrombocytosis, which haematological entity is it?
3. Are there any complications of thrombocytosis?

1. Reactive Thrombocytosis

Platelets are an acute phase reactant; very high levels can be seen in acute inflammation (the degree of thrombocytosis is not useful in distinguishing reactive vs. clonal disorders). Aetiologies include:

- **Infection**: Acute sepsis or chronic infections, for example, TB.
- **Inflammation**: Acute stress (e.g., trauma and surgery), cancer, autoimmune disease.
- **Haematological disease**: Anaemia (blood loss, haemolysis, iron deficiency), asplenia, transient rebound from thrombocytopenia.
- **Drugs**: Growth factors (e.g., GCSF), cytokines, some chemotherapy.

---

[1] In addition to JAK-2 testing, bone marrow aspiration is also performed in most cases.

Workup: A reactive aetiology may be obvious. If not, begin with careful history taking and examination. In the absence of localising signs and symptoms, it is reasonable to repeat the platelet count, exclude anaemia, screen for infection, do age-appropriate cancer screening and serology for autoimmune disorders (antinuclear antibody [ANA], etc.).

2. Primary Thrombocytosis

In persistent thrombocytosis without a secondary cause, the next step is to look for and classify a haematological disorder. This usually requires bone marrow biopsy, cytogenetic studies and JAK-2 mutation studies. Positive JAK-2 makes a haematological disorder likely (essential thrombocytosis [ET], PV or MF). On the other hand, negative JAK-2 does not rule out ET, as it is positive in only 50% of cases.[2]

Thrombocytosis is common to many of the myeloproliferative diseases; the diagnosis of ET requires exclusion of other myeloproliferative diseases.[3] Clinically, the presence or absence of splenomegaly is a useful way of classifying these disorders.

Splenomegaly typical (and often massive):

- **Chronic myeloid leukaemia (CML)**: Usually presents with neutrophilia, but it can sometimes present as isolated thrombocytosis (see page 333).

- **Primary myelofibrosis (MF)**: A leukoerythroblastic blood film (nucleated RBC and WBC forms) and bone marrow aspirate showing abnormal bone marrow megakaryocytes ± marrow fibrosis.

Splenomegaly may be absent:

- **Polycythaemia vera (PV)**: Splenomegaly is often absent, and where present, usually small. Polycythaemia is the key to diagnosis (page 330).

- **Myelodysplastic syndromes (MDS)**: May occasionally have raised platelets.[4]

- **Essential thrombocytosis (ET)**: Diagnosed after ruling out reactive thrombocytosis and other myeloproliferative disorders. Giant platelets and megakaryocyte clusters are sometimes seen.

3. Are There Any Complications?

These are more likely in primary thrombocytosis; reactive thrombocytosis does not increase risk beyond that of the underlying disease (e.g., cancer).

- **Thromboembolic disease**: Arterial (stroke, myocardial infarction, digital ischaemia) and venous (DVT/pulmonary embolism, Budd–Chiari syndrome, portal vein thrombosis).

---

[2] Some patients with JAK-2 wild type essential thrombocytosis exhibit other genetic defects (e.g., calreticulin, MPL-1 mutation) associated with essential thrombocytosis.

[3] There are detailed WHO diagnostic criteria for each disorder; these will not be covered in detail.

[4] Isolated del(5q) or RARS-T subtypes.

- **Vasomotor symptoms**: Headache, visual changes, light-headedness, atypical chest pain, erythromelalgia.
- **Bleeding**: Especially if thrombocytosis is extreme (e.g., $> 1500 \times 10^9/\text{L}$).
- Transformation to secondary MF (splenomegaly, low platelets) or acute leukaemia.

Leucocytosis

Leucocytosis is most commonly a response to systemic disease. It may also be a clonal disorder (i.e., abnormal overproduction of a single mutant 'clone'), which is more likely if other cell lines (red cells, platelets) are affected, or if white cell counts are extremely high.

Begin by looking at the white cell differential and blood film. Proceed based on the dominant white cell type: neutrophils, lymphocytes, eosinophils, monocytes, blast cells ($\geq 20\%$), or a leukoerythroblastic picture (immature cells, e.g., nucleated red cells, myelocytes, metamyelocytes; Figure 34.2):

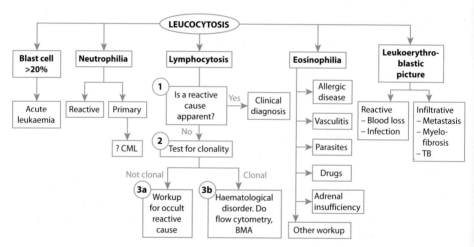

BMA, bone marrow aspirate; CML, chronic myeloid leukaemia; TB, tuberculosis.

Figure 34.2. Approach to leucocytosis.

Blast Cell Dominant

A full blood count (FBC) or bone marrow with predominantly blasts ($\geq 20\%$) is **acute leukaemia** until proven otherwise. Suppression of other cell lines is common. Workup entails blood film, bone marrow aspiration, flow cytometry, cytogenetic and molecular tests. There are various subtypes (and a differential: chronic myeloid leukaemia in blast crisis).

In the acute setting, exclude acute promyelocytic leukaemia (promyelocytes on the blood film), which has good prognosis if treated, but high early mortality if treatment is delayed.

Neutrophilia

Reactive: The most common cause of neutrophilia. Blood film may show band forms and toxic granulation.

- **Acute bacterial infection or inflammation**: In the absence of chronic illness, acute-onset neutrophilia usually means infection or inflammation. The task is then to localise the infection (symptoms, signs and septic workup). Non-infective causes should be apparent from the clinical context, for example, surgery, burns, trauma, thyroid storm. If these are obvious then no further workup is necessary; neutrophilia should resolve once the cause is treated.

- **Chronic inflammatory state**: This is usually known rheumatologic or autoimmune disease. Cigarette smoking can also cause chronic neutrophilia.

- **Bone marrow stimulation**: Secondary to haemolytic anaemia, immune thrombocytopenia or splenectomy.

- **Drugs**: For example, steroids, granulocyte colony-stimulating factor (GCSF), lithium.

- **Solid organ tumour**: Can cause a paraneoplastic neutrophilia even without infection or GCSF use.

Primary causes: This may be apparent with a classic FBC picture, or only pursued when a reactive cause is not found. Except for rare hereditary causes and syndromes, this is usually a clonal disorder.

- **Chronic myelocytic leukaemia (CML)**: Patients may be asymptomatic or complain of non-specific symptoms such as fatigue, night sweats, abdominal fullness and early satiety (due to splenomegaly). Splenomegaly is usually present, and can be massive. The differential WBC count often has a characteristic mix of eosinophils, basophils, immature cells (e.g., metacytes, myelocytes), and a small number (< 10%) of blasts. Mild anaemia, thrombocytopenia or thrombocytosis may be found. Perform bone marrow examination, and confirm the diagnosis by cytogenetic analysis for the Philadelphia chromosome (t9,22 translocation), or PCR testing for BCR–ABL fusion gene.

- **Other myeloproliferative diseases**: While the textbook blood findings of PV, MF and ET are quite distinct (another cell line usually increased), in practice there can be some overlap with CML. BCR–ABL testing will resolve any doubt.

- Chronic neutrophilic leukaemia: Rare.

Lymphocytosis

1. **Is a reactive cause apparent?** Start by looking for the obvious:
   - **Virus**: Acute viral infection (classically Epstein–Barr virus [EBV], also cytomegalovirus [CMV], influenza and many other viruses) is the commonest cause of lymphocytosis. A history of viral symptoms (upper respiratory symptoms, myalgia, malaise) is usually present, and atypical lymphocytes may be seen (in EBV).

- **Pertussis**: This bacterium is unusual in giving lymphocytosis rather than neutrophilia. Cough ≥ 2 weeks or a characteristic whoop should prompt suspicion. This can be confirmed on culture and PCR. Tuberculosis is a differential.

- **Splenectomy**.

- **Drug allergy**: Drug reaction with eosinophilia and systemic symptoms (DRESS; page 335) may present with marked atypical lymphocytosis, in addition to eosinophilia.

2. **Testing for clonality**: If a reactive cause is obvious, further workup is unnecessary. If none can be found and lymphocytosis persists, or if there is concern for a clonal disorder, begin with blood film and flow cytometry. Blood film may find distinctive features corresponding to specific diagnoses. Flow cytometry is very informative; in the first instance, it identifies whether lymphocytosis is clonal—an abundance of cells with identical cytogenetic and molecular signatures imply that they arose from a single precursor which underwent neoplastic proliferation.

3a. **Not clonal—workup for occult reactive causes**

- **Viral illnesses**: Do HIV and hepatitis serology.

- **Tuberculosis**: Inquire for symptoms, do chest X-ray.

- **Other atypical infections**: Cat scratch disease, toxoplasmosis, rickettsia. Consider serology.

- Cigarette smoking is associated with mild increases in polyclonal B cells.

3b. **Clonal—identify haematological disorder**: This includes chronic lymphocytic leukaemia (CLL), its pre-malignant state (monoclonal B-cell lymphocytosis), as well as various non-Hodgkin lymphomas. Differential diagnosis may be determined by flow cytometry, but definitive diagnosis generally requires immunohistochemistry from a lymph node biopsy (preferred) or a bone marrow biopsy.

Isolated Eosinophilia

Initial approach: Begin by looking for apparent causes of eosinophilia through clinical evaluation and simple tests. Consider:

- **Allergic disease**: Mild eosinophilia may be present in allergy-driven respiratory (allergic rhinitis, asthma), skin (e.g., atopic dermatitis) or renal (drug-induced acute interstitial nephritis, transplant rejection) disease. A careful history should reveal symptoms, for example, pruritus, nasal congestion, wheezing, cough. Initial tests include chest X-ray and a renal panel.

- **Vasculitis**: Eosinophilia, asthma and otolaryngological symptoms is typical for eosinophilic granulomatosis with polyangiitis (Churg–Strauss), and may less commonly be found in other connective tissue disease. If suspected, test antineutrophil cytoplasmic antibodies (ANCA).

- **Parasites**: These can be asymptomatic. Origin from or recent travel to a developing country increases likelihood of parasitic disease, but its absence does not exclude parasites—some parasites (e.g., strongyloides) can persist for decades. Consider stool ova/cyst/parasites and various serologies (e.g., strongyloides, toxocariasis, trichinella, hookworm, schistosomiasis).

- **Drugs**: Review all prescription drugs and complementary medicine. Eosinophilia is a feature of various drug reactions. Perhaps the most serious is drug reaction with eosinophilia and systemic symptoms (DRESS), which should be considered if there is eosinophilia, rash (classically a confluent morbilliform eruption or exfoliative dermatitis) and organ involvement. Typical culprits are antiepileptics, allopurinol and antibiotics (sulphonamides, dapsone, vancomycin).

- **Adrenal insufficiency**: Eosinophilia is associated with loss of endogenous glucocorticoids. If not a known diagnosis and symptoms are present, consider doing a short synacthen test.

- **Solid organ cancers**: Various solid organ neoplasms can cause reactive eosinophilia, often in advanced disease. Exclude occult malignancy in cases of unexplained eosinophilia.

- **Other haematological neoplasms**: Eosinophilia can be part of a myeloproliferative neoplasm (CML, PV, ET, MF), lymphoma and lymphoid leukaemia—in these conditions eosinophilia is not an isolated finding, and the conditions should be recognised based on their other abnormalities (see previous sections and Chapter 45).

Further workup: If simple tests are unrewarding, and eosinophilia persists, further workup may be necessary. This is too specialised for detailed coverage in this text; broadly, consider both primary (clonal) and secondary (reactive) causes. Workup falls into the following tracks:

- **Haematological**: Blood film, then bone marrow aspirate for clonal eosinophils (whether part of another neoplasm or isolated—rare aetiologies: acute or chronic eosinophilic leukaemia).

- **Infectious diseases**: For more occult parasites.

- **Allergy and rheumatology**: Workup for possible autoimmune disease, immunoglobulin disorders and trial of drug discontinuation.

Leukoerythroblastic Picture

The leukoerythroblastic reaction refers to a peripheral blood finding of immature RBCs (nucleated RBCs) and WBCs (myelocyte, metamyelocytes and blasts). There may also be thrombocytosis.

(a) **Reactive causes**: First exclude these stressors, which may press immature cells into service to meet needs:
- **WBC consumption**: Infection, often severe.
- **RBC destruction**: Haemorrhage, haemolysis.
- Recovery from severe myelosuppression.

(b) **Bone marrow infiltration**: Then look for these aetiologies in which the lack of marrow space 'pushes out' immature cells into circulation.
- **Metastatic cancer** with bone marrow replacement (e.g., breast, thyroid, lung, prostate, renal). The primary cancer is usually obvious by this time.

- **Myelofibrosis (MF):** Large splenomegaly and a leukoerythroblastic FBC are hallmarks. There may also be hepatomegaly, anaemia, leucocytosis or leuko-penia, thrombocytosis or thrombocytopenia and raised LDH. Bone marrow aspirate often yields a 'dry tap', trephine reveals marked fibrosis, megakaryocyte proliferation and atypia.

- **Other infiltration:** For example, tuberculosis and sarcoidosis.

 Using what you have learnt, **pen down your approach** to the Clinical Case at the start of the chapter **BEFORE reading the discussion** below.

Case Discussion

This lady has striking leucocytosis, which is mainly neutrophilic. With a 3-month history of non-specific symptoms and splenomegaly, it is highly suggestive of chronic myeloid leukaemia (CML), although reactive causes of neutrophilia should be ruled out (including chronic infections, autoimmune disease and steroids, for example, in complementary medicine and supplements). Pay attention to the white cell differential—eosinophilia, basophilia and immature cells lend support to a diagnosis of CML. A small number of blasts may be present, with >10% defining CML accelerated phase, and >20% defining CML blast crisis (an emergency). Further investigations include a bone marrow aspirate and either PCR or cytogenetic testing for the BCR–ABL fusion gene.

Key Lessons	
	1. There are three key questions in polycythaemia—(a) Is there haemocon-centration? (b) Is there tissue hypoxia? (c) What are the erythropoietin levels? This distinguishes polycythaemia vera from secondary causes.
	2. Thrombocytosis is most often reactive. If a secondary cause is not found, pursue bone marrow biopsy, cytogenetic studies and JAK-2 mutation studies to identify a myeloproliferative disease.
	3. The approach to leucocytosis begins by excluding acute leukaemia (blasts > 20%) and identifying the main type of white cell—neutrophils, lympho-cytes or eosinophils. Each has a number of reactive causes including infec-tions, inflammatory states (autoimmune diseases, allergy) and drugs (steroids and allergies). Each may also be due to a primary clonal process, in which case diagnosis requires bone marrow aspiration, flow cytometry and other testing.

Common Pitfalls	
	1. Full blood counts are routinely ordered but not everyone looks at the dif-ferential counts. Cases of acute leukaemia and neutropenic sepsis have been missed.
	2. Most cases of high cell counts are reactive. Do not be impatient to pursue advanced tests, unless there is strong clinical suspicion of a primary haema-tological disorder. Consider repeating the full blood count at a later date, aiming to investigate if the abnormality persists.

Questions

1. **REFLECT!** Have you ever seen a first presentation of acute leukaemia? What were the presenting symptoms, and was the patient well or sick?

2. **EXPLORE!** The myeloproliferative diseases can be confusing. Fill in the following table (some boxes have been filled in for you).

	Polycythaemia vera	Chronic myeloid leukaemia	Essential thrombocytosis	Myelofibrosis
Haemoglobin	>16.5 g/dL (male) >16 g/dL (female)	Normal or slightly low		
White cell count			Usually normal	
Platelet levels				
Spleen size				Enlarged
Characteristic gene abnormality		BCR–ABL Philadelphia chromosome		
Other characteristic features	Aquagenic pruritus			

3. **GO FURTHER!** Blasts, promyelocytes or neutropenia are worrisome findings on a differential FBC count. Why are these findings haematologic emergencies, and what must be done?

Endocrine and General Physiological Disturbances

Chapter 35

An Approach to Fever

Clinical Case

A premorbidly well 55-year-old gentleman was admitted for an 8-day history of fever and lethargy. There were no other symptoms such as cough, dyspnoea, dysuria, abdominal pain, nausea, vomiting, jaundice, headache or rash. He was given co-amoxiclav by a general practitioner 4 days prior to admission, however his fever persisted. On admission, his inflammatory markers were markedly raised (white blood cell [WBC] 17, 85% neutrophils, procalcitonin 4.5 µg/L, CRP 83 mg/L). Chest X-ray, urine microscopy, liver enzymes, one set of blood culture and a urine culture were unremarkable.

This is his fifth day of admission and twelfth day of fever. In spite of IV co-amoxiclav, he is still having spiking fevers up to 39.3°C. How would you approach his fever?

Fever is a resetting of the hypothalamic set point to an elevated body temperature > 37.5°C, often associated with chills, rigours, malaise and tachycardia. Its aetiologies include infective, inflammatory, malignant and central entities. Fever is not always a straightforward infection for which standard antibiotics is the correct reflex. The approach depends on the clinical picture (Figure 35.1).

- **Sepsis and septic shock**: These are conditions with high mortality, requiring urgent resuscitation and aggressive treatment.

- **Fever with apparent clinical localisation**: The majority of patients admitted for fever have a likely source of infection (e.g., pneumonia or urinary tract infection), and do not pose excessive diagnostic difficulty.

- **Fever in immunocompromised host**: These patients are vulnerable to serious forms of common infectious, along with opportunistic and unusual infections. Any fever has to be taken seriously and managed aggressively.

- **Pyrexia of unknown origin** (PUO): Classically, pyrexia ≥ 3 weeks with no identified cause after inpatient evaluation for 3 days or three outpatient visits. In practice, cases are labelled 'PUO' when initial investigations are inconclusive. The imperative is to embark on a more systematic search for less common infectious and non-infectious causes.

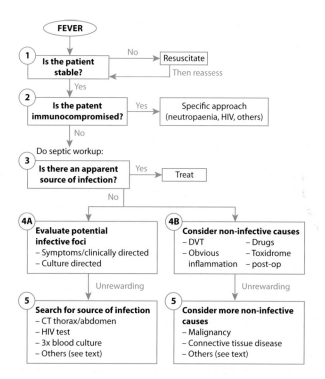

Figure 35.1. Approach to fever.

1–3. Initial Approach

1. Is the Patient Stable?

Look for the following:

- **Sepsis**: 'Life-threatening organ dysfunction caused by a dysregulated host response to infection' (Sepsis-3 definition). At the bedside, look for altered mental status, systolic blood pressure ≤ 100 mmHg or respiratory rate ≥ 22/min (the qSOFA criteria). With experience, most clinicians can pick up at the bedside which patients 'do not look good'.

- **Septic shock**: Sepsis and hypotension (BP < 90/60).

- **Cryptic shock**: Raised lactate (> 4 mmol/L) implies anaerobic metabolism from insufficient tissue perfusion. Levels above 4 mmol/L, even with normal blood pressure, has a mortality rate comparable to overt septic shock. Lactate is especially valuable to look for cryptic shock in moderately unwell patients.

These patients must receive aggressive supportive therapy and empirical antibiotics, even as workup for a source continues.

2. Is the Patient Immunocompromised?

Next, ask whether the patient is immunocompromised. These include those on chemotherapy or immunosuppressive drugs, and transplant or HIV patients. These patients are unique because (a) common infections are likely to be more severe and complicated, (b) a wider range of infective aetiologies have to be considered and (c) they may not mount a fever or inflammatory response—physical findings may be subtle, for example, absence of erythema in serious line infection.

Specific forms of immunocompromise:

- **Neutropenia**: All patients on chemotherapy should get an early full blood count (FBC) for any fever—even a simple flu. Neutropenia is defined as a decrease in absolute neutrophil count (ANC)—cut offs vary, but the highest risk patients have ANC < 0.5×10^9/L. Most neutropenic patients will require broad-spectrum IV antibiotics as per local protocol, except for selected low-risk patients.[1] Please *avoid per-rectal exam* as trauma to fragile rectal mucosa may result in bacterial translocation.

- **HIV**: Various opportunistic infections (OI) correlate with the extent of immunocompromise. OIs are unlikely with CD4 > 400, possible with CD4 < 200 and become prominent at CD4 < 100. The workup for specific OIs depends on the clinical presentation. For example, a HIV patient with pulmonary symptoms should be worked up for pneumocystis pneumonia (PCP, especially if there is hypoxaemia), tuberculosis (which may be atypical) and other OIs in addition to the usual bacterial pneumonias. A full discussion of HIV infective syndromes is beyond the scope of this text.

- **Immunosuppression**: The approach needs to be tailored based on the net state of immunosuppression, prior infections or colonisation with resistant organisms, and prior antibiotic exposure. Consider fungal and viral aetiologies in the appropriate clinical context. Do galactomannan (for aspergillosis) and cryptococcal antigens if there is clinical suspicion. BK viraemia may be suspected in renal transplant patients, or immunocompromised hosts presenting with haemorrhagic cystitis. If there are persistent cytopenias, viral aetiologies such as CMV and parvovirus (classically anaemia) come to mind.

3. Is There an Apparent Source of Infection?

Every infection has a causative organism(s) and a source. The commonest sources are lung, urine, gastrointestinal tract, lines and skin and soft tissue; but remember endocarditis, abscesses and osteomyelitis. For many patients, history, examination and a basic 'septic workup' will suffice to identify a source. Begin with these:

At the bedside: Try to localise by eliciting.

- **Localising symptoms**: Organ-specific symptoms (e.g., cough, dyspnoea, dysuria, abdominal pain) direct you to a source.

---

[1] Risk calculators, for example, Multinational Association for Supportive Care in Cancer (MASCC) Risk Index score, can be used to stratify risk.

- **Underlying conditions**: Consider the patient's premorbids, which may increase the risk of certain infections. An old stroke predisposes to aspiration pneumonia, untreated gallstones predisposes to biliary sepsis and splenectomy increases risk of infection by encapsulated bacteria (pneumococcus, meningococcus and *Haemophilus*).

- **Exposures**: Contact with healthcare services (e.g., recent hospitalisation and hae-modialysis) offers a microbiology that is relatively more resistant to common antibiotics. Travel to exotic destinations may prompt consideration of the weird and wonderful.

- **Examination**: Be directed yet thorough, covering all organ systems including lymph nodes. Skin, eyes, ears, mouth and perineum are often missed. Examine lines and wounds. Describe the pattern and distribution of rashes (see Chapter 40).

Initial septic workup:

- **FBC** can be very informative. Look not only for leucocytosis, but also at the differential count—neutrophilia with left shift suggests bacterial infection, lymphocytosis suggests viral infection and eosinophilia suggests parasitic infection or other IgE-associated autoimmune pathology. Ensure that no blasts are seen. Cytopenias are equally helpful. Viral infections may be associated with lymphopenia or even pancytopenia, and thrombocytopenia is classic in dengue.

- **Inflammatory markers**: Elevated WBCs and C-reactive protein (CRP) reflect an acute phase reaction, which may be infective or inflammatory. Procalcitonin > 0.5 µg/L is supposedly more specific for bacterial infection, but may also be elevated in fungal infection and renal insufficiency.

- **Blood cultures**: Generally taken in most patients, unless the patient is well with a clear, benign source of fever (such as viral upper respiratory tract infection).

- **Localising investigations**: These include a chest X-ray and urine microscopy and cultures. These should be pursued if there are symptoms, risk factors (e.g., urinary catheter—which should be removed and reinserted with cultures taken from the new catheter) or in patients who may not be able to complain of symptoms (e.g., elderly patients with non-specific symptoms, uncommunicative patients, etc.).

4. Further Investigation

If initial workup is unrewarding, continue to interrogate potential foci of infection, and consider non-infective causes.

4a. Evaluate Potential Infective Foci

Clinical suspicion directed: Symptoms and risk factors prompts further investigation.

- **Respiratory**: Patients with cough should have sputum sent for gram stain and culture ± acid fast bacilli (AFB) smear, culture and TB-PCR, ± respiratory viral swab. Pleural effusions should be tapped and cultured. Certain patients (e.g., immunocompromised) may require CT thorax (if there is high clinical suspicion of pneumonia despite 'normal' chest X-ray).

- **Lines**: Patients with intravascular lines (e.g., central venous catheters, dialysis catheters, peripherally inserted central catheters) should have blood cultures taken from both line and peripheral blood. Look for positive cultures with organisms typical for line sepsis (e.g., staphylococcus aureus), and look for the differential time to positivity (if the line caused sepsis, its cultures turn positive first).

- **Hepatobiliary**: Deranged liver function tests lead to suspicion of a hepatobiliary source of sepsis. Raised aspartate aminotransferase (AST) and alanine aminotransferase (ALT) may be due to viral hepatitis, other infective aetiologies (such as dengue, leptospirosis) or ischaemic hepatitis. A predominant elevation in ALP suggests cholangitis or hepatic abscess (see Chapter 10). Mild elevations of liver function test (LFTs) (e.g., ×2) may occur in systemic infections and are not specific for a liver source.

- **Intra-abdominal**: Recent abdominal surgery, perforated viscus or intra-abdominal symptoms raises the question of intra-abdominal abscesses. Contrasted CT abdomen/pelvis is the investigation of choice, renal function permitting.

- **Endocarditis**: Suspect endocarditis if there are risk factors (IV drug use, intracardiac prosthesis including heart valves, ventricular assist devices and pacemaker leads), a new murmur, co-occurrence of fever and heart failure or embolic phenomena (neurological deficits, septic emboli seeding abscesses in multiple organs). Classic signs (e.g., Janeway lesions, Osler nodes, splinter haemorrhages, clubbing) are not commonly seen. Obtain three sets of blood cultures and an echocardiogram.

- **Dengue**: Certain patients present without the classical findings of thrombocytopenia, confluent blanching erythematous rash with islands of sparing, myalgia and retro-orbital pain, or only develop them later. Consider testing if a febrile patient later develops thrombocytopenia. Dengue NS1 antigen turns positive early (from day 1), IgM later (day 5 onwards). Both are part of the 'dengue duo' rapid kit. Look for warning signs (abdominal pain, persistent vomiting, third spacing, e.g., pleural effusion, bleeding, lethargy) and features of severe dengue (shock, bleeding, severe transaminitis, altered mental state).

- **Chikungunya**: Compared to dengue, there is marked arthralgia (*break-bone fever*) and minimal thrombocytopenia. Order PCR for diagnosis.

- **Travel history**: If there is a travel history to tropical countries, send thick and thin blood films for malaria parasites. The travel destination may prompt consideration of exotic organisms (see page 348).

- **Central nervous system**: Altered mental state, headache, photophobia and meningism suggest meningitis. Encephalitis may be subtle; a high index of suspicion is necessary. Consider lumbar puncture (see page 215 for interpretation of lumbar puncture results).

- **Soft tissues**: Examine carefully—Fournier's gangrene and deep perianal abscesses have been missed. Skin swabs should be done selectively. Swab for varicella-zoster and herpes simplex in vesicular rashes and suspected herpetic ulcers. Swab pus from abscesses, but surface swabs of chronic ulcers (e.g., sacral sores) may identify colonisers rather than pathogens.

Blood culture directed: Positive cultures prompt investigation for specific sources. Diagnosing bacteraemia does not suffice—you must identify and control its source. For example:

- **Staphylococcus aureus** (methicillin-sensitive or resistant): This bacterium enters the bloodstream from soft tissue infections or vascular catheters (especially dialysis lines), and has a propensity to cause infective endocarditis. Do transthoracic echocardiography (TTE)—if this finds valvular vegetations, endocarditis is likely (see the modified Duke criteria). As TTE is insufficiently sensitive, a negative result does not rule out endocarditis; if there is sufficient clinical suspicion, pursue trans-oesophageal echocardiography (TEE).

- **Gram negative organisms** (e.g., *Escherichia coli*, *Proteus*, *Klebsiella*): these are intra-abdominal organisms and may be isolated in urinary infections, biliary tract infections or gastrointestinal infections (e.g., perforations and abscesses). In addition to urine cultures and liver enzyme levels, abdominal imaging (e.g., CT or ultrasound abdomen) is warranted in many cases, looking for gallstones, abscesses and so forth.

- **Contaminants**: Coagulase-negative Staphylococci,[2] Corynebacterium and Bacillus species are often contaminants—unless cultured from a central line, or if there is prosthetic intravascular material.

4b. Consider Non-Infective Causes

While most acute fevers are infective, consider these non-infective causes early (common ones marked *):

Inflammatory:

- **Deep vein thrombosis*/pulmonary embolism**: Examine lower limbs for swelling and erythema, work up further if suspecting deep vein thrombosis (see Chapter 47).

- **Allergies**: Consider reactions to drugs, vaccines and blood transfusion. Look for manifestations of histamine release, for example, urticarial rash.

- **Gout***: May present as a painful swollen joint with fever—but beware, septic arthritis can present in an identical fashion. Joint aspiration differentiates the two (see Chapter 48).

- **Tissue destruction**: Usually clinically obvious, for example, rhabdomyolysis, pancreatitis or tumour necrosis.

Central: This is hyperthermia (failure of central thermoregulation) rather than fever (resetting of the hypothalamic set-point). Antipyretics do not work.

- **Heat stroke**: Measure rectal temperature (see page 297).

- **Endocrine**: Consider thyrotoxicosis (see Chapter 36) and phaeochromocytoma.

---

[2] Exception: *Staphylococcus lugdunensis* is pathogenic and should usually be managed similarly to *Staphylococcus aureus*.

- **Drugs**: Review the drug chart and consider:
  - **Neuroleptic malignant syndrome (NMS)**: Seen in patients treated with antipsychotics (e.g., haloperidol) and dopamine antagonists (e.g., metoclopramide). Patients present with fever, altered mental state and autonomic dysfunction (e.g., tachycardia, labile blood pressure), usually over 1 to 3 days. There may be rhabdomyolysis with elevated creatine kinase.
  - **Serotonin syndrome**: This is a syndrome of increased central nervous system serotoninergic activity due to serotonin agonists (e.g., serotonin reuptake inhibitors, monoamine oxidase inhibitors, tricyclic antidepressants and the antibiotic linezolid), especially if multiple such agents are taken. It resembles NMS in its fever, tachycardia and altered mental state; unlike NMS, serotonin syndrome has a more acute onset (within 24 hr) and neuromuscular hyper-reactivity (clonus, tremor, hyperreflexia) rather than rigidity.
  - **Drug fever***: Anticonvulsants (phenytoin, carbamazepine, etc.), antibiotics (especially beta lactams, cotrimoxazole) and allopurinol may cause fever.
  - **Malignant hyperthermia**: Due to inhalational anaesthetics or succinylcholine in patients with an inherited abnormality of the sarcoplasmic reticulum.
- **Toxins**:
  - **Psychostimulants**: For example, cocaine.
  - **Anticholinergic toxicity**: A classic toxidrome of hyperthermia (hot as a hare), pupil dilation (blind as a bat), dry skin (dry as a bone), vasodilation (red as a beet), agitation (mad as a hatter), urinary retention (full as a tick) and tachycardia (the heart goes on alone). Culprit drugs include tricyclic antidepressants, atropine and antihistamines.
  - **Sympathomimetic toxicity**: Fever, dilated pupils, diaphoresis and excitement/ agitation. Drugs here include cocaine, methamphetamine and ecstasy (MDMA).

Post-op: In the post-operative patient, fever may be nothing more than an inflammatory response to surgery, but investigate anything more than a slight temperature, or anything that does not resolve after a few days. Note that wound infections usually present only after a week or more, except Streptococcus pyogenes and Clostridium perfringens.

If these investigations and considerations are unrewarding, proceed to step 5.

5. Common Causes Exhausted

The impetus now is to be meticulous and thorough. Consider whether any of the previous-mentioned causes have been missed, and other less common causes of fever. Embark on a thorough search of the patient's past medical history, travel and sexual exposures. Create a detailed timeline of the patient's fever trend (spikes and pattern), interventions that have been carried out (e.g., antibiotics) and their impact on the fever. Pattern recognition is key and experience counts. Try not to 'carpet bomb'—but go by clinical suspicion. By now an infectious disease specialist should be on board. Consider:

Infective Fever

- **Bacterial infections in sources not previously evaluated**: Consider each source not previously evaluated—especially intra-abdominal sepsis, for example, hepatic abscess, any prosthetic joint, osteomyelitis (e.g., if there is back pain). These may evade initial workup and are rather commonly missed. If genitalia were previously not examined, now is a good time to do so. It is reasonable to obtain a CT thorax and abdomen, plus specific imaging (e.g., MRI spine) where guided by symptoms.

- **Infective endocarditis**: Keep in mind as symptoms are vague and cultures may be negative. Ensure that at least three sets of cultures are done. Inform the lab to keep cultures for 2 weeks for fastidious organisms.

- **Viruses**: Primary HIV infection can present as PUO, a mild flu-like illness or even encephalitis. HIV screen should be performed. Test for dengue and Chikungunya, if there is the slightest clinical suspicion.

- **Tuberculosis**: Search hard for lymph nodes, look for changes on CT thorax (CXR may be subtle especially if there is concomitant lung disease or HIV).

- **Rickettsia**: Classic pentad is fever, headache, rash, eschar and arthralgia; all five features are rarely present. There may be tick/louse/flea exposure or a history of construction work, and an eschar at the site of tick bite. Rickettsial infection may progress to pneumonitis or meningoencephalitis, and will improve with trial of doxycycline (fever should improve within 48–72 hr after doxycycline is initiated, if fever does not improve, rickettsia is unlikely).

- **Leptospirosis**: This can range from a mild illness to severe multi-organ failure. Presentations include hepatitis, pulmonary haemorrhage, aseptic meningitis, acute kidney injury and coagulopathy. Conjunctival suffusion is classic and not commonly seen in other causes of PUO. This is a rat-borne illness. PCR for diagnosis is available, but takes time to return.

Malignant Fever

Consider constitutional symptoms, personal and family history.

- **Haematological cancers** (lymphoma, leukaemia) are particularly prone to causing fever (a *B symptom*). Ensure that there are no blasts on FBC. Pan-CT may identify non-palpable lymphadenopathy, which should be biopsied. Consider protein electrophoresis for myeloma, and bone marrow aspiration if FBC is deranged.

- **Solid organ tumours**: Most tend not to present with fever, except renal cell carcinoma, hepatocellular carcinoma or liver metastases.

Inflammatory Causes

- **Connective tissue disease**: The two commonest rheumatologic diseases to present with PUO are adult Still's disease and giant cell (temporal) arteritis (GCA). The former presents with fever, arthritis and rash, with markedly elevated erythrocyte sedimentation rate (ESR), C-reactive protein (CRP) and ferritin. Consider GCA if the patient has visual problems, jaw claudication or headache; ESR is elevated. Other autoimmune diseases including lupus, ANCA vasculitis or autoimmune hepatitis may also present with fever.

- **Deep vein thrombosis/pulmonary embolism** is worth a second look.
- **Granulomatous disorders**: Sarcoidosis.

Diagnoses of Exclusion

- **Neurological**: Brainstem dysfunction can cause autonomic dysfunction and fever. Aetiologies include traumatic brain injury, pontine haemorrhage or degenerative disease, for example, multiple system atrophy. This should be a diagnosis of exclusion.
- **Factitious fever**.
- **Periodic fever syndromes**: For example, familial Mediterranean fever.

In some patients, extensive workup may not reveal any diagnosis. The majority of such patients do well.

 Using what you have learnt, **pen down your approach** to the Clinical Case at the start of the chapter **BEFORE reading the discussion** below.

Case Discussion

This is a 55-year-old gentleman with pyrexia of unknown origin, who did not respond to IV Augmentin. Generally, there are a few reasons why a patient may not respond to antibiotics: (1) inadequate dosage of antibiotics, (2) the infecting bacteria is not sensitive to the antibiotic used, (3) failure to achieve source control, (4) infection is not bacterial or (5) it is not an infection.

Given markedly raised inflammatory markers and procalcitonin, infection remains more likely than a non-infective cause of fever. The impetus is to search for the source of infection. Examine carefully for any perianal abscess, lymphadenopathy, organomegaly or soft tissue infective focus; ask about any travel history. As a start, he should receive two more sets of blood cultures (unfortunately pre-treatment with antibiotics decreases diagnostic yield), a HIV test and CT thorax/abdomen. A number of intra-abdominal abscesses (e.g., hepatic abscess, perianal abscess, sealed diverticular perforations) present in this manner. Echocardiogram for endocarditis should also be considered, particularly if blood cultures are positive for an organism typical of endocarditis. If these investigations are unremarkable, additional causes of infection and non-infective causes of fever should be considered.

Key Lessons	1. Two categories of febrile patients need to be handled differently: the haemodynamically unstable, and the immunocompromised.
	2. The evaluation for infective fever is in the first instance guided by clinical signs and symptoms, risk factors (e.g., prosthetic valve, dialysis catheter, recent abdominal surgery, travel history) and basic workup. If these are unrewarding, consider three sets of blood cultures, HIV testing, CT thorax/abdomen, echocardiogram and further investigations (see text).
	3. Non-infective causes of fever include drugs, inflammatory disorders (deep vein thrombosis, gout, connective tissue disease) and malignancies.
Common Pitfalls	1. Empiric antibiotics are unhelpful in patients with pyrexia of unknown origin, as they merely suppress occult infective processes, and diminish the diagnostic yield of various investigations.
	2. Infective sources are missed if the patient is not examined head-to-toe (including perineum and extremities).
Questions	1. **REFLECT!** Have you ever seen a patient with pyrexia of unknown origin? What workup was performed, and what was the eventual diagnosis?
	2. **EXPLORE!** Many patients have central lines or dialysis catheters; they can develop both central line related bloodstream infections (CLABSI) and unrelated infections (e.g., pneumonia). How do you decide if the line is the cause of infection, or if it is merely a bystander?
	3. **DISCUSS!** Should all patients with acute-onset fever and no clear infective source receive empiric antibiotics?
	4. **GO FURTHER!** Why are blood cultures persistently negative in some patients with infective endocarditis? What should be done for such patients?

An Approach to Thyroid Abnormalities

Clinical Case

A 22-year-old lady presents with a 1-month history of heat intolerance, palpitations and weight loss. She is afebrile, with a blood pressure of 109/62 mmHg and heart rate of 111/min. Examination reveals an anxious young lady with rest tremor and lid lag. She has a smooth, soft midline neck mass that ascends on swallowing. How would you approach her presentation?

Thyroid disease presents with signs and symptoms of hyperthyroidism, hypothyroidism or goitre. This chapter will first discuss some general principles, then approaches to hyperthyroidism ± goitre, hypothyroidism ± goitre and thyroid nodules.

General Principles

The approach to thyroid abnormalities begins with assessing thyroid structure and thyroid function.

Assessing Thyroid Structure: A thyroid is a midline lower neck mass that ascends with swallowing but not tongue protrusion. Consider and exclude other neck lumps (see Chapter 44). Diagnostically, thyroid structure may be classified into four groups: (1) no goitre, (2) diffuse goitre, (3) multinodular goitre or (4) a solitary thyroid nodule.

Assessing Thyroid Function: Classical symptoms of hyper- and hypothyroidism are recognisable (Table 36.1); however, because of the wide variation in clinical presentation and the non-specificity of these symptoms, the diagnosis is usually biochemical (i.e., elevated or reduced T_4). Rare patients present with extreme hyperthyroidism (thyroid storm) or extreme hypothyroidism (myxoedema coma).

Correlating Structure and Function

The diagnosis can usually be found at the intersection of structure and function (Table 36.2).

Table 36.1. Functional Assessment of the Thyroid

	Hyperthyroid	Thyroid storm[a]	Hypothyroid	Myxoedema coma[a]
Metabolic	Heat intolerance Weight loss Irritability, insomnia	Hyperpyrexia	Cold intolerance Weight gain Lethargy	Hypothermia
Cardiac	Palpitations Atrial fibrillation	Tachycardia Cardiac failure	Bradycardia	Pericardial effusion Cardiac failure
Gastrointestinal	Diarrhoea	Vomiting, diarrhoea Jaundice	Constipation	
Neurological	Anxiety Rest tremor Lid lag Proximal myopathy Brisk reflexes	Delirium Seizure Coma	Proximal myopathy Slow relaxing reflexes Nerve entrapment, e.g., carpel tunnel Impaired cognition	Altered mental status Hypoventilation
Skin	Sweaty, warm		Coarse, smooth	
Gynaecologic	Oligomenorrhoea		Menorrhagia Infertility	

[a] Thyroid storm and myxoedema coma should be thought of as exaggerations of the clinical manifestations of hyper- and hypothyroidism. *Burch–Wartofsky scoring*, while not diagnostic, is used as a tool to predict the likelihood of thyroid storm.

Table 36.2. Thyroid Disease as the Intersection of Structure and Function

		Thyroid function		
		Hyperthyroid	Euthyroid	Hypothyroid
Thyroid structure	**No goitre**	Thyroiditis (early) Drugs	[normal]	Thyroiditis (late) RAI, thyroidectomy, drugs Secondary hypothyroidism
	Diffuse goitre	Graves' disease Secondary hyperthyroidism	I_2 deficiency goitre	Hashimoto's thyroiditis (late) I_2 deficiency goitre
	MNG	MNG (toxic)	MNG (compensated)	MNG (with I_2 deficiency)
	Solitary nodule	Toxic adenoma Carcinoma (rare) MNG with toxic nodule	Benign: adenomas, cysts Carcinoma MNG dominant nodule	

I_2, iodine; MNG, multinodular goitre; RAI, radioactive iodine.

The natural history of some conditions takes them through various states of hyper- and hypothyroidism. For example:

- In thyroiditis, thyroid inflammation first causes release of pre-formed hormones (hyperthyroid phase), then gland damage (hypothyroid phase); with continued antibody stimulation (as in Hashimoto's disease), a goitre grows.

- Longstanding iodine deficiency stimulates thyroid growth, and goitre develops with time. It may or may not compensate well for iodine deficiency, so patients can be euthyroid or hypothyroid. This goitre is initially diffuse, but because some thyroid follicles grow faster than others, it may become multinodular with time (similar to idiopathic multinodular goitres [MNG], which are unrelated to iodine deficiency).

- Some MNGs develop autonomous T_4 secretion (toxic MNG, if there is no iodine deficiency)—these patients are hyperthyroid. MNGs are usually multinodular, as their name suggests, but one nodule may be more prominent than others (dominant nodule). They may also undergo malignant change, and not necessarily from the dominant nodule.

Interpretation of Thyroid Function Tests

Table 36.3. Interpretation of Thyroid Function Tests

	↓ TSH	Normal TSH	↑ TSH
↓ T_4	Secondary hypothyroidism[a] Sick euthyroid[d]	Secondary hypothyroidism[a]	Primary hypothyroidism[a] Sick euthyroid[d]
Normal T_4	Subclinical hyperthyroidism[b] T_3 toxicosis[c]	[Normal]	Subclinical hypothyroidism[b]
↑ T_4	Primary hyperthyroidism[a] Pregnancy[e]	Secondary hyperthyroidism[a] T_4 resistance[f]	Secondary hyperthyroidism[a]

Explanatory notes: Understand the principles behind these derangements.

[a] Understand the hypothalamic–pituitary–thyroid axis. Primary thyroid disease results in appropriate pituitary responses—hyperthyroidism suppresses thyroid-stimulating hormone (TSH) while hypothyroidism stimulates TSH. An abnormal TSH response, including 'inappropriately normal' levels, suggests pituitary disease (i.e., secondary hyper- or hypothyroidism).

[b] TSH has the highest sensitivity and specificity in diagnosing thyroid disorders. Normal TSH makes a thyroid disorder unlikely. If TSH is abnormal, measure T_4 (± T_3) to distinguish between overt hyper- or hypothyroidism (abnormal T_4) and subclinical hyper- or hypothyroidism (normal T_4).

[c] If the patient is clinically hyperthyroid but T_4 is 'normal', test for T_3 thyrotoxicosis.

[d] Thyroid function is difficult to interpret in non-thyroidal illness, especially in the critically ill (sick euthyroid syndrome), as well as during recovery from hyper- or hypothyroidism (thyroid in transition). There can be any pattern of thyroid function tests, with low T_4 and T_3 being the most common. TSH is often low, but can be high during recovery. However, extreme values of TSH (undetectable or > 20 mU/L) suggests permanent hyper- or hypothyroidism.

[e] Pregnancy: Human chorionic gonadotropin (hCG), the basis of pregnancy tests, mimics TSH and stimulates the TSH receptor. This leads to an increase in T_4 and reduction in TSH. Trimester-specific reference ranges should be used for interpreting thyroid hormone values.

[f] Resistance to thyroid hormone is a rare condition in which patients are clinically euthyroid in spite of elevated T_4.

Hyperthyroidism ± Goitre

The causes of hyperthyroidism may be distinguished based on clinical features, antibody testing, thyroid ultrasound and radioactive iodine (RAI; Figure 36.1).

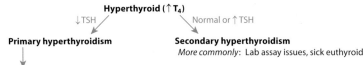

Hyperthyroid ($\uparrow T_4$)

↓TSH   Normal or ↑TSH

Primary hyperthyroidism   **Secondary hyperthyroidism**
More commonly: Lab assay issues, sick euthyroid

Aetiology	Clinical features	Goitre and ultrasound	TRAb	RAI
Graves' disease	Graves' eye signs	Diffuse goitre, ↑ blood flow	Positive	Diffuse uptake
Toxic MNG Toxic adenoma		Nodular goitre	Negative	Focal uptake
Thyroiditis	Usually transient	Diffuse or nil, ↓ blood flow	Usually negative[a]	Low uptake
Drug-induced	Suggestive history	No goitre	Negative	
Paraneoplastic	hCG positive			

[a] Fine print: Thyroid blocking antibodies may be present in Hashimoto's thyroiditis. Therefore, an assay measuring total TRAb (without specificity for thyroid stimulating antibodies) may be positive in Hashimoto's thyroiditis.

hCG, human chorionic gonadotropin; MNG, multinodular goitre; RAI, radioactive iodine; TRAb, TSH-receptor antibody; US, ultrasound.

Figure 36.1. Approach to hyperthyroidism.

Primary Hyperthyroidism

Clinical features:

- **Graves' disease**: This is the commonest cause of hyperthyroidism. The classical presentation is a young lady with clinical hyperthyroidism, diffuse goitre (± bruit), exophthalmos, pretibial myxoedema and thyroid acropachy (clubbing). About 25% of patients with Graves' disease have ophthalmopathy; this arises because the TSH-receptor antibody (TRAb) in Graves' disease also binds retro-orbital tissue, causing retro-orbital inflammation. Severe cases can be complicated by ophthalmoplegia, diplopia, chemosis and corneal ulceration. These eye signs are specific to Graves' disease; in contrast, lid lag is a manifestation of sympathetic overdrive and also found in other causes of hyperthyroidism. The absence of eye signs does not rule out Graves' disease.

- **Toxic MNG or adenoma**: Long-standing thyroid nodules may become autonomous and produce T_4 independent of TSH stimulation.

- **Thyroiditis**: Patients can be hyperthyroid in early thyroiditis, as thyrocyte destruction leads to release of preformed hormones. Subacute (De Quervain's) thyroiditis presents in the post-viral setting as a painful goitre, hyperthyroidism, fever and malaise. Pain is absent in the other causes of thyroiditis—Hashimoto thyroiditis, transient painless thyroiditis and postpartum thyroiditis.

- **Drug-induced**: There are a number of mechanisms. Amiodarone, lithium, tyrosine kinase inhibitors and interferon can cause thyroiditis (both hyper- and hypothyroidism). Excessive iodine exposure occurs in patients given iodine, CT contrast agents or contaminated food. Excess exogenous thyroid hormone can be iatrogenic or factitious (some patients hear that it is a good weight loss drug—and it is). The diagnosis of these causes rests on clinical history.

- **Paraneoplastic**: Some tumours produce human chorionic gonadotropin (hCG; testicular germ cell tumour, hydatidiform mole, choriocarcinoma), which resembles TSH, stimulating TSH receptors. hCG is positive in these conditions.

Further testing: If there are overt clinical manifestations of Graves' disease, TRAb testing generally suffices. In their absence, either TRAb + thyroid ultrasound or RAI uptake are acceptable strategies for further evaluation (Figure 36.1).

- **TRAb or thyroid stimulating immunoglobulin (TSI)**: Elevated TRAb or TSI (these are alternative assays) generally confirm a diagnosis of Graves' disease; a small minority of Graves' patients are antibody negative.

- **Thyroid ultrasound**: This identifies thyroid nodules (toxic adenoma or MNG), diffuse goitre with increased blood flow (Graves' disease) and decreased blood flow with or without goitre (thyroiditis).

- **RAI uptake**: Diffuse increased uptake is consistent with Graves' disease. Focal uptake is seen in toxic adenoma and toxic MNG. The other causes of hyperthyroidism generally have low RAI uptake. RAI studies are contraindicated in pregnancy.

Secondary Hyperthyroidism

$\uparrow T_4$ with $\uparrow$ TSH (or inappropriately normal TSH) is the textbook picture of a TSH-producing pituitary adenoma, but this is very rare. Such a biochemical picture is more commonly due to lab assay issues, sick euthyroid and thyroid in transition. Entertain the diagnosis of a TSH-producing adenoma if the patient is clinically hyperthyroid, especially if there are other pituitary hormone abnormalities or known pituitary disease.

Hypothyroidism ± Goitre

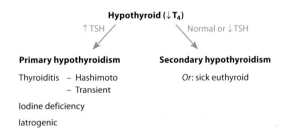

Figure 36.2. Approach to hypothyroidism.

Primary Hypothyroidism

Causes:

- **Hashimoto thyroiditis** (chronic autoimmune thyroiditis): After a transient hyperthyroid phase (either manifest or subclinical), patients become *permanently* hypothyroid. This is the most common cause of hypothyroidism in iodine-sufficient regions.

- **Transient thyroiditis:** Subacute thyroiditis (painful), painless thyroiditis and postpartum thyroiditis present with transient hyperthyroidism, followed by hypothyroidism, then recovery. These disorders *do not lead to permanent hypothyroidism*.

- **Iodine deficiency:** Iodine is an essential component of T_4, and deficiency can result in hypothyroidism (which may form a goitre or eventually become MNG). This affects large parts of the developing world, where salt is not always fortified with iodine.

- **Iatrogenic:** Thyroidectomy and neck radiation are obvious causes of thyroid destruction. Many patients treated with RAI for Graves' disease (not diagnostic doses of RAI) eventually develop hypothyroidism. Some drugs (amiodarone, lithium, tyrosine kinase inhibitors and others) cause thyroiditis and either hyper- or hypothyroidism.

Antibody testing: Anti-thyroid peroxidase (anti-TPO) antibodies are usually positive in Hashimoto thyroiditis. In patients with a clinical history of thyroiditis (i.e., hyperthyroid then hypothyroid), positive anti-TPO antibodies predict the development of chronic hypothyroidism (i.e., Hashimoto disease) as opposed to eventual recovery (i.e., subacute thyroiditis).

Secondary Hypothyroidism

- **Panhypopituitarism:** Deficiencies in multiple pituitary hormones may arise after cranial radiotherapy (e.g., for nasopharyngeal cancer), infiltrative diseases of the pituitary, trauma and postpartum haemorrhage.

- **Pituitary adenoma with suppression of TSH:** A large pituitary adenoma (functional or non-functional) may suppress other pituitary hormones. The gonadotropins are lost first, with TSH only being suppressed very late (therefore reproductive-aged patients would have complained of amenorrhea or loss of libido before hypothyroidism becomes manifest).

Further workup entails assessment of other pituitary hormone function (prolactin, follicle stimulating hormone (FSH), luteinising hormone (LH), adrenocorticotropic hormone (ACTH) and cortisol) and pituitary imaging.

Thyroid Nodules

The main concern in a thyroid nodule is to exclude malignancy. Benign differentials include MNGs, adenomas, cysts and others.

Clinical Assessment

The clinical assessment may increase or decrease the suspicion of malignancy:

- **Local symptoms and signs**: Large goitres may have compressive symptoms—dyspnoea, stridor, dysphagia and tracheal deviation; these are not specific for cancer. In contrast, a *hoarse voice* suggests malignant infiltration of the recurrent laryngeal nerve until proven otherwise. *Regional lymphadenopathy* is worrisome for papillary thyroid cancer.

- **Hyperthyroidism**: Overt or subclinical hyperthyroidism (suppressed TSH) suggests a toxic adenoma or MNG, and makes cancer less likely.

- **Systemic features**: Weight loss (in the absence of hyperthyroidism), bone pain or dyspnoea raise concern for metastatic cancer.

- **Cancer risk**: Risk factors include family history of thyroid and related cancers (e.g., familial adenomatosis polyposis), radiation (papillary thyroid cancer), history of Hashimoto thyroiditis (thyroid lymphoma) or neck radiation.

Workup to Exclude Malignancy

Euthyroid patients:

- **Thyroid ultrasound**: This identifies thyroid nodules (including non-palpable ones) and characterises them. Suspicious sonographic features include microcalcifications, irregular margins, invasion and nodules that are deeper than wide. Purely cystic nodules are likely benign.

- **Fine needle aspiration cytology (FNAC)**: FNAC should generally be offered for nodules ≥ 1 cm (except purely cystic nodules), especially those with suspicious features. The most suspicious nodule(s), as identified on ultrasound, should be targeted for sampling.

Hyperthyroid patients: Two strategies are employed:

- **RAI uptake scan**: RAI scans may demonstrate that a hyperthyroid patient's nodule is 'hot' (high uptake) and therefore functional and less likely malignant; some clinicians do not offer FNAC for hot nodules.

- **Thyroid US + FNAC**: Other clinicians omit RAI scans and proceed directly to ultrasound and FNAC.

Interpretation of FNAC results:

- Benign lesion—follow up with interval ultrasound.

- Suspicious or malignant—cancer staging and surgery. There are different histologic subtypes of thyroid cancer (follicular, papillary, anaplastic, medullary and thyroid lymphoma; each with different behaviour).

- Follicular lesion—this is either adenoma (no capsular invasion) or follicular carcinoma (with capsular invasion), and FNAC cannot distinguish the two. Excision is indicated; the eventual diagnosis of adenoma vs. carcinoma can only be made after pathologic examination of the excised nodule.

Using what you have learnt, **pen down your approach** to the Clinical Case at the start of the chapter **BEFORE reading the discussion** below.

Case Discussion

This young lady has clinical hyperthyroidism and a diffuse goitre. Hyperthyroidism should be confirmed biochemically; T_4 will be elevated and TSH suppressed.

Look for ophthalmopathy (exophthalmos and ophthalmoplegia)—if present, the diagnosis is almost certainly Graves' disease (note that lid lag can be found in other causes of hyperthyroidism). Positive TRAb confirms Graves' disease.

If ophthalmopathy is absent, the differential diagnosis includes both Graves' disease and other causes of hyperthyroidism. Explore a history of viral illness, drugs and other precipitants of hyperthyroidism. Send TRAb, anti-TPO and beta-hCG. If anti-TPO is positive, she is probably in the hyperthyroid phase of Hashimoto thyroiditis; if negative, and there are no other identifiable causes of hyperthyroidism, she is likely to have transient thyroiditis; with time, she may enter a hypothyroid phase, then recover.

Key Lessons	1. The assessment of thyroid disease begins with an assessment of thyroid structure and function. Thyroid function tests should be interpreted with an understanding of the hypothalamic–pituitary–thyroid axis, and an awareness of the impact of non-thyroidal illness on these tests.
	2. Graves' disease is the most common cause of primary hyperthyroidism; patients have a diffuse goitre with increased blood flow, positive TSH-receptor antibodies (TRAb) and diffuse radioactive iodine (RAI) uptake. There may be characteristic eye signs. Other causes of hyperthyroidism include early thyroiditis, toxic nodules and drugs.
	3. In non-iodine-deficient areas of the world, thyroiditis is the most common cause of primary hypothyroidism. This may be permanent (Hashimoto thyroiditis) or transient.
	4. The main concern with thyroid nodules is to exclude malignancy. Euthyroid patients should receive thyroid ultrasound and fine needle aspiration cytology.
Common Pitfalls	1. Do not do thyroid function tests in critically ill patients unless thyroid disease is clinically suspected; T_4 and TSH are often abnormal in these patients.
Questions	1. **DISCUSS!** Apart from patients who present with overt hyper- or hypothyroidism, what are the clinical circumstances in which thyroid function testing is indicated?
	2. **EXPLORE!** 'Subclinical' hypo- or hyperthyroidism, by definition, is asymptomatic. What is the clinical significance of subclinical thyroid disease—is it an entirely benign condition?

3. **GO FURTHER!** A 30-year-old gentleman is evaluated for a firm midline neck lump. Fine needle aspiration cytology reveals medullary thyroid carcinoma. He is incidentally found to have hypercalcaemia. What is the unifying diagnosis, and what is the most appropriate next test?

Chapter **An Approach to**

37 **Hyper- and Hypoglycaemia**

Clinical Case

A 16-year-old boy presents with a 1-day history of fever, cough, vomiting and lethargy. He has been complaining of increased thirst, frequent urination and weight loss in the past few days. On examination, he appears tachypneic and unwell. His vitals are: BP 104/70 mmHg, HR 112/min, Temp 38.5°C, SpO2 98% on room air. Examination finds crackles in his right lung base and a soft abdomen. A capillary blood glucose reads 'HI'. He has no other past medical history. What is the next test you would do?

Physiologic homoeostasis maintains blood glucose between 4.0 and 11.0 mmol/L (4.0–6.0 mmol/L when fasting). Unfortunately, these homoeostatic processes can malfunction, occasionally in life-threatening ways. Bedside capillary blood glucose testing makes hyper- or hypoglycaemia easy to confirm. This chapter presents an approach to (1) acute severe hyperglycaemia, (2) chronic hyperglycaemia and the metabolic syndrome and (3) hypoglycaemia.

Acute Severe Hyperglycaemia

Capillary blood glucose screening picks up severe hyperglycaemia relatively often. The main concern is to identify life-threatening diabetic emergencies—diabetic ketoacidosis (DKA) and the hyperglycaemic hyperosmolar state (HHS); patients need not have a prior diagnosis of diabetes to present with DKA/HHS.

1. What Do Clinical Symptoms Suggest?

The clinical picture is usually helpful.

- **DKA**: An acute history (< 24 hr) of polyuria, polydipsia and lethargy, then nausea and vomiting, abdominal pain and dyspnoea (respiratory compensation for metabolic acidosis). Delirium is less common and less severe than in HHS. Physical examination may find dehydration, Kussmaul (deep, laboured) breathing and a fruity breath odour (ketones). DKA classically occurs in undiagnosed or non-compliant type 1 diabetics, but can also occur in type 2 diabetes.

- **HHS**: A more insidious onset (days) of osmotic symptoms (polyuria and polydipsia), lethargy and often marked delirium (due to the effect of hyperosmolarity on cerebral neurons). On examination, marked hypovolaemia is apparent, but there should not be Kussmaul breathing.

- In the absence of DKA/HHS, symptoms are less marked. Asymptomatic severe hyperglycaemia is quite common; most of these patients just have poorly controlled (or previously undiagnosed) diabetes.

2. Laboratory Diagnosis

If DKA/HHS is suspected, send arterial blood gas or venous bicarbonate, and serum ketones. DKA is a ketogenic state perpetuated by insulin deficiency; there is ketosis and ketoacidosis (Table 37.1), but glucose is not always very high. In contrast, HHS is a state of severe hyperglycaemia causing osmotic diuresis and marked dehydration, therefore glucose, sodium and osmolality are markedly elevated (Table 37.1). Occasionally there is both ketoacidosis and hyperosmolality; such patients are described to have a DKA–HHS overlap.

Table 37.1. Laboratory Parameters in DKA and HHS

	Non-DKA/HHS	DKA	HHS	Comment
Plasma glucose (mmol/L)	Variable	$\geq 14^a$	≥ 33	
Arterial pH	> 7.3	< 7.3	> 7.3	Anion gap elevated in DKA (see Chapter 16)
Venous HCO_3^- (mmol/L)	> 18	< 18	> 18	
Serum beta-hydroxybutyrate (mmol/L)	< 0.6	> 3	< 0.6	Urine ketones also ++
Effective serum osmolality (mOsm/kg)	< 320	< 320	> 320	Calculate as 2 [Na$^+$] + glucose

[a] Fine print: patients on SGLT-2 inhibitors (e.g., Dapagliflozin and Empagliflozin) can develop ketoacidosis without hyperglycaemia, or with uncharacteristically mild hyperglycaemia (euglycaemic DKA).

DKA, diabetic ketoacidosis; HHS, hyperglycaemic hyperosmolar state.

3. Identify a Precipitant

Episodes of severe hyperglycaemia, especially DKA/HHS, are often precipitated by intercurrent illness (such as infection) or non-compliance to insulin or oral hypoglycaemic therapy. Search for and treat this precipitant.

Chronic Hyperglycaemia

Chronic hyperglycaemia is the pathologic hallmark of diabetes mellitus. This is mainly a management challenge, but some issues pertaining to diagnosis and assessment are reviewed here.

Diagnosis of Diabetes

Most patients are asymptomatic and are diagnosed on screening, or when they present with a complication (e.g., recurrent infections, chronic kidney disease, etc.) A minority present with osmotic symptoms (polyuria, polydipsia, weight loss), and some in extremis with DKA. The glucose thresholds for diagnosis are presented in Table 37.2.

Table 37.2. Diagnostic Criteria for Diabetes Mellitus

	Normal	Pre-diabetes	Diabetes[a]
Fasting glucose (mmol/L)	≤6.0	6.1–6.9 (impaired fasting glucose)	≥7.0
Oral glucose tolerance test (mmol/L)	≤7.8	7.8–11.0 (impaired glucose tolerance)	≥11.1
Serum HbA1c (%)[b]	≤5.6	5.7–6.4 (elevated risk)	≥6.5
Random glucose (mmol/L)			≥11.1

[a] Two positive tests are required for diagnosis in an asymptomatic patient, but only one in a symptomatic patient.

[b] HbA1c is not accepted for diagnosis of diabetes in some countries. Values are influenced by red blood cell turnover and can be falsely low in anaemia, iron deficiency and chronic kidney disease.

Look for Secondary Causes of Hyperglycaemia

These factors may contribute to hyperglycaemia and are possibly reversible. Diabetes should not be diagnosed in the presence of a potentially short-lived, reversible cause.

- **Drugs**: For example, corticosteroids, supplements and traditional medicines (many of which contain steroids, unknown to the consumer).
- **Critical illness**: Stress hyperglycaemia.
- **Endocrine disease**: Cushing's disease and acromegaly (see Chapter 38), may contribute to hyperglycaemia.
- **Pancreatic disorders**: Beta cell destruction may occur in hemochromatosis (primary or secondary, e.g., due to repeated transfusions), chronic pancreatitis, cystic fibrosis and surgical pancreatectomy.

If Primary Diabetes, Which Type?

Type 1 and 2 diabetes were historically thought of as two polar opposites—type 1 presenting as fulminant DKA in young, thin individuals, while type 2 presenting insidiously in older, overweight patients (Table 37.3).

Table 37.3. Classic Type 1 and Type 2 Diabetes

	Classic Type 1 Diabetes	Classic Type 2 Diabetes
Pathophysiology	Insulin deficiency from autoimmune beta-cell destruction	Initially, peripheral insulin resistance. Later, insulin deficiency due to beta-cell destruction from chronic hyperglycaemia
Patient profile	Young, thin, associated with other autoimmune disease	Middle-aged to elderly. Overweight, with other features of the metabolic syndrome
Presentation and course	Fulminant presentation, e.g., DKA Insulin dependant Brittle, tips over into DKA	Insidious presentation, often asymptomatic Can often manage with oral agents Less brittle
Antibodies	Anti-islet cell, anti-GAD[a]	None
C-peptide levels	Low	High initially[b]

[a] Specific but not sensitive.

[b] C-peptide levels reflect endogenous glucose production. Levels are low in type 1 diabetes, high in early type 2 diabetes, but fall in late type 2 diabetes.

DKA, diabetic ketoacidosis; GAD, glutamic acid decarboxylase.

We now know that the polar dichotomy between type 1 and 2 diabetes is an over-simplification. In late type 2 diabetes, beta cells are progressively destroyed by the toxic effect of chronic hyperglycaemia. Therefore, in addition to insulin resistance, patients develop insulin deficiency and a clinical picture which mimics type 1 diabetes—more insulin dependent, more brittle and more ketosis-prone. Other types of diabetes have been characterised, including latent autoimmune diabetes in adults (LADA) and maturity-onset diabetes of the young (MODY); these will not be detailed here.

Other Tasks

- Patients with diabetes are likely to have other metabolic risk factors, including hypertension, hyperlipidaemia and obesity. Screen for and address these risk factors.
- Assess for complications. Diabetic foot screening (for neuropathy), eye screening (for retinopathy) and albuminuria screening (for nephropathy) are standard in most diabetic monitoring programmes.

Hypoglycaemia

Hypoglycaemia presents with sympathetic activation (diaphoresis, palpitations, anxiety), and when severe, neurological symptoms (weakness, seizure, coma). The majority of patients with hypoglycaemia are diabetics on treatment (especially insulin), and they may develop hypoglycaemic unawareness if episodes of hypoglycaemia are frequent.

As a Complication of Diabetic Treatment

Hypoglycaemia is the predictable cause of insulin–carbohydrate mismatch. This is often multifactorial. Contributory factors include:

- **Drugs**: Excessively high doses of insulin or insulin secretagogues (e.g., glipizide and gliclazide). Other oral hypoglycaemic agents (e.g., metformin and DPP4-inhibitors) are less likely to cause hypoglycaemias.

- **Reduced carbohydrate intake**: Reduced intake and meal timing mismatch.

- **Increased carbohydrate expenditure**: For example, unusual physical activity.

- **Renal impairment**: Renal impairment (acute kidney injury or progressive diabetic nephropathy) leads to reduced insulin clearance; if patients are maintained on the same doses of insulin or oral hypoglycaemic agents, hypoglycaemia will occur.

Other Causes of Hypoglycaemia

These causes should be considered in non-diabetics, or in diabetics in whom there is no overt insulin–carbohydrate mismatch.

- **Critical illness**: Impairment of glucose homoeostasis occurs in critical illness, including hepatic failure and sepsis.

- **Cortisol deficiency**: For example, adrenal insufficiency, panhypopituitarism. This can be evaluated with a short synacthen (adrenocorticotropic hormone (ACTH) stimulation) test.

- **Drugs**: Alcohol binge coupled with limited food intake (inhibits gluconeogenesis), oral supplements or traditional medicine spiked with oral hypoglycaemic agents, and factitious hypoglycaemia (self-induced hypoglycaemia due to insulin injection). A careful drug history is important, although patients may not be forthcoming in factitious hypoglycaemia.

- **Insulinoma** and other endogenous causes of insulin overproduction.

In most cases, the cause is clinically overt. If no apparent cause is found, further workup for insulinoma entails a 72-hr fast with biochemical testing at the point of hypoglycaemia. This will not be discussed in detail (see 'GO FURTHER' on page 365).

 Using what you have learnt, **pen down your approach** to the Clinical Case at the start of the chapter **BEFORE reading the discussion** below.

Case Discussion

This teenager presents with severe hyperglycaemia, following a short history of osmotic symptoms. This is a typical history of diabetic ketoacidosis (DKA); measure venous glucose and confirm DKA by sending blood gases (acidosis), electrolytes (high anion gap) and ketones (positive). His DKA seems to have been precipitated by a respiratory infection (fever and cough)—do a CXR and treat infection. He is likely to have underlying type one diabetes, which will require long-term insulin therapy.

Key Lessons	1. Diabetic ketoacidosis (DKA) and hyperglycaemic hyperosmolar state (HHS) are the two hyperglycaemic emergencies. DKA is marked by ketosis and acidosis, while HHS is marked by severe dehydration, hyperosmolality and markedly elevated glucose.
	2. Secondary causes of hyperglycaemia include drugs, critical illness, Cushing's disease, acromegaly and pancreatic disease. Patients with primary diabetes may fit into classic type 1 or type 2 phenotypes, or may have a more nuanced presentation.
	3. Hypoglycaemia is usually a complication of diabetic treatment. Other causes include critical illness, cortisol deficiency, drugs and insulinoma.
Common Pitfalls	1. Tachypnoea and apparent respiratory distress is not always due to lung pathology. Acidotic patients, such as those with DKA, will also have deep, laboured breathing.
Questions	1. **REFLECT!** Have you ever managed a patient with HHS? How did the patient present and what differentials for delirium were considered?
	2. **EXPLORE!** What electrolyte abnormalities, apart from hyperglycaemia and acidosis, may be found in DKA/HHS, and why are these abnormalities significant?
	3. **GO FURTHER!** How is a 72-hr fast conducted and interpreted? How might biochemical testing distinguish between factitious hypoglycaemia (exogenous insulin) and insulinoma (endogenous insulin)?

Chapter

38

An Approach to Obesity and the Cushing's Syndrome

Clinical Case

A 33-year-old lady sees her dermatologist. She has had mild acne since her teens, but it has become unusually severe in the past year. She is also troubled by her face looking perpetually red and puffy, even without sun exposure. She has been trying various creams, oral medications and 'anti-acne' supplements to no avail. She is also concerned that she has gained 7 kg in the past 6 months and developed abdominal stretch marks. How would you approach her complaint?

The World Health Organization defines obesity as a body mass index (BMI) > 30, and overweight as a BMI of 25 to 30. It is a disease of epidemic proportions, with irrefutable morbidity and mortality risk. While few patients see a doctor complaining of excess weight, the physician can 'size up' every patient who walks through the door, even for a simple upper respiratory tract infection; patients seen for metabolic diseases (e.g., diabetes and gout) should have their BMI measured. There is much the physician can and ought to do to prevent the downstream complications of obesity. The diagnostic aspects, but not management details, are discussed here.

Obesity

The majority of obese patients have a mismatch of energy intake and expenditure due to lifestyle factors, such as dietary excess and lack of exercise (smoking cessation also causes weight gain). A minority will have a medical reason for weight gain. Recent or rapid weight gain should prompt suspicion for a secondary cause.

Medical Causes of Weight Gain

These are identified clinically:

- **Fluid retention:** Some patients gain weight because of fluid retention. Peripheral oedema will be apparent on examination, and there may be other cardiac, renal or hepatic symptoms (see Chapter 47).

- **Drug-induced weight gain:** Weight gain is a side effect of some antipsychotics (e.g., olanzapine), tricyclic antidepressants, antiepileptics (valproate and carbamazepine), insulin and sulphonylurea drugs. Take a drug history for all patients.

- **Endocrine causes:**

  - **Hypothyroidism:** Screening thyroid function is worthwhile (see Chapter 36).

- **Cushing's syndrome**: A distinct clinical picture of corticosteroid excess including centripetal obesity, thin skin, abdominal striae, proximal myopathy and other organ involvement (see the following).

- **Polycystic ovarian syndrome (PCOS)**: A young to middle-aged lady with obesity, oligomenorrhoea and hyperandrogenism (hirsutism, hair loss, acne) (see Chapter 54).

- **Hypothalamic**: Damage to hypothalamic regulatory centres causes hyperphagia. This occurs in the Prader–Willi syndrome and hypothalamic trauma (rare).

Look for Comorbids

There are many comorbids associated with obesity, which need to be individually addressed. Look for:

- Cardiovascular risk factors: Diabetes, hypertension, hyperlipidaemia.

- Other complications of obesity: Obstructive sleep apnoea, non-alcoholic fatty liver disease, gallstones, exacerbation of osteoarthritis and so forth.

The Cushing's Syndrome

The Cushing's syndrome is a clinically recognisable manifestation of corticosteroid excess, with centripetal obesity (facial and abdominal obesity with thin extremities, supraclavicular and dorsocervical fat pads) and skin abnormalities (thin skin, abdominal striae, plethora, easy bruising, hirsutism and acne). Multiple organs may be affected, causing proximal myopathy, glucose intolerance, hypertension, irritability and menstrual irregularities (less prominent than in PCOS). There may be hypokalaemia as cortisol has some mineralocorticoid effect.

Cushing's syndrome should be recognised clinically, confirmed biochemically and worked up for an aetiology—exogenous steroids, a pituitary tumour, adrenal tumour or ectopic ACTH secretion (Figure 38.1).

1. Exclude Exogenous Steroids

The first step is to exclude exogenous steroid use—either prescribed or in bogus supplements. Unfortunately, this is the most common cause of Cushing's syndrome. This diagnosis hinges on clinical history, not biochemical tests. Take a full drug history including traditional medicine and supplements (some of which do not truthfully declare their steroid content). Inhaled corticosteroids (e.g., for asthma) and topical steroids (e.g., for eczema) generally do not cause Cushing's syndrome.

2. Confirm Endogenous Hypercortisolism

Confirmatory testing requires two positive tests (as they individually have inadequate sensitivity and specificity):

- **24-hour urine cortisol**: Elevated.

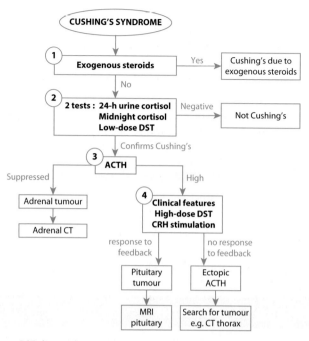

DST, dexamethasone suppression test.

Figure 38.1. Approach to Cushing's syndrome.

- **Midnight cortisol levels** (blood or salivary): Cortisol secretion follows a circadian rhythm, peaking at 8 am and reaching a nadir around midnight, therefore, elevated midnight cortisol levels suggests hypercortisolism. However, collection of midnight cortisol is problematic—waking the patient to draw blood is not a stress-free sample!

- *Low-dose* **dexamethasone suppression test (DST)**: 8 am cortisol is measured after administering 1 mg dexamethasone at midnight (overnight protocol) or 0.5 mg dexamethasone QDS × 2/7 (2-day protocol). Dexamethasone is expected to suppress cortisol secretion; failure to suppress supports a diagnosis of Cushing's syndrome.

3. ACTH Independent vs. ACTH Dependent

Cortisol overproduction may be driven by adrenocorticotropic hormone (ACTH) over-production, or independent of ACTH stimulation. These can be distinguished based on:

(a) **Clinical features**: Some clinical features are signs of a specific aetiology of Cushing's syndrome—hyperpigmentation is seen in ACTH-dependent Cushing's (as the ACTH precursor has a melanocyte stimulating component), while virilisation (male-pattern balding, deepening voice, clitoris hypertrophy) suggests an adrenal tumour.

(b) **Biochemical**: Interrogate the hypothalamic–pituitary–adrenal axis by measuring ACTH levels (usually drawn together with 8 am cortisol if a low-dose DST is done).

- **ACTH levels suppressed**: This indicates autonomous cortisol production, delinked from pituitary stimulation. The pathology is in the adrenal gland—usually an adrenal adenoma, less commonly adrenal carcinoma. Do a contrasted CT adrenals (also see Chapter 54).

- **ACTH levels high or inappropriately normal**: This indicates that ACTH overproduction is driving cortisol production. The next step is to identify whether ACTH is secreted by the pituitary, or by an extra-pituitary site.

4. Pituitary vs. Ectopic ACTH Secretion

ACTH may be secreted by a pituitary tumour (Cushing's disease), or by an extra-pituitary site (most commonly a lung, pancreas or thymus carcinoma). These can be differentiated based on:

- **Clinical features**: Bitemporal hemianopia or cavernous sinus syndrome (cranial nerves III, IV, VI, V_1 and V_2 palsies) suggests mass effect from a pituitary tumour. In ectopic ACTH secretion, patients may have symptoms from the primary tumour (e.g., cough, weight loss, haemoptysis). Many patients have no clinical features of either.

- *High-dose* DST: Pituitary adenomas, arising from normal pituitary tissue, generally retain *some* response to negative feedback. In contrast, tumours with ectopic ACTH secretion do not respond. Therefore, suppression of 8 am cortisol by high doses of dexamethasone (8 mg overnight, in contrast with the 1 mg low-dose test) favours a pituitary adenoma over ectopic ACTH secretion.

- **Corticotropin-releasing hormone (CRH) stimulation test**: Similarly, pituitary adenomas retain some response to CRH stimulation. If CRH administration results in a rise in ACTH and cortisol levels, pituitary adenoma is more likely.

Next step:[1]

- **Likely pituitary tumour**: Obtain MRI pituitary to visualise the tumour. Assess other pituitary hormone function (prolactin, follicle stimulating hormone/luteinising hormone [FSH/LH], thyroid-stimulating hormone [TSH]).

- **Likely ectopic ACTH**: Search for a tumour, usually beginning with CT thorax.

---

[1] There is a role for petrosal venous sinus sampling in selected patients, especially in cases of diagnostic difficulty, in those who do not have a clear-cut pituitary adenoma, or before pituitary surgery (to confirm a functioning adenoma). This is an invasive test involving insertion of a catheter into the venous drainage of the pituitary gland, with attendant risks of stroke and bleeding. It allows demonstration of elevated ACTH levels in the venous drainage from the pituitary gland (compared to peripheral blood ACTH levels), confirming an ACTH-producing pituitary adenoma.

Using what you have learnt, **pen down your approach** to the Clinical Case at the start of the chapter **BEFORE reading the discussion** below.

Case Discussion

This young lady has Cushing's syndrome, with weight gain, abdominal striae, facial plethora and acne. Examine for the other features of Cushing's syndrome. A differential to consider would be the polycystic ovarian syndrome—ask about oligomenorrhoea and examine for marked hirsutism; this can also cause acne and weight gain.

The most likely cause of Cushing's syndrome is undeclared exogenous steroids in the supplements that she has been taking (so much for being 'anti-acne'). If exogenous steroids are ruled out, confirm Cushing's syndrome by doing 24-hr urine cortisol and a low-dose dexamethasone suppression test. Then determine the aetiology of Cushing's syndrome (pituitary, adrenals or ectopic ACTH), beginning with ACTH levels.

Key Lessons	1. Most obesity is due to lifestyle factors, but consider medical reasons for weight gain such as fluid retention, drugs and endocrine disease (hypothyroidism, Cushing's syndrome and polycystic ovarian syndrome).
	2. The most common cause of Cushing's syndrome is exogenous steroids. Endogenous hypercortisolism can be confirmed with 24-hr urine cortisol, midnight cortisol or low-dose dexamethasone suppression testing (two tests).
	3. Cushing's syndrome may be due to a pituitary tumour, adrenal tumour or ectopic ACTH secretion, most commonly by lung cancer. These are differentiated based on clinical features, ACTH levels and ACTH response to high-dose dexamethasone and corticotrophin.
Common Pitfalls	1. Patients may not volunteer a history of taking traditional medicine and supplements, as they do not consider these 'medicines'. They have to be asked specifically whether they use these products.
Questions	1. **REFLECT!** Have you ever seen a patient with Cushing's syndrome? Why did he/she seek medical attention, and which clinical manifestation was the most troubling?
	2. **DISCUSS!** What disorders may mimic the clinical features of Cushing's syndrome? What features are more specific for Cushing's syndrome, and which are less specific?

Chapter

39

An Approach to Falls in the Elderly

Clinical Case

An 80-year-old Chinese lady seeks medical attention after having fallen in the toilet. She was unable to get up, and was found only when her son came home from work in the evening. She had been lethargic in the 2 days preceding the fall. On examination, she is fully alert and orientated, but her right leg is externally rotated and shortened.

At baseline, she is activities of daily living (ADL)-independent and community ambulant with a quad-stick. She has had at least three falls in the last 2 months—one when getting up from the bed, another while walking on level ground and a third after she tripped over a stack of newspaper placed at the door of her bedroom. Her past medical history includes: long-standing diabetes, hypertension, hyperlipidaemia, chronic kidney disease, ischaemic heart disease, atrial fibrillation and osteoarthritis of the knees. Her medications include: Aspirin 100 mg OM, Atorvastatin 40 mg OM, Bisoprolol 5 mg OM, Diclofenac 50 mg BD PRN, Glipizide 5 mg BD, Losartan 50 mg OM, Nifedipine 60 mg OM, Metformin 1 g BD and Warfarin 3 mg OM. In addition, she was started on hydrochlorothiazide 2 months ago for poorly controlled hypertension.

How would you approach her fall(s)?

Falls are common in the frail elderly and threaten functional independence. One-year mortality after a hip fracture is ~25%. It may occur together with other geriatric syndromes, for example, functional decline and delirium. Think through the following questions:

1. Are there any acute medical precipitants?
2. Are there any complications from the fall?
3. How is this patient's baseline like?
4. What are this patient's risk factors for falls and which of them are reversible?

Initial Management

In the acute setting, the imperative is to deal with any acute medical issues, and complications from the fall.

1. Are There Any Acute Medical Precipitants?

Falls may be the initial presentation of systemic disease in an elderly patient with limited functional reserve. Recognise any acute medical emergency or intercurrent illness that may have precipitated the fall. Elicit the circumstances surrounding the fall (pre, during, post-fall)—exploring if it is something more than a simple mechanical fall; a collaborative history is helpful here.

- Red flag symptoms—for example, syncope, loss of consciousness, chest pain, palpitations, sudden weakness or facial droop prior to the fall.

- Lateral tongue bite mark or drowsiness post-fall raises concern for an unwitnessed seizure.

- Fall while attempting to get up from a chair/bed suggests postural hypotension.

- Lethargy, malaise or functional decline over a recent duration implies an intercurrent illness, for example, infection, which may not present with apparent infective symptoms in the elderly. Consider screening chest and urine.

- Some long-standing symptoms, such as chronic non-specific giddiness or functional decline over a long duration, are less likely to be acute medical precipitants. However, they merit attention as they can contribute to falls.

2. Are There Any Complications from the Fall?

Assess for injuries, in particular:

- **Head injury**: Ask for any history of hitting the head or loss of consciousness; examine Glasgow coma scale (GCS), pupils, neurology and look for any scalp bruises or haematoma. Consider CT brain, particularly if there is drowsiness, vomiting, amnesia, a dangerous mechanism of fall (e.g., from height), or signs of basal skull fracture (e.g., 'raccoon eyes', mastoid ecchymosis).[1]

- **Musculoskeletal injury**: Ask about any localising pain, and examine for long bone and joint deformities, including range of motion—hip fractures have been missed because the patient did not complain of pain, and range of motion was not examined. Ability to bear weight post injury is a good indicator that all is well; inability to bear weight may be due to fracture or soft tissue injury alone.

- **Rhabdomyolysis**: Screen creatinine kinase. Patients with a prolonged lie post-fall may suffer rhabdomyolysis, which may lead to renal impairment if not addressed.

Optimisation and Risk Reduction

After stabilising acute medical issues, the focus shifts to optimising the patient's overall function and reducing risk of recurrent falls.

---

[1] Which head injuries require a CT brain? Generally, the threshold is low in the elderly. Various clinical decision rules are available—the Canadian CT Head rule is well known.

3. How Is This Patient's Baseline Like?

Assess the patient's baseline function, for example:

- History of falls
- Baseline function and ambulation status (Table 39.1). Also consider:
  - **Get up and go test**: The time taken to rise from a chair, walk 3 metres, turn around, walk back to the chair and sit down. > 10 s is abnormal.
  - **Functional reach test**: Reaching forward while upright without taking a step forward or losing balance.
- Screen of cognition, mood and social setup.
- Look for concomitant geriatric syndromes, for example, functional decline, delirium/ dementia, incontinence, polypharmacy.

Table 39.1. Functional Assessment of the Elderly

Basic activities of daily living (BADL)		Instrumental activities of daily living (IADL)	
D	Dressing	S	Shopping
E	Eating	H	Housework
A	Ambulation	A	Accounting (managing money)
T	Transfer (e.g. from bed to wheelchair)	F	Food preparation (cooking)
H	Hygiene—toileting	T	Take medicine
S	Showering	T	Telephone use
		T	Transport (e.g., able to take a bus)

4. What Are the Risk Factors for Falls?

Identify the patient's risk factors for falls through a comprehensive review of the patient's medical history, drugs and environment. Of these risk factors, explore which are potentially modifiable, such that intervention might reduce the risk of recurrent falls. A helpful mnemonic is 'BEDBOUND':

- *Blood pressure*: Postural hypotension: Do a good supine-standing postural blood pressure. Postural hypotension may be due to medications (e.g., diuretics), dehydration, diabetic autonomic neuropathy and so forth.
- *Environment*: Environmental hazards, for example, slippery floors, trip hazards (e.g., carpets and loose wires), poor lighting, clutter, objects placed on high areas.
- *Discernment of environment*: Sensory impairment, for example, cataracts, hearing impairment.
- *Brain*: Cognitive impairment or delirium (see Chapter 31).
- *Other medical conditions*: For example, hyponatraemia, chronic giddiness, urinary urgency, anaemia.
- *Unsafe practice*: Poor safety awareness, inappropriate footwear, inappropriate mobility devices.

- **Neurological**: Impairment in strength or balance, for example, prior stroke, Parkinson's disease, cervical myelopathy, normal pressure hydrocephalus, foot drop.

- **Drugs**: Causing hypoglycaemia (e.g., insulin, oral hypoglycaemic agents), hypotension (e.g., anti-hypertensives), or sedation (e.g., antihistamines, anticholinergics, orphenadrine in anarex, opioid analgesics). Attempt to reduce polypharmacy, which increases adverse events and reduces compliance, and be wary of drug–drug and drug–disease interactions.

Also look for risk factors for injury after fall, including:

- **Osteoporosis**: Osteoporosis screening (bone mineral density, fracture risk assessment) and treatment can reduce the risk of hip fracture.

- **Vitamin D** levels.

- **Bleeding risk**: Antiplatelet and anticoagulant agents.

Having identified the risk factors, consider which are modifiable. Intervention strategies to reduce fall risk are necessarily multi-modal, and should target the most modifiable risk factors.

 Using what you have learnt, **pen down your approach** to the Clinical Case at the start of the chapter **BEFORE reading the discussion** below.

Case Discussion

This is an elderly patient with frequent falls. Her latest fall seems to have resulted in a hip fracture—pelvic X-ray will confirm the diagnosis. She has had a prolonged lie and may have rhabdomyolysis—check creatinine kinase and potassium. Her 2-day history of lethargy is concerning for a precipitating cause of fall—for example, an intercurrent infection (screen urine, chest and inflammatory markers). Very commonly, infections in the elderly present not with localising symptoms, but as diminished function, falls or delirium. Other precipitating causes of fall should also be considered.

Having stabilised her acute medical issue (fix fracture, treat infection, etc.), attention shifts to reducing her risk of falling. In this lady, risk factors that can be identified from the vignette include: postural hypotension (falling when getting up), home environment (newspaper placed in doorway), chronic knee pain and diabetic neuropathy (likely as she already has nephropathy). Her falls seem to have started after thiazide was added—a drug notorious for hyponatraemia and postural hypotension. Neurological examination may reveal evidence of prior stroke or cervical myelopathy.

Medication reconciliation is important—in particular, consider stopping thiazide and reducing blood pressure medications (with a less stringent blood pressure target), re-examining the risk-benefit ratio of warfarin in light of recurrent falls, and stopping NSAIDs—she has chronic kidney disease, and in any case the first painkiller should be paracetamol.

Key Lessons	1. Acute management of falls in an elderly patient includes searching for precipitants of the fall, and complications from the fall.
	2. After stabilising acute medical issues, aim to reduce the risk of falls. Evaluate the patient's baseline function, and look for risk factors—think 'BEDBOUND': *b*lood pressure, *e*nvironment, *d*iscernment (sensory), *b*rain (cognition), *o*ther medical conditions, *u*nsafe practices and aids, *n*eurological disease and *d*rugs.
Common Pitfalls	1. Try not to diagnose 'mechanical fall' in elderly patients. There are usually acute precipitants and/or chronic predisposing factors, which can be addressed.
	2. Take the initiative to perform medication reconciliation. Many patients are still on drugs that they no longer need, or no longer benefit from.
Questions	1. **REFLECT!** Have you ever been on an orthopaedic fracture service? How many of your patients with hip fractures manage to regain full functional independence?
	2. **DISCUSS!** Would it be possible to create and implement a preventive 'fall/fracture risk reduction' bundle for all elderly patients admitted to hospital? What would be some of the challenges?
	3. **GO FURTHER!** What are some protective factors against falls in the elderly? How might we reinforce these factors so as to mitigate fall risk?
	4. **EXPLORE!** The Canadian CT Head Rule is a risk-stratification system to help decide which patients with minor head injury merit a CT brain. What does this rule say, and is it a good clinical decision aid?

Skin and Subcutaneous Tissues

Chapter **An Approach to**
40 **Rash**

Clinical Case

A previously well 23-year-old student presents with fever and a generalised rash. She had a bad flu a week ago, which got better after taking some medicines. On examination, she appears unwell with 1 cm to 2 cm red spots on her trunk and limbs. Some of the spots are raised, and some are confluent. What are the differential diagnoses? What are the 'danger signs' to look for?

We often wonder how dermatologists take one look at a rash, glance at the clinical context and make a spot diagnosis. Few other approaches rely as heavily on gestalt and pattern recognition; there is no replacement for clinical experience. Nonetheless, it is helpful to begin with a few differentials for each morphology of rash, and be aware of key distinguishing features to look for. Rashes are discussed in this chapter, growths and lumps in the next.

Note: This approach offers a simple framework to start recognising typical presentations of common rashes. It is helpful to look up pictures as you read through the chapter (e.g., use a dermatology atlas, or www.dermnetnz.org)—there is no shortcut to recognise morphology. Familiarity with the vocabulary to describe morphology is assumed; note also that atypical presentations and less common rashes are omitted.

Initial Approach

If you recognise the rash, zoom in on the spot diagnosis but consider the differential diagnosis. If you do not recognise the rash, identify broad morphologic groups (Figure 40.1).

- **Eczematous and scaling rashes**: Pruritic rashes ± excoriations, scaling (light-coloured skin flakes that fall off easily) and lichenification (thick epidermis with accentuated skin markings).

- **Vesicles, bullae and pustules**: Intra-epidermal fluid-filled or pus-filled papules. These lesions may also leave crust—adherent dried serum and debris, which can be scraped off (less easily than scales) to leave a weeping base.

- **Erythematous non-scaly rash**: Erythematous non-scaly macules and papules that blanch on pressure.

- **Dark non-blanchable rash**: Hyperpigmented non-blanchable macules and papules.

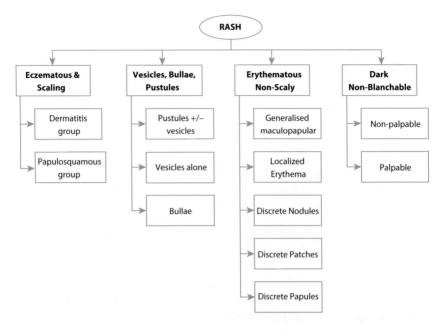

Figure 40.1. Morphologies of a rash.

Eczematous and Scaling Rashes

Eczematous and scaling rashes can be divided into two overlapping groups (if unsure consider both):

- **Dermatitis group**: Intensely pruritic eczematous rashes with *indistinct borders*. The hallmark of chronic dermatitis is lichenification—visible, palpable epidermal thickening with accentuated skin markings.

- **Papulosquamous group**: *Scaly* papules, plaques and patches; usually *well-demarcated* and pruritic (pruritus may range from mild to severe). Be sure to distinguish *scale* from *crust* (seen in broken vesicles, bullae and pustules).

Dermatitis Group

1. **Is there a secondary cause?** Look for these causes because they can be treated.
   - **Contact dermatitis**: Any dermatitis that takes a specific pattern (e.g., linear, rectangle, distinct borders) or which may conform to areas of contact (e.g., beneath a wristwatch) should prompt suspicion of contact dermatitis. Contact dermatitis may be irritant or allergic in nature. Take an exposure history for these causes, and consider patch testing to confirm:
     - Hands: Occupational/household chemicals, gloves.
     - Wrist, ears, belt line: Jewellery, watch, belt.
     - Face and neck: Cosmetics, aerosolised fragrances (e.g., perfumes and air fresheners).

- Others: Creams, topical medications.
- Perineum: Moisture, especially if on diapers.

- **Stasis dermatitis**: Venous hypertension can result in lower limb eczema, hyper-pigmentation and even venous ulcers. This is most marked above the medial malleoli (see Chapter 46).

- **Scabies**: Always consider in the right demographic group (e.g., nursing home resident, elderly, less privileged, recent hospitalisation), or if finger and toe webs, wrists, axillary and pubic folds are particularly affected. Scabies classically presents as pruritic papules in web spaces and skin folds, sometimes with visible burrows, but can resemble dermatitis after extensive scratching. Ask for a contact history (is anyone else at home scratching?).

2. **If no secondary cause found, consider idiopathic aetiologies.**

- **Atopic dermatitis (eczema)**: This starts in childhood and has a chronic relapsing course. It especially affects the flexor surfaces (cubital and popliteal fossa), and often extends beyond. The patient often has atopic comorbids (i.e., atopic dermatitis, asthma, allergic rhinitis) and a positive family history.

- **Xerotic eczema**: Dry with craquele (fish-scale) appearance, can fissure with resultant pain and erythema and superimposed secondary infection.

- **Nummular (discoid) eczema**: Coin-shaped patches and plaques, usually multiple on limbs, which start erythematous and turn dry and scaly.

- **Seborrheic dermatitis**: Affecting mainly the T-zone of the face and the scalp (page 382).

Papulosquamous Group

1. **Can this be fungal?**

- **Dermatophyte fungi (tinea, ringworm)**: Annular patches with elevated, well-defined, serpiginous borders ± central clearing. This may affect the groin (tinea cruris), foot (tinea pedis, athlete's foot), face (tinea faciale) or elsewhere on the body (tinea corporis) and are usually asymmetrical. Always consider dermatophyte infection in an itchy patch—skin scraping and potassium hydroxide (KOH) smear may find spores and hyphae.

2. **Attempt to identify based on morphology and distribution.**

- **Psoriasis**: Skin-coloured or erythematous papules and plaques with silvery scales, classically affecting scalp, elbows and knees. These may be few and large (e.g., chronic plaque psoriasis) or small and many (e.g., guttate psoriasis), and is usually more symmetrical than tinea. Removal of scales reveals small bleeding points (Auspitz sign), and skin trauma aggravates lesions (Koebner phenomenon). Nails involvement is common (pitting, onycholysis, discoloration), and there may also be arthritis (see Chapter 48). This is a chronic long-standing disease.

- **Nummular (discoid) eczema**: Oval, weeping patches and plaques with crusted papulovesicles (exudative acute discoid eczema) or multiple dry, erythematous, well-circumscribed oval plaques (dry discoid eczema).

- **Pityriasis rosea**: This starts as a herald patch on the trunk (resembling tinea). Two to five days later, the patient develops tan or salmon-coloured oval scaly papules and patches with collarette scales (arranged in a ring) on the trunk and proximal limbs, in a 'Christmas tree' distribution (following skin cleavage lines). This is thought to be an immune reaction to herpes viruses 6 and 7, which self-resolves in 6 to 8 weeks.

- **Pityriasis lichenoides** et varioliformis acuta (PLEVA) and Pityriasis lichenoides chronica (PLC): Crops of erythematous papules on trunk and limbs appearing over weeks–months; with central necrosis and haemorrhagic crusting (in PLEVA), or central mica-like scales (in PLC), or hyper/hypo-pigmentation (post-inflammatory) or any combination of lesions.

- **Seborrheic dermatitis**: Ill-defined erythematous patches with course greasy scales, mainly affecting sebaceous gland-rich areas—scalp, eyebrows, creases around the nose and behind the ears; sometimes also the upper trunk and skin folds (axilla, groin, inframammary folds).

- **Lichen planus**: Pruritic purple planar polygonal papules and plaques, or white mucosal patches with white lines (see page 388).

3. **Consider systemic disease and sinister causes.**

- **Discoid lupus**: These plaques begin purplish-red and scaly, then turn depressed and *atrophic* (often with a hyperpigmented border). These are usually found on sun-exposed skin (face, trunk, arms). If involving scalp or hairline, it may also cause scarring alopecia. Lupus may be skin-limited or systemic—look for manifestations of possible systemic lupus erythematosus (SLE), test antinuclear antibody (ANA), dsDNA and consider biopsy.

- **Malignant and premalignant causes**: The first clue is often that the lesion looks 'atypical' or thick, and does not respond to topical treatment. A biopsy is necessary to confirm or exclude.

  - **Mycosis fungoides**: A cutaneous T-cell lymphoma, initially indistinguishable from psoriasis or eczema (may be irregular or look atypical to an experienced eye), which gradually becomes elevated, indurated, then nodular or ulcerative.

  - **Extramammary Paget's disease**: Suspect this in a chronic 'eczematous rash', 'lichen simplex' or 'psoriatic plaque' in the groin that does not improve with steroids. This is an intraepithelial adenocarcinoma that may arise from skin cancer or from underlying anorectal or bladder adenocarcinoma.

  - **Bowen's disease** (squamous cell carcinoma *in situ*): An irregular, asymmetrical, erythematous scaly or crusted plaque.

  - **Actinic keratosis**: A scaly, erythematous patch or papule on sun-exposed skin (usually face).

- **Secondary syphilis**: A great mimic; consider especially if palms and soles are involved. Take a sexual history, do VDRL and a treponemal test (e.g., TPPA).

- **Drug eruptions**: For example, antimalarials (chloroquine), lithium, beta-blockers.

Vesicles, Bullae, Pustules

Decide if these papules are filled with pus (**pustules**) or clear fluid. Clear blisters are sorted by size as **vesicles** (small < 0.5 cm) and **bullae** (larger > 0.5 cm).

Pustules ± Vesicles

Pustules are neutrophil collections representing infection or inflammation. Their distribution is key.

Predominantly face:

- **Acne**: Usually a young person with papules and pustules, open and closed comedones (black- and whiteheads) in the face and upper trunk. Rule out secondary causes, for example, cosmetics, drugs (steroids, phenytoin, lithium) and Cushing's disease. A lady with particularly bad acne should be examined for other signs of hirsutism (see Chapter 54).

- **Rosacea**: Often a middle-aged patient with chronic erythema and telangiectasia of the central third of the face (nose and medial cheeks). There may be papules and pustules, blepharitis, conjunctivitis and frequent flushing; comedones are absent.

Asymmetrical, localised: More likely an infective cause.

- **Herpes zoster** (shingles): Vesicles and pustules on an erythematous base, in a *dermatomal distribution*, often with pain and pruritus. Send vesicle smear for varicella-zoster virus (VZV) PCR. Zoster in the CN V_1 dermatome can cause sight-threatening corneal involvement—urgent ophthalmology consult is indicated. Zoster in the immunocompromised can be disseminated and life-threatening.

- **Impetigo (non-bullous)**: *Staphylococcus aureus* skin infection can present *anywhere* as pustules, which quickly break to form a honey-coloured crust. Scraping crust away leaves a non-ulcerated glistening base. Gram stain of the crust finds gram positive cocci.

Symmetrical, generalised—angry looking pustules with a background of erythematous skin:

- **Acute generalised exanthematous pustulosis** (AGEP): An acute generalised eruption of pinpoint superficial non-follicular pustules on a background of erythematous skin, which may coalesce to become lakes of pustules. Triggers include drugs (antibiotics, e.g., beta-lactams, carbamazepine, etc.) and viruses.

- **Pustular psoriasis**: The morphology is identical to AGEP—but there is usually a history of psoriasis, and often a superimposed trigger (e.g., steroid withdrawal, sepsis, stress or hypocalcaemia). This is potentially life threatening.

Symmetrical, generalised—without angry skin:

- **Varicella zoster** (chickenpox): A generalised pruritic eruption. Lesions develop rapidly from macules, to papules, vesicles, then pustules and crusting; *lesions of all stages are present at the same time*. This is a disease of childhood, but may occur in adults who have neither had chickenpox nor vaccination.

- **Folliculitis**: Papules and pustules formed in hair follicles (hair seen at the centre of lesions). This may be due to *Malassezia furfur* (pustules appear monomorphic), gram positive skin commensals or gram negative bacteria (especially in patients on antibiotics). Do gram stain and skin scraping.

- **Pseudofolliculitis barbae**: 'Folliculitis' of a dense beard may not be infective, but an inflammatory response to a curved ingrowing beard.

Vesicles Alone

The key is to recognise these monomorphic vesicles, filled with clear fluid. Distinguish by their distribution:

- **Acute contact dermatitis**: May present initially as vesicles in the area of contact, before becoming an eczematous rash. Look for classic sites of contact dermatitis and take a contact history (see page 380).

- **Herpes simplex virus (HSV)**: HSV infection presents as grouped vesicles on an erythematous base, affecting the lips (HSV-1), genitals (HSV-2: screen for other STDs) or hands (herpetic whitlow); autoinoculation of distant sites can also occur. Primary infection results in more extensive disease ± systemic fever and malaise, while recurrent lesions occur in the same site and are milder. HSV infection can be severe in the immunocompromised, or on eczematous skin (eczema herpeticum). Viral swabs can be taken by scraping the base of a fresh blister; virus can be proven by PCR or immunofluorescence, and Tzanck smear may show multinucleated giant cells.

- **Hand–foot–mouth disease** (coxsackievirus and enterovirus): Erythematous macules, vesicles and ulcers affecting hand, foot and mouth. There may be sore throat and fever.

Bullae

Bullae arise from disruption of adhesion molecules or epidermal cell injury. Intra-epidermal bullae are flaccid and easily ruptured, but sub-epidermal bullae are tense and less easily broken. Very often, patients present with bullae already broken, leaving the skin with erosions or crusts and the clinician with no clue. Some differentials:

- **Stevens–Johnson syndrome and toxic epidermal necrolysis (SJS–TEN)**: This is the first differential to consider in a sick patient—bullae and erosions occur late in its course (see page 385).

- **Bullous impetigo**: While impetigo usually presents with pustules and thick crusts, *S. aureus* strains that produce exfoliative toxins can present with bullous impetigo—*flaccid* clear or cloudy bullae, which rupture to leave a thin crust. One bulla can become multiple after autoinoculation.

- **Pemphigus vulgaris**: Large *flaccid* blisters, which rupture to leave weeping/crusted erosions. There is extensive mucous membrane involvement, and Nikolsky's sign is positive (pressure applied laterally to the bulla results in extension). This is an autoimmune disease occurring in middle-aged to elderly patients, and may rarely be a paraneoplastic syndrome.

- **Pemphigus foliaceus**: *Flaccid* blisters with positive Nikolsky's sign, similar to pemphigus vulgaris, but without mucosal involvement.
- **Bullous pemphigoid**: *Tense* pruritic blisters on normal or erythematous skin, negative Nikolsky's sign and mucosal sparing. This is an autoimmune disease occurring in elderly patients, associated with neurologic disease.

Workup: Skin biopsy and immunofluorescence is essential for diagnosis of bullous diseases.

Erythematous Non-Scaly Rash

Erythema is a sign of hyper-vascularity from local inflammation. Broad subgroups are:

- **Generalised maculopapular rash**: Generalised erythema or erythematous macules and papules, symmetrically distributed over large areas of skin.
- **Localised erythema**: Unique morphologies with a specific distribution.
- **Discrete erythematous nodules**: Isolated subcutaneous nodules.
- **Discrete erythematous plaques and patches**: Isolated erythematous to dark plaques and patches.
- **Discrete erythematous papules**: Small pruritic papules that do not become confluent.

Generalised Maculopapular Rashes

First rule out Stevens–Johnson syndrome/toxic epidermal necrolysis (SJS–TEN). Drug and viral rashes are hard to tell apart; toxic erythemas and erythroderma look classic.

Distinctive:

- **SJS–TEN**: Begins as fever + a *painful* diffuse symmetrical rash (erythema, dusky patches, coalescing erythematous ± purpuric macules; may also include papules and other morphologies), starting in the face and thorax then spreading elsewhere. Later, bullae form and skin sloughs to give large erosions; the extent of body surface area sloughed distinguishes SJS (< 10%), SJS–TEN overlap (10–30%) and TEN (> 30%). Mucous membranes are almost always involved—causing painful mucositis, ulcers, conjunctivitis or urethritis. Patients are systemically ill with fever, anaemia, leucocytosis or leukopenia, fluid loss with electrolyte imbalances and secondary bacterial infection. Aetiologies of SJS/TEN are drugs (the same list below) and infection (especially mycoplasma). Biopsy is usually done.
- *Erythema *multiforme*:*[1] Erythematous lesions of *m*ultiple *f*orms, including erythematous papules and plaques, target lesions, vesicles and bullae. Target lesions are

---

[1] **Note**: 'Erythema multiforme major' refers to SJS; this term is discouraged as they are thought to be distinct diseases and not a continuum.

diagnostic but not always present—these have *three zones* of colour: an (1) erythematous halo around (2) a middle pale area, within which an (3) erythematous or dark centre. Lesions develop acutely (< 24 hr), starting in the peripheries and spreading centripetally, and persist for about 2 weeks. They may be pruritic and involve mucous membranes. Aetiology is most commonly infectious (e.g., HSV, mycoplasma) or drug-related.

Mainly maculopapular rash:

- **Drug rash**: Sudden-onset symmetrical rash; may or may not be pruritic, and may exfoliate. *Drugs can cause many rash morphologies; always consider drugs in any acute-onset rash.* Take a careful drug history (including over-the-counter, traditional medicines and supplements) to assess the likelihood of a drug rash, and identify the likely culprit based on:

  (1) Known propensity of the drug to cause rashes: Especially beta-lactams, NSAIDs, sulphonamides (e.g., bactrim), allopurinol, antivirals and antiepileptics.

  (2) Temporal course: Usually a new drug initiated several days ago (not immediately). Exception: DRESS (drug reaction with eosinophilia and systemic symptoms) is a delayed reaction 2 to 6 weeks after drug initiation. Drawing a drug chart helps.

- **Viral exanthem**: Itself indistinguishable from drug rashes, but there may be accompanying viral symptoms (fever, upper respiratory symptoms, etc.). The classic viral exanthems include measles, rubella, roseola (fifth disease, herpes virus 6), enteroviruses and erythema infectiosum (parvovirus B19)—but many other viruses can cause exanthems too. Viral exanthems are most common in children; take a vaccination and contact history.

- **Secondary syphilis**: Consider especially if palms and soles are involved.

Mainly erythema:

- **Toxic erythemas**: Generalised erythema with a sandpaper feel ± desquamation, fever and mucous membrane involvement. Each cause of toxic erythema has unique features:

  - **Scarlet fever**: Sore throat and strawberry tongue (initially white exudate with red papillae, then beefy red). This is due to toxin secretion by erythrogenic strains of *Streptococcus pyogenes.*

  - **Staphylococcal scalded skin syndrome**: Red, blistering skin (that looks like a scald) due to a local staphylococcus infection (abscess, cellulitis, otitis). Mucous membranes are spared.

  - **Toxic shock syndrome**: Typically, a patient with cutaneous staphylococcus infection who abruptly develops fever, hypotension, *diffuse erythroderma with subsequent desquamation*, mucosal hyperaemia and multiorgan involvement (gastrointestinal, muscular, renal, hepatic, neurological and haematological).

  - **Kawasaki disease**: A child with fever exceeding 5 days, bilateral non-suppurative conjunctivitis, mucosal erythema, cervical lymphadenopathy, truncal rash, erythema and oedema of palms/soles then desquamation. Not all features may be present but one clue is that children with Kawasaki disease are always irritable.

This is a vasculitis and important to diagnose because of the propensity for coronary artery aneurysm formation (and medicolegal complications).

- **Erythroderma**: Erythema and exfoliation affecting almost the entire skin (>90%)—multiple causes: psoriasis, severe atopic dermatitis, drug (e.g., vancomycin), Sezary syndrome (cutaneous T-cell lymphoma) and so forth.

Localised Erythema

These have unique morphologies and are spot diagnoses.

- **Urticaria (hives) and angioedema**: Urticaria is seen as pruritic oedematous wheals with red borders and pale centres. Angioedema also involves mucosa (e.g., eyelids, lips), and may be tender. Rule out anaphylaxis (stridor, dyspnoea or hypotension).

  - Acute urticaria is transient (<24 hr, or <72 hr for angio-oedema) and triggered by acute viral infections, drugs (antibiotics, NSAIDs, opiates, CT contrast, etc.), food allergy or insect stings. If urticaria is painful, resolves slowly (>24 hr), or leaves a bruise or hyper-pigmentation, suspect urticarial vasculitis and do biopsy.

  - Chronic urticaria (>6 weeks, each wheal <24 hr) may be due to physical (heat, cold, pressure, sunlight, exercise) or contact (e.g., latex) triggers, occult infection (e.g., *Helicobacter pylori*), autoimmune disease (e.g., thyroid) or idiopathic. Also consider urticaria due to ACE-inhibitors (bradykinin pathway) and hereditary angio-oedema (due to C1 inhibitor deficiency).

- **Cellulitis**: A febrile patient with an erythematous, warm, swollen and tender patch of skin (most commonly in the lower limbs). Watch out for necrotising fasciitis if pain is unusually severe, erythema progresses rapidly or the patient is toxic.

- **Systemic autoimmune diseases**: Photosensitive erythematous rashes characteristically occurring on sun-exposed areas (e.g., face, neck and shoulders in a 'shawl' distribution, etc.), with other characteristic features:

  - **Lupus**: 'Butterfly' malar facial rash sparing the nasolabial folds, oral ulcers, discoid rash and systemic involvement (see Chapter 48).

  - **Dermatomyositis**: Violaceous macules around the eyelids (heliotrope rash), hyperpigmented papules over the knuckles (Gottron's papules) and proximal myopathy.

Discrete Erythematous Nodules

- **Erythema nodosum**: Acute-onset tender nodules on bilateral shins. This has multiple disease associations, including infection (streptococcal throat infection, viruses, mycoplasma, tuberculosis), autoimmune disease (inflammatory bowel disease, sarcoidosis), haematological malignancies and drugs (oral contraceptives, sulphonamides, NSAIDs).

- **Prurigo nodularis**: Intensely pruritic erythematous and firm nodules (1–3 cm), often with excoriations and scratch marks. There will often be a history of the patient repeatedly scratching the nodule, which contributes to its persistence.

- Consider the various causes of skin lumps (see Chapter 41).

Discrete Erythematous Plaques and Patches

- **Lichen planus**: Pruritic *p*urple *p*lanar (flat) *p*olygonal *p*apules and *p*laques, with a reticulate pattern of white lines on its surface (Wickham's striae). This classically affects flexors of wrists and shins, but can involve any site, including mucosa (white patches with reticulated white lines) and scalp (scarring alopecia). Trauma aggravates lesions (the Koebner phenomenon), and lichen planus can occur in streaks (it spreads along where the patient has scratched). Lichen planus is idiopathic or secondary to drugs (take a drug history). Most lesions resolve spontaneously in 1 to 2 years but 10% remain chronic.

- **Candidiasis**: A confluent, beefy red eruption with indistinct borders, satellite papules and pustules. This usually occurs in a moist area, for example, the groin. Fungal scrapings are positive.

- **Fixed drug eruption**: Sharply demarcated red, violet or dusky plaques, appearing 24 to 48 hr after exposure to an offending drug; the centre of the plaque can blister, fading when the drug is discontinued, and recurring at the same spot when re-exposed to the drug.

- **Erythema migrans**: This cutaneous lesion of Lyme disease is an erythematous patch that expands over days to weeks, giving a macular non-scaling border (fungal scrapings negative) and clearing centre. Consider in patients with a travel history to grassy areas in temperate countries—where ticks may be found.

Discrete Erythematous Papules

- **Insect bites**: The diagnosis is usually obvious—a pruritic hive with a central punctum ± excoriations, usually on exposed skin. Consider mosquitoes, bedbugs (bites in threes—breakfast, lunch and dinner) and head lice (nits may be found).

- **Scabies**: Intensely pruritic papules in the finger and toe webs, wrists and elbows, axillae, feet and pubic region. Small burrows may be visible as snaking thread-like lines; these are diagnostic. Skin scrapings of the papules and burrows will find mites and eggs. Many patients with scabies are from nursing homes and deprived socioeconomic environments; as it can affect close contacts, ask about itching in family members and family pets—all of whom must be treated.

- **Folliculitis**: Papules and pustules formed in hair follicles (page 384).

- **Pruritic papular eruption of HIV**: Intensely pruritic papules with a symmetrical and diffuse distribution, which mimics folliculitis and prurigo nodularis. Patients presenting with 'folliculitis' should be tested for HIV.

- **Miliaria (heat rash)**: Multiple pruritic small papules (dewdrops) on the trunk, caused by occlusion of sweat ducts in a hot and humid environment.

- **Keratosis pilaris**: Small 'rough bumps' on upper arms, thighs and sometimes face. This is due to keratinised hair follicles.

Dark Non-Blanchable Rash

Identify if a dark rash is palpable or non-palpable.

Non-Palpable Dark Macules

Hyperpigmentation arises from either melanin or blood.

Purpuric: Purpura are *dark* and *non-blanchable* (purpura are intradermal bleeds, pressure cannot return extravasated blood into circulation, so they do not blanch).

- **Bleeding diathesis**: For example, disseminated intravascular coagulation (DIVC), immune thrombocytopenia (ITP), dengue, over-warfarinisation (see Chapter 33).

- **Rule out SJS/TEN**: Look for erosions and mucosal involvement (see page 385).

- **Senile purpura**: Most commonly bruises at IV cannula and phlebotomy sites in elderly patients with thin skin.

Non-purpuric: Mostly due to melanin overproduction.

- **Freckles**: A hyperpigmented macule found on sun-exposed skin, appearing before 3 years of age, darkening with sunlight.

- **Melasma**: Patchy hyperpigmented facial macules, often in women, associated with sunlight, pregnancy and birth control pills.

- **Actinic (solar) lentigos, nevus (moles) and melanomas**: A solar lentigo is a brown to dark macule occurring on sun-exposed areas in adulthood. A nevus usually presents as a growth, but may also be a flat macule. An asymmetrical, variegated and progressively enlarging dark macule should raise concern for melanoma (see Chapter 41).

- **Fixed drug eruption**: This may appear dark (see page 388).

- **Diabetic dermopathy**: Multiple red–brown or hyperpigmented papules, usually on anterior shins.

Palpable Purpura

Palpable purpura implies vasculitis—inflammatory changes cause oedema and elevate the lesion such that it is palpable. These most commonly present on the lower limbs. Aetiologies include:

- **Infections**: A febrile and toxic patient with palpable purpura has meningococcal sepsis until proven otherwise. Other bacterial (Staphylococcus, Streptococcus, Pseudomonas, Gonococcus), and viral (HIV, hepatitis) infections can also cause palpable purpura.

- **Drugs**: A drug history is important. Frequently blamed drugs include beta-lactam antibiotics (penicillin and cephalosporins), sulphonamides (including loop and thiazide diuretics), phenytoin, allopurinol and aspirin.

- **Systemic autoimmune disease**: Many, including lupus, ANCA vasculitis (e.g., granulomatosis with polyangiitis), polyarteritis nodosa and Henoch–Schonlein purpura. Look for systemic manifestations of these diseases.

- **Malignancy**: Usually haematological, for example, lymphoma and myeloma.

- **Idiopathic cutaneous small vessel vasculitis**: A diagnosis of exclusion; may be precipitated by mild viral infection but usually self-limiting.

Workup for palpable purpura: First rule out bacterial sepsis; if suspected, culture and treat urgently. Do a careful systemic review for systemic features of infection, autoimmune disease and malignancy; do a drug chart and rule out drug causes. Confirm vasculitis by biopsy and immunofluorescence. If the patient is otherwise well, an option is to wait 2 weeks for transient viral causes to resolve. If persistent, workup based on clinical and immunofluorescence findings, for example, send autoimmune serology (ANCA, ANA, etc.), viral tests (e.g., Hepatitis B/C), screen for systemic organ involvement (e.g., creatinine), myeloma and cryoglobulins.

 Using what you have learnt, **pen down your approach** to the Clinical Case at the start of the chapter **BEFORE reading the discussion** below.

Case Discussion

The morphology described is a generalised maculopapular rash. The most dangerous differential is SJS–TEN. Danger signs which would favour SJS–TEN over a more benign cause include: dusky-looking rash, epithelial sloughing, pain over the rash, mucosal involvement (gingival sloughing, oral ulcers, conjunctivitis and urethritis), and a systemically ill patient. Other differentials include erythema multiform, drug rash and viral exanthem.

She has had an antecedent flu-like illness and has also received medicines. Construct a drug chart—beta-lactam antibiotics (especially if she has never taken them before) are potential culprits, while antihistamines and cough suppressants would be less likely; drugs used for a long time or those only started after the rash began are less likely to be the cause of her rash. Infection (mycoplasma, viruses) may also the cause of her exanthem. Stop any culprit drug, but exercise caution before labelling an allergy as this has long-term consequences—the more severe the drug reaction, and the more certain that a drug is the culprit, the more inclined one should be to label it as an allergy.

Key Lessons	1. Most rashes can be identified by classifying into broad morphologic groups (see flowchart).
	2. Few rashes are true emergencies: Stevens–Johnson's syndrome, meningococcal sepsis, pustular psoriasis and acute generalised exanthematous pustulosis. Always consider these emergencies early.

3. Red flags for systemic disease include an isolated atypical psoriatic plaque (malignancy), palpable purpura (vasculitis), symmetrical pruritic papules in a compatible demographic group (HIV) and involvement of palms and soles (syphilis).

Common Pitfalls

1. Do not rush to guess a spot diagnosis if you are unfamiliar. Instead, carefully observe the rash and describe its morphology. Then match morphological description to diagnosis, and diagnosis to aetiology.

2. There is no hurry to make a diagnosis. Many rashes self-resolve, watchful waiting is in itself a diagnostic tool as long as the patient remains well.

Questions

1. **REFLECT!** Have you ever had a patient whose rash was a diagnostic mystery? What was the eventual diagnosis, and how was it clinched?

2. **EXPLORE!** Look up pictures of common rashes—photos of different rashes, as well as different photos of the same rash. It is helpful to have a 'mental photo library' of the common rashes against which you can compare a new, unknown rash.

3. **DISCUSS!** 'Knowing the exact diagnosis of a rash is usually not critical, because one can simply give a combination cream (e.g., Triderm® or Combiderm®, a 3-in-1 preparation of betamethasone, clotrimazole and gentamicin)'. Do you agree?

Chapter

41 An Approach to Skin Growths and Lumps

Clinical Case

A 40-year-old Italian lady is troubled by a 'mole' on her inner thigh. It had been there all her life but has been enlarging in size recently. Examination reveals an 8 mm × 9 mm irregularly shaped plaque. It is darkly pigmented with intervening areas of lighter pigmentation. What is the next step?

Patients who present with skin growths or lumps are usually concerned about either malignancy or cosmesis. Even if you are unable to pinpoint an exact diagnosis, it is important to identify red flags (e.g., irregular margins or fixation to deep structures). First narrow down the category:

- **Epidermal growths**: Growths arising solely from the epidermis, appearing as localised epidermal thickenings, fixed to skin and mobile over subcutaneous tissues.

- **Lumps**: Palpable lumps deep to the skin; they may or may not be associated with overlying skin changes.

- **Lumps in specific locations**: Consider specific differentials—see the approaches to breast lumps (see Chapter 43), groin lumps (see Chapter 42), neck lumps (see Chapter 44) and lymphadenopathy (see Chapter 45).

Epidermal Growths

Diagnosis hinges on recognising morphology. First dichotomise into pigmented and unpigmented growths.

Unpigmented Epidermal Growths

Malignant and premalignant:

- **Basal cell carcinoma (BCC), nodular type**: A pearly nodule with a rolled border, with irregular margins, surface telangiectasia, central depression or ulceration (rodent ulcer).

- **Squamous cell carcinoma (SCC)**: A hard, flesh-coloured or erythematous nodule. There may be surface necrosis, crusting, ulceration or fixation to deep tissue. SCC tends to occurs on the head and neck, on mucous membranes and in areas of chronic injury (e.g., chronic ulcers and burn scars).

- **Keratoacanthoma:** This resembles SCC but grows rapidly over 4 to 6 weeks. It has an irregular crater with a central keratin plug. Can be difficult to distinguish from SCC, and is managed similarly.

- **Actinic (solar) keratosis:** A rough-textured and crusty, erythematous, scaling patch or papule occurring in sun-exposed areas. This is pre-malignant; if thick and indurated, consider malignant change.

Others:

- **Corn:** A white–grey, well-circumscribed hard papule or nodule with preservation of skin lines. This usually occurs on skin exposed to chronic friction or pressure, for example, on feet or fingers. On paring, skin lines are preserved.

- **Wart:** A flesh-coloured, hyperkeratotic, firm papule or nodule, with a corrugated (common wart) or flat surface (flat wart). If on the sole (plantar wart), it may be painful and covered with thick callus. Paring down with a scalpel reveals the underlying wart with interruption of skin lines and black puncta (these are thrombosed capillaries).

- **Molluscum contagiosum:** A smooth, hard, flesh-coloured small dome-shaped papule with central umbilication.

- **Adnexal structures:** Skin-coloured growths *on the face* may arise from sweat glands (syringoma—especially around the eyelids), hair follicles (trichoepithelioma—especially around the nasolabial fold) or from sebaceous gland hyperplasia (yellow umbilicated papules on cheeks and forehead).

- **Skin tag (squamous papilloma):** A soft, flesh coloured, pedunculated fleshy papule.

Pigmented Epidermal Growths

Pigmented macules (flat) are covered in Chapter 40. Obvious growths include:

- **Melanoma:** Suspicious features (ABCDE) in any pigmented growth (*a*symmetry, *b*order irregularity, *c*olour variegation, *d*iameter > 6 mm and *e*levation) should prompt consideration of melanoma. May be found not only on skin but also on palms or soles (acral lentiginous melanoma), on nails and on oral/genital mucosal surfaces.

- **Pigmented BCC:** Mimics a melanoma, but with a pearly rolled margin seen when viewed side-on.

- **Nevus (mole):** Pigmented macule (junctional naevi) or papule (dermal naevi) with uniform colour, regular border and a smooth or verrucous surface.

- **Seborrheic keratosis:** Multiple greasy, 'pasted on' plaques or papules, with sharp margins. This starts skin-coloured but slowly darken and can turn black.

Workup

All lesions with suspicion of malignancy should be biopsied for definitive diagnosis.

Skin Lumps

Diagnosis hinges on careful physical examination. Look at site, size, shape, margins and surface or scars. Feel for temperature, tenderness, consistency and fluctuance. Attempt to move the lump, assessing fixation. Ask about time course and symptoms. Rapid increase in size, necrosis or ulceration are red flags for malignancy.

The various lumps can be divided into non-tender (a) soft, (b) firm and (c) hard lumps; as well as (d) tender and erythematous lumps. Lumps appearing only at specific sites (breast, groin, neck) are discussed in their relevant chapters.

(a) Soft Skin Lumps

The colour of the lump is a helpful guide.

- **Lipoma**: A soft, mobile, compressible lump with a smooth surface, positive slip sign and *intact overlying skin*. Some lipomas feel lobulated.

- **Dermoid cyst**: A soft, mobile, fluctuant (non-compressible) lump with a smooth surface, negative slip sign and *intact overlying skin*. These are usually found along lines of skin fusion, for example, along the eyebrows or in the midline.

- **Neurofibroma**: Soft, *flesh-coloured* papules/nodules, which, with pressure, can be invaginated into the skin, forming a 'button-hole' defect. Look for other neurofibromas, café-au-lait spots (> 15 mm is significant in post-pubertal individuals) and axillary or inguinal freckling that would suggest neurofibromatosis.

- **Haemangioma**: A *red* (superficial) to *blue* (deep) nodule, often blanchable.

- **Kaposi sarcoma**: *Purple* macule, plaque or nodule; may be multiple. Examine for lymphadenopathy and hairy leucoplakia in the mouth. Biopsy and test for HIV— Kaposi's sarcoma occurs in AIDS and immunosuppressed individuals.

(b) Firm Skin Lumps

- **Sebaceous cyst (epidermal inclusion cyst)**: A firm flesh-coloured nodule, often tense and fluctuant. The overlying skin shows a *central punctum* and may have a blue hue. It may produce a greasy yellow foul smelling discharge.

- **Dermatofibroma**: A small (0.5 cm) firm lump with variable skin colour; pinching the lump results in central dimpling (dimple sign).

- **Keloid**: A flesh-coloured, firm nodule or plaque arising after a surgical incision or skin trauma. A keloid extends beyond the limit of the inciting trauma, while a hypertrophic scar does not.

- **Xanthoma**: Yellowish papules, plaques or nodules. They may also occur on the eyelids (xanthelasmas) or tendons (tendon xanthomas). These are actually cutaneous lipid deposits seen in familial hyperlipidaemia and primary biliary cirrhosis.

On the hands also consider:

- **Ganglion cyst**: A fluid-filled outpouching of the synovial membrane of a joint or tendon sheath. They are firm, smooth, fluctuant, transilluminable and fixed to underlying joint or tendon. Classical sites include dorsum and radial palmar side of wrist, flexor sheaths and on the distal interphalangeal joints (myxoid cysts) where they are associated with osteoarthritis of the underlying joint.

- **Giant cell tumour of tendon sheath** (pigmented villonodular tenosynovitis): A firm (usually firmer than a ganglion cyst), fixed, non-transilluminable lump most commonly found on the palmar aspect of the fingers. This is benign and slow-growing, but may destroy underlying bone.

(c) Hard Skin Lumps

- **Skin metastasis**: Skin metastases from internal malignancies (e.g., leukaemia and lymphoma) can present as hard lumps. All hard dermal lumps should be biopsied.

- **Bony lumps**: A rock-hard lump, located where skin is thin over bone, may arise from underlying bone.

(d) Tender and Erythematous Lumps

- **Infective**: Acute, erythematous, painful lumps. An **abscess** is a tender, fluctuant, erythematous nodule, often with visible pus pointing. A **furuncle** (boil), an infected hair follicle, presents as a small abscess atop an inflamed, erythematous, tender nodule. Multiple furuncles coalesce into a **carbuncle**, with purulent discharge from several follicular openings.

- **Inflammatory—erythema nodosum**: Multiple deep, tender erythematous nodules usually on the lower limbs, which look like bruises when resolving. They are poorly demarcated, which is often the first clue to their depth. This may be idiopathic, or due to infection (streptococcal throat infection, viruses, mycoplasma, tuberculosis), autoimmune disease (inflammatory bowel disease, sarcoidosis), haematological malignancies and drugs (oral contraceptives, sulphonamides, NSAIDs).

- **Pyogenic granuloma**: A shiny red papule with a raspberry-like surface, which grows rapidly (days–weeks) often after minor trauma. This bleeds easily (often the presenting complaint) and may become crusted or ulcerated later.

 Using what you have learnt, **pen down your approach** to the Clinical Case at the start of the chapter **BEFORE reading the discussion** below.

Case Discussion

The description of this 'mole' is concerning for melanoma; it is relatively large, elevated and irregular. In patients with multiple nevi, a pigmented lesion that is enlarging in size, or is obviously different from the others (an 'ugly duckling') should be deemed suspicious. The next step is to offer biopsy of the lesion.

Key Lessons	1. There are many epidermal growths; some are critical to recognise—for example, malignancies (melanoma, squamous cell carcinoma, basal cell carcinoma) and warts (can progress if untreated).
	2. The skin lumps are recognised based on their colour, consistency and other unique features. Rapid increase in size, necrosis or ulceration are red flags for malignancy.
Common Pitfalls	1. Try not to fixate on your first impression of a growth, lump or rash. This is a source of diagnostic error (premature closure; see Chapter 1). Always consider differentials and be prepared to revise the initial diagnosis as additional information becomes available.
Questions	1. **EXPLORE!** Look up pictures of the lesions described in this chapter, so that you may recognise them.
	2. **GO FURTHER!** The neurocutaneous syndromes each have unique cutaneous features. What are the distinctive skin signs in (a) neurofibromatosis, and (b) tuberous sclerosis? In which scenarios might it be important to recognise these conditions?

Chapter

42

An Approach to
Groin Lumps

Clinical Case

A 50-year-old taxi driver complains of a right scrotal swelling, which had been present for many years but has gotten bigger in the last 3 months. It used to only be a problem when he stood up, but recently has been present whether he is standing or sitting. He is keen to get it fixed because it is uncomfortable when he sits for long hours in the taxi. His only other medical history is a chronic smoker's cough and obesity. What is examination likely to find, and how would you distinguish between the key differentials?

In addition to the usual causes of skin lumps (see Chapter 41), a number of lumps are unique to the groin. Most of these lumps can be diagnosed on careful examination, without imaging studies.

Begin by distinguishing inguinal from scrotal lumps (Figure 42.1):

- **Inguinal lump**: Confined to the inguinal region, testes are separately palpable.

- **Scrotal lump**: Confined to the scrotum, with a distinct upper border (can get above it) and a palpable spermatic cord. The testes are not separately palpable.

- **Inguino-scrotal lump**: Appears to involve both the inguinal and scrotal regions, or may appear to be a scrotal mass. However, there is no distinct upper border (cannot get above it) and the testes is separately palpable.

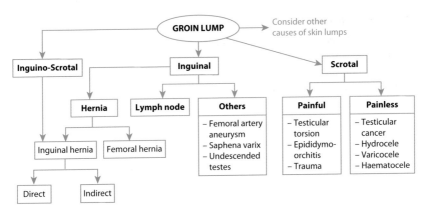

Figure 42.1. Approach to groin lumps.

Inguinal Lump

Examination and Differentials

Examine the patient standing.

- **Hernia**: A soft, compressible lump with an expansile cough impulse (unless too large or incarcerated). Due to gravity, a hernia can become more apparent on standing, and reduce in the supine position—but it may also become irreducible (i.e., incarcerated).

- **Inguinal lymph nodes**: Firm, discrete lumps with no cough impulse. Tender nodes suggest infection, while lobulated hard nodes suggest malignancy. Look for other lymphadenopathy, local infection or malignancy in the limbs, lower abdomen and perineum (including per-rectal and per-vaginal examinations; see Chapter 45).

- **Femoral artery aneurysm**: An expansile, pulsatile mass located at the mid-inguinal point. Be especially suspicious in intravenous drug users who may use femoral vessels for vascular access.

- **Saphena varix**: This is a venous dilation at the junction of the long saphenous vein and femoral vein, which appears in patients with extensive lower limb varicosities. They empty with minimal pressure and refill on release.

- **Undescended testes**: This will not be missed if the scrotum is examined—an empty scrotum should prompt suspicion of undescended testes.

- Other skin lumps: Lipoma, sebaceous cyst, groin abscess, neuroma of femoral nerve and so forth (see Chapter 41).

The approach to a hernia is further discussed.

Further Questions in a Hernia

Which type of hernia?

(a) **Femoral vs. inguinal**: Carefully palpate bony land-marks. An inguinal hernia reduces to a point above and medial to the pubic tubercle, but a femoral hernia reduces inferior and lateral. Due to their narrow neck, femoral herniae may not demonstrate a cough impulse, are usually incarcerated, and are at higher risk of strangulation.

(b) **If inguinal, direct vs. indirect**: This distinction is somewhat academic as treatment is similar. Clinically, reduce the hernia and apply pressure over the deep inguinal ring[1]—an indirect inguinal hernia may be controlled by this manoeuvre,

---

[1] The deep ring is located 2 cm above the *midpoint of the inguinal ligament,* that is, the midpoint of a line connecting anterior superior iliac spine to pubic *tubercle.* This is not the same as the *mid-inguinal point,* the landmark for the femoral artery, which is the midpoint of a line connecting anterior superior iliac spine to pubic *symphysis.*

while a direct hernia will not. At surgery, the neck of an indirect inguinal hernia appears lateral to the inferior epigastric artery, while that of a direct hernia appears medial.

Identify any complications:

- **Incarceration**: An irreducible hernia. Incarcerated herniae may be mildly uncomfortable, but there should not be the severe pain of strangulation.

- **Obstruction**: Bowel loops within a hernia may become obstructed, leading to symptoms of intestinal obstruction—abdominal pain, distension, nausea and vomiting and lack of passage of stool or flatus (see Chapter 12).

- **Strangulation**: When vascular supply to the loop of incarcerated bowel is compromised, the hernia becomes irreducible, tender and warm. Operation is urgent to save ischaemic bowel.

Inguino-Scrotal Lump

Inguino-scrotal lumps are almost always inguinal herniae, as long as the testes are separately palpable. Indirect herniae are more likely than direct herniae to descend into the scrotum. Approach as per an inguinal hernia.

Scrotal Lump

Painful Scrotal Lump

	Workup
• **Testicular torsion**: Usually a young man with acute scrotal or abdominal pain. Examination reveals a tender, high-riding testes, which lies transversely. The cremasteric reflex is lost. Operation is urgent to save the testes.	− High probability: Urgent surgery − Low probability: Doppler ultrasound for testicular blood flow
• **Epididymo-orchitis**: Pain and tenderness on palpation of the epididymis (on the posterior aspect of the testes); there may also be fever, dysuria and urethral discharge. This should only be diagnosed if torsion is excluded.	− UFEME and culture − PCR for chlamydia and gonorrhoea
• **Torsion of appendix testes** (cyst of Morgagni): The torted appendage may be palpable as a localised tenderness or nodule (a blue dot sign).	
• **Trauma**: Exclude trauma to the testes (e.g., due to a saddle injury).	− Ultrasound testes

Painless Scrotal Lump

	Workup
• **Testicular tumour**: Painless progressive testicular swelling ± a sensation of heaviness. On examination, the testis is enlarged, hard and non-tender.	− Scrotal ultrasound − Tumour markers: alpha feto-protein (AFP), lactate dehydrogenase (LDH), beta-hCG
• **Hydrocele**: A non-tender, fluctuant swelling which transilluminates. The testes may not be palpable as it is buried under fluid. This may be idiopathic, secondary to testicular pathology (e.g., tumour), or secondary to ascites (e.g., from nephrotic syndrome) in the presence of a patent processus vaginalis.	− Ultrasound scrotum to exclude secondary hydrocele − Examine for ascites
• **Varicocele**: A 'bag of worms' of dilated veins, which reduces on lying supine. Varicoceles may be idiopathic, but an acute-onset right sided varicocele, as well as varicoceles that do not empty when supine, are suspicious for obstructed testicular venous drainage (e.g., by a renal cell carcinoma with renal vein tumour thrombus).	− Ultrasound scrotum and kidney; may require CT abdomen
• **Haematocele**: A tense, tender, non-transilluminable swelling after scrotal injury.	

 Using what you have learnt, **pen down your approach** to the Clinical Case at the start of the chapter **BEFORE reading the discussion** below.

Case Discussion

This gentleman's history is most suggestive of a long-standing inguinal hernia, which has now become incarcerated. He has chronic cough and obesity, both of which increase intra-abdominal pressure and predispose to hernia formation.

Examination is most likely to find a soft inguino-scrotal lump with or without a cough impulse. It should not be possible to 'get above' the lump—if so, it may be a scrotal lump instead of a hernia. It should not be firm or hard—if so, consider lymph nodes or testicular tumour. It should not be pulsatile—unlike a femoral artery aneurysm. There may be discomfort but exquisite tenderness would suggest strangulation—a surgical emergency.

Key Lessons	1. Inguinal or inguino-scrotal lumps may be herniae (inguinal or femoral), lymph nodes, vascular structures or other skin lumps. If a hernia descends into the scrotum, its upper border cannot be distinctly palpated.

2. Scrotal lumps may be painful or painless. The acutely painful scrotum is testicular torsion until proven otherwise. A hard, painless scrotal lump is likely a testicular tumour.

Common Pitfalls	1. Before performing a procedure on any groin lump, ensure that is NOT an aneurysm. Partially thrombosed aneurysms may not be very pulsatile. Inguinal 'lymph nodes' have mistakenly been biopsied, only to result in torrential arterial bleeding! In doubt, do ultrasound first.
Questions	1. **REFLECT!** Have you ever encountered a patient with an inguinal hernia? Why did he/she seek treatment, and what differentials were considered before making the diagnosis of a hernia?
	2. **DISCUSS!** How would the patient's age influence the diagnostic approach to an inguinal or scrotal lump? Compare the likely differentials in a young (teenage) boy vs. a middle-aged to elderly man.

Chapter

43 An Approach to Breast Lumps and Complaints

Clinical Case

A 50-year-old housewife presents with a 6-month history of an itchy rash around her right nipple. She had tried topical steroids with some improvement but the rash recurred after she stopped applying steroids. Examination finds a 2 cm × 2 cm firm mass, 2 cm from the nipple at the 7 o'clock position. What is the next step?

Breast cancer is well publicised. Behind every breast complaint, is usually the fear of cancer. Excluding cancer is the clinician's main task.

Presenting Complaints

Patients may complain of a breast lump, skin changes, nipple discharge and breast pain. The differentials to consider are discussed.

Breast Lumps

- **Cancer**: Features suspicious for cancer include—large size, irregular borders, hard consistency, fixation to skin or underlying muscle, skin changes and limb swelling (suggesting lymphatic obstruction). Examine for axillary and cervical lymphadenopathy, which would be suspicious.

- **Fibroadenoma**: One or more firm, mobile, discrete lumps. This is more common in younger patients and may fluctuate in size with the menstrual cycle.

- **Cyst**: A smooth, spherical, very well-circumscribed lump. Consistency varies, ranging from soft to tense. Cysts can appear rapidly, at times with pain.

- **Breast abscess**: A painful, warm and erythematous lump, usually associated with breastfeeding. There may be fever and other signs of systemic infection.

- **Fat necrosis**: Breast trauma may cause fat necrosis, then a fibrotic reaction, which presents weeks later as a hard irregular lump with skin tethering. The initial trauma may be small and forgotten.

Skin Changes

Any skin changes overlying the breast should prompt suspicion for malignancy.

- Skin dimpling (Peau d'Orange) and nipple retraction suggests breast cancer.

- An eczematous rash around the nipple is worrisome for Paget's disease, which is associated with an underlying breast cancer (*in situ* or invasive). All eczematous nipple rashes merit biopsy.
- Surface ulceration is a late sign of malignancy.
- Skin erythema is usually infection, but may also occur in inflammatory breast cancer.

Nipple Discharge

Bilateral discharge is usually non-sinister. A clear discharge is physiological. Milky discharge, suggesting galactorrhoea, may be physiological or due to hyperprolacti-naemia (e.g., pituitary tumour or anti-dopaminergic drugs).

Unilateral discharge is more suspicious.

- **Breast cancer**: This may present with uniductal bloody discharge.
- **Intraductal papilloma**: This benign condition may cause uniductal spontaneous straw-coloured discharge.
- **Duct ectasia**: This is a benign condition in which lactiferous ducts shorten and dilate, causing multiductal cream to blue–green discharges.

Breast Pain

Breast cancer is typically painless.[1] Mild cyclical mastalgia is physiological (it has been attributed to fibrocystic changes). Mastitis (infection) is usually painful; it is associated with breastfeeding.

Assessment for Breast Cancer

The standard workup for all breast lumps is '**triple assessment**', that is, physical exam, imaging and biopsy. The goal of each step is to evaluate for cancer.

1. History and Examination

Assess the clinical risk of cancer. In particular, consider:

- **History**: A progressively enlarging, painless lump is suspicious. Look also for systemic symptoms (e.g., weight loss).
- **Examination** of the breast (including the axillary tail) for any breast lump (as earlier) and lymph nodes.
- **Risk factors**: For example, family history, known BRCA-1 or BRCA-2 mutation, oestrogen exposure (early menarche, late menopause, nulliparity, use of oestrogen-containing contraceptives or hormone replacement therapy).

---

[1] **Exception**: Inflammatory breast cancer presents as a rapidly enlarging, warm and painful breast. This is rare.

2. Imaging

- **Mammogram** (cranio-caudal and medial–lateral-oblique views): This is the mainstay of breast imaging. Suspicious features include a spiculated mass, microcalcifications and architectural distortion. Large coarse or homogenous calcifications suggests a benign aetiology.

- **Ultrasound**: This is a useful adjunct (not a replacement for mammography) to identify malignant features and guide biopsy. For a solid mass, any irregular margin, spiculation, or lump that is taller than wide is suspicious. In contrast, fibroadenomas are regularly shaped and well circumscribed. Breast cysts appear anechoic and very well circumscribed; purely cystic lesions do not require biopsy but those with solid components do.

- **Breast MRI**: Of limited general use, but helpful in younger women in whom dense breasts limit the sensitivity of mammogram.

3. Histopathology

Biopsy solid or solid-cystic breast lumps. Cysts may be aspirated, unless there is a solid component, or the aspirate is bloody (possible malignancy). In terms of choice of biopsy:

- **Suspicious lesion—Core biopsy**: A core biopsy preserves tissue architecture for assessment of vascular and capsular invasion, and yields sufficient material for immunochemical analysis (i.e., hormone receptor status determination).

- **Likely benign lesion—Excision biopsy**: The entire lesion is removed, with or without a margin of normal breast tissue. This removes and cures benign lesions. However, if the lesion turns out to be malignant, re-operation to obtain wider margins is needed.

- **For Paget's disease**: Punch, wedge or excisional biopsy of the nipple-areolar complex for histopathological examination.

- **Not ideal—Fine needle aspiration cytology** (FNAC): FNAC is not ideal as only cells are aspirated and tissue architecture cannot be visualised, and there is insufficient material for hormone receptor status and other genetic testing.

Based on the information from (1), (2) and (3), a final diagnosis of malignancy or benign disease can be made.

 Using what you have learnt, **pen down your approach** to the Clinical Case at the start of the chapter **BEFORE reading the discussion** below.

Case Discussion

This middle-aged lady presents with Paget's disease and a breast lump. This is suspicious for breast cancer, and illustrates the point that a nipple rash should never be written off as 'eczema'. Examine the lump for suspicious features (e.g., irregularity and fixation), not forgetting its axillary tail. Take a history for systemic symptoms and risk factors. Next, offer mammogram and core biopsy.

Key Lessons	1. The most important goal in approaching any breast complaint is to rule out cancer. Assessment of any breast lump involves history, examination, imaging (usually mammography) and biopsy (ideally a core biopsy).
	2. Apart from a breast lump, breast complaints suspicious for malignancy include—overlying skin changes, especially skin dimpling, nipple retraction, and rashes around the nipple, as well as unilateral uniductal bloody nipple discharge. Breast pain is usually non-malignant.
Common Pitfalls	1. Breast examination includes an examination of the axillary tail; lumps in the axillary tail are easily missed.
Questions	1. **DISCUSS!** Why is a single test (mammography) sufficient for breast cancer screening, when patients with breast lumps require 'triple assessment' with examination, imaging and biopsy?
	2. **GO FURTHER!** Approximately 5% to 10% of breast cancers are attributed to BRCA-1 or BRCA-2 mutations.
	(i) When would you suspect a BRCA mutation?
	(ii) Genetic testing raises complex issues, both for the patient and family members. What are some considerations raised in pre- and post-testing genetic counselling?

An Approach to Neck Lumps

Clinical Case

A 70-year-old gentleman, who is a chronic smoker, presents with a painless neck lump which has grown larger over the past 3 months. On examination, there is a hard lump, just beneath the left earlobe. He is unable to close his left eye as tightly as his right, but has no facial droop. What is the likely diagnosis?

There are many structures in the neck, and therefore many differentials to consider when a patient presents with a neck lump. This is in addition to the general causes of a skin lump (see Chapter 41).

Localising Neck Lumps

The anatomical location of the lump is of utmost diagnostic importance (Figure 44.1):

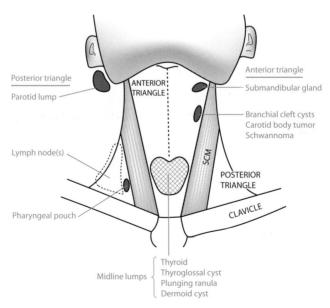

Note: Lymph nodes may actually be found in any location.

SCM, sternocleidomastoid.

Figure 44.1. Anatomical localisation of common neck lumps.

- **Posterior triangle lump**: Lateral to the sternocleidomastoid (the posterior triangle is bounded by the sternocleidomastoid, trapezius muscle and clavicle).
- **Anterior triangle lump**: Medial to the sternocleidomastoid (the anterior triangle is bounded by the sternocleidomastoid, lower jaw and the midline).
- **Multiple lumps**: Either lymph nodes or a multinodular goitre.

Anterior Triangle Lump

Identify if the lump (i) moves with swallowing, and (ii) is midline or off-centre.

Moves with Swallowing

- **Thyroid**: An inferior neck lump that ascends with swallowing, but not with tongue protrusion. This may be a soft diffuse goitre (as in Graves' disease), or a hard and fixed nodule (as in thyroid cancer). A diffuse or multinodular goitre is usually found in the midline, but a single nodule (e.g., adenoma or cancer) may be found in either left or right thyroid lobes (see Chapter 36).
- **Thyroglossal cyst**: A persistent thyroglossal duct arising from the foramen cecum. This presents as a firm-to-hard lump that ascends on swallowing *and* on tongue protrusion. It is found at the level of the hyoid (i.e., more superior than a thyroid lump). Fluctuance and transilluminance may be present, but are unreliable.

Does Not Move with Swallowing—Midline

- **Plunging ranula**: A mucus retention cyst arising from an obstruction in the sublingual glands. It more commonly appears as a blue–grey swelling at the floor of the mouth, but may also 'plunge' below the mylohyoid to give a midline lump above the hyoid.
- **Dermoid cyst**: A mobile, firm mass arising from entrapment of epithelium in deeper tissue.

Does Not Move with Swallowing—Off Centre

- **Cervical lymph nodes**: May be found in both anterior and posterior triangles (see Chapter 45).
- **Submandibular gland**: A small soft gland palpable just under the mandible. Bilateral small submandibular glands may normally be palpable. An unusually prominent, unilateral, hard lump is suspicious for cancer.
- **Carotid body tumour (paraganglioma)**: This arises from the carotid body chemoreceptor tissue and is located at the carotid bifurcation (above and lateral to the hyoid). It is pulsatile (transmitted pulse from carotid), mobile side-to-side but not vertically (i.e., the carotid artery can move perpendicularly to its direction of

travel), and may have be a bruit. About 10% have malignant potential, and some secrete catecholamines like a phaeochromocytoma.

- **Schwannoma/neuroma**: This arises from nerve fibres around the carotid vessels. Its characteristics are similar to a carotid body tumour in location and mobility, but without pulsatility.

- **Branchial cleft cysts**: This second branchial cleft remnant may present in young adults. It is found in the upper neck, deep to the anterior edge of the sternocleidomastoid. It is firm, fluctuant and may or may not transilluminate. It enlarges slowly and painlessly, or rapidly and painfully if infected. Rarely it becomes a draining sinus.

Workup

The majority of anterior triangle lumps may be confirmed based on characteristic features and anatomical relationships on a CT/MRI neck. Some (e.g., thyroid nodules and submandibular gland swelling) may require biopsy for definitive diagnosis. The approach to a goitre is further discussed in Chapter 36.

Posterior Triangle Lump

Causes of a Posterior Triangle Lump

- **Lymph nodes**: Discrete nodules, single or multiple, found anywhere in the neck. Its characteristics vary depending on the underlying aetiology—for example, soft tender nodes due to infection, vs. hard fixed nodes due to cancer. Identify *why* the lymph node is enlarged (see Chapter 45).

- **Parotid gland**: This lump is found at the angle of the mandible, lifting the earlobe (see the following). A normal parotid gland should not be palpable.

- **Pharyngeal pouch** (Zenker's diverticulum): A pseudodiverticulum formed by pharyngeal mucosa above the upper oesophageal sphincter. This may appear as a soft, indentable, deep and non-mobile lump at the posterior sternocleidomastoid border below the thyroid cartilage. There may be symptoms of regurgitation and dysphagia.

Approach to Parotidomegaly

Painful parotidomegaly:

- **Sialolithiasis**: Salivary duct calculi may cause episodic pain and swelling triggered by eating. On examination, small stones may be visible at Stensen's duct (opposite the upper second molar), and these may be bimanually palpable.

Workup

− Ultrasound or CT parotid

- **Acute sialadenitis**: Infection of an obstructed salivary duct causes pain, swelling and fever. Examination may reveal severe parotid tenderness and pus draining from its duct.
  - Ultrasound or CT parotid
  - Septic workup including blood cultures

- **Mumps**: Bilateral (or less often unilateral) parotid swelling, preceded by a viral prodrome. Ask about vaccination history, and look for complications, for example, orchitis.
  - Usually a clinical diagnosis
  - Serology available

Painless parotidomegaly: This requires careful evaluation for malignancy.

Workup

- **Parotid carcinoma**: Red flags include (i) a hard, fixed mass, (ii) facial nerve palsy suggesting nerve invasion, (iii) rapid growth and (iv) concomitant lymphadenopathy. Do not be fooled by the long-standing parotid lump that suddenly grows rapidly — it may be malignant transformation of a pleomorphic adenoma.
  - CT/MRI parotid
  - Biopsy

- **Parotid adenoma**: These include pleomorphic adenomas and Warthin's tumour. They are more likely to be firm (not hard) and there should not be facial nerve palsy; carcinoma must be excluded.
  - CT/MRI parotid
  - Biopsy

- **Sjogren's syndrome**: In addition to dry eyes and dry mouth, Sjogren's syndrome may present with progressive bilateral parotid swelling and destruction. This may be primary or secondary (to other rheumatologic disease).
  - Look for other manifestations— MRI parotid (there are Sjogren's-specific changes)
  - Anti-Ro, Anti-La

- **Sarcoidosis**: This occasionally infiltrates the parotid glands (Heerfordt's syndrome: parotitis, uveitis, facial paralysis and fever).
  - Look for other manifestations
  - Biopsy

 Using what you have learnt, **pen down your approach** to the Clinical Case at the start of the chapter **BEFORE reading the discussion** below.

Case Discussion

This elderly gentleman presents with a painless hard parotid mass and facial nerve palsy (in him, only the zygomatic branch of the facial nerve is affected—hence the importance of examining all branches of the facial nerve individually, not just a cursory glance for facial droop). This is worrisome for parotid cancer. Examine for lymphadenopathy. He should receive further imaging (CT or MRI) and ultrasound-guided biopsy.

Key Lessons	1. The key to diagnosing anterior triangle neck lumps is visualising the deep structures of the neck—think of the thyroid (and related structures) in the midline, structures along the carotid vessels laterally, and the submandibular glands superiorly.
	2. The most common posterior triangle neck lumps are lymph nodes and an enlarged parotid gland. Painless parotidomegaly prompts consideration of a parotid tumour.
Common Pitfalls	1. Neck lumps are missed if palpation is done carelessly. One technique is to palpate from behind, using three fingers of each hand to 'roll' the skin over underlying structures. Be sure to cover all areas, reaching the midline.
Questions	1. **EXPLORE!** The location of malignant cervical lymphadenopathy correlates with the location of its primary tumour. Where is the most likely primary, if the following lymph nodes are enlarged? (a) posterior triangle (b) upper jugular chain (high anterior triangle) (c) supraclavicular
	2. **DISCUSS!** Most neck lumps are asymptomatic. What symptoms might a neck lump cause, and under what circumstances do these symptoms develop?

Chapter
45

An Approach to Lymphadenopathy

Clinical Case

A 32-year-old foreign domestic worker presents with a 2-month history of progressively enlarging right cervical lymphadenopathy. Examination reveals two firm 2 cm × 2 cm cervical lymph nodes. There are no other enlarged lymph nodes and no hepatosplenomegaly. What are your differentials? What other information will you like, and what investigations will you pursue?

Enlarged lymph nodes may be palpable in the cervical, supraclavicular, axillary and inguinal regions. Some deeper nodes (para-aortic, mediastinal, central compartment of neck) are not palpable. The causes of lymphadenopathy may be classified by aetiology or by distribution (Table 45.1).

Table 45.1. Causes of Lymphadenopathy

	Localised	Generalised
Infective	Local bacterial infection in drainage region Tuberculosis	Viral infection, e.g., EBV Acute HIV infection
Neoplastic	Cancer in drainage region	Lymphoma
Inflammatory	Kikuchi, Kimura Sarcoidosis	Lupus Sarcoidosis

EBV, Epstein–Barr virus.

Localised Lymphadenopathy

First ascertain that the palpable masses are indeed lymph nodes, considering other differentials (see Chapters 42 and 44). Examine all other lymph node groups, liver and spleen. If only localised lymphadenopathy is detected, proceed as follows.

1. What Do the Lymph Nodes Feel Like?

Clinical palpation gives some idea of the likely aetiology of lymphadenopathy. Time course is helpful but not always reliable—a newly noticed node may have been present for months.

- **Acute bacterial infection**: Acute-onset, small, soft, mobile ± tender nodes.

- **Neoplastic**: Painless, large (> 2 cm) or progressively enlarging, hard and fixed nodes raises suspicion of nodal spread from malignancy.

- **Tuberculosis (TB)**: These start as discrete cold, non-tender, mobile, node(s), which enlarge over weeks or months to become rubbery and matted, but still non-tender. Eventually, they may caseate into a 'cold abscess', which can discharge. TB may mimic both infective and neoplastic nodes. Pulmonary symptoms are absent in extrapulmonary TB.

2. Is There a Clinically Apparent Local Source?

As each group of lymph nodes drains a particular anatomical region, begin by searching for infection or malignancy in its draining site:

- **Cervical lymph nodes**: These drain the head and neck region. Local infection (e.g., upper respiratory tract infection, sinusitis, pharyngitis, otitis media) will give obvious symptoms. Ask for symptoms of head and neck cancers, for example, naso-pharyngeal carcinoma (blood-stained saliva, hearing loss from otitis media with effusion, cranial nerve palsy) and thyroid cancer (e.g., hoarseness of voice). Examine skin, scalp, the oral cavity and the ear (via otoscopy) carefully for growths or abscesses, palpate thyroid and salivary glands, and check cranial nerves. If all the above is unrewarding, consider lung or gastrointestinal (GI) sources as well.

- **Supraclavicular lymph nodes**: These are associated with malignancy of the stomach (e.g., the classic left supraclavicular 'Virchow's' node), lung or oesophagus. Elicit symptoms of these cancers and examine carefully.

- **Axillary lymph nodes**: Examine *both* breasts for signs of breast cancer (see Chapter 43). Also examine the ipsilateral arm (including interdigital spaces and skin creases) and chest wall for local infection. Ask about insect bites, pet scratches, outdoor activities and travel history.

- **Inguinal lymph nodes**: Examine lower limbs, lower abdomen and lower back for a skin and soft-tissue infection (e.g., cellulitis, ulcers, or dermatophyte infection especially in toe webs) or a skin cancer. Take a sexual history and ask for symptoms of sexually transmitted disease (e.g., penile or vaginal discharge, genital ulcers). Examine perineum (including a per-rectal and per-vaginal exam), looking for cancers and signs of sexually transmitted disease including discharge, ulcers and cervical excitation. Note that testicular cancers spread to deep para-aortic nodes instead of inguinal nodes, due to their embryological origin.

Source found: If a clinical diagnosis can be made:

- **Known local infection**: Culture, treat and address underlying factors (e.g., poorly controlled diabetes, etc.).

- **Likely local cancer**: Workup as for that cancer (tissue diagnosis, staging, etc.).

Source not apparent: Proceed to (3).

3. Is Further Workup Necessary?

Soft small (< 1 cm) asymptomatic nodes, especially in a young or thin patient, may be physiological. Reactive nodes due to local infection can be observed for resolution, and re-examined after an interval. If further workup is necessary, continue as follows:

(a) **Consider: What else are we suspecting?**

- **Cancer**: Based on the risk profile (e.g., smoking, family history, constitutional symptoms). Localising signs and symptoms may not be present.

- **TB** and non-tuberculous mycobacteria: This is an important differential. Look for constitutional symptoms (e.g., fever, weight loss, night sweats), exposure to or personal/family history of TB.

- **Inflammatory causes**: Kikuchi disease presents as fever and cervical lymphadenopathy in young women. Kimura disease causes cervical lymphadenopathy and eosinophilia. These are rare, and usually diagnosed only after biopsy.

- **Causes of generalised lymphadenopathy**: See page 414.

(b) **Directed investigation of local sources**: As per clinical suspicion, especially for suspected malignancy.

- **Cervical lymph nodes**: Flexible nasoendoscopy in the first instance; triple endoscopy (nasoendoscopy, oesophagogastroduodenoscopy [OGD], bronchoscopy) if strongly suspecting cancer (e.g., hard fixed nodes). Obtain chest imaging to exclude pulmonary TB.

- **Supraclavicular lymph nodes**: Based on clinical suspicion, imaging of the lung and GI tract may include chest X-ray, CT thorax and abdomen. Consider OGD especially in an enlarged Virchow's node.

- **Axillary lymph nodes**: As per the workup for breast cancer, including mammograms, ultrasound and core biopsy (see Chapter 43).

- **Inguinal lymph nodes**: No specific workup.

(c) **Consider lymph node biopsy**: Unless there is an obvious aetiology of lymphadenopathy (e.g., local infection), which is expected to resolve with treatment, most persistently enlarged lymph nodes should be biopsied.

- **Suspect TB**: Fine needle aspiration cytology (FNAC), the least invasive option, is generally sufficient for diagnosing TB.

- **Suspect malignancy**: If a suspected primary has been identified, either the primary or the lymph node can be biopsied—whichever is more accessible. Excision biopsy is preferred as this allows complete sampling, architectural assessment and obtains sufficient tissue for ancillary tests. Core biopsy is an alternative, but may be inadequate. FNAC is generally not ideal, as it does not permit proper assessment of architecture.

Generalised Lymphadenopathy

Enlargement of multiple lymph nodes, or the presence of hepatosplenomegaly, implies a more systemic cause.

Differentials

Infective:

- **Acute viral infection**: For example, Epstein–Barr virus (EBV), cytomegalovirus (CMV), herpes simplex virus (HSV). There may also be fever and pharyngitis.

- **Acute retroviral syndrome**: Primary HIV infection may present as lymphadenopathy ± fever, sore throat, headache, myalgia and rash. Symptoms are non-specific and a high index of suspicion is necessary, especially in patients with a high risk profile, or who have features unusual in other viral infections (e.g., a folliculitis-type rash, mucocutaneous ulcers).

- **Other infections** (including fungi, protozoa): For example, toxoplasmosis, secondary syphilis and Lyme disease.

Neoplastic:

- **Lymphoma**: Usually multiple non-tender, rubbery, matted, mobile nodes. Aggressive lymphomas may present with rapid lymph node enlargement, splenomegaly, 'B' symptoms (fever, night sweats, weight loss) or as complications (e.g., cord compression, superior vena cava obstruction, hypercalcaemia). Indolent lymphomas may present with longstanding waxing and waning lymphadenopathy.

Inflammatory:

- **Lupus**: SMultiple soft, non-tender, discrete nodes may be present, especially during lupus flares. However, do consider superimposed infection (especially if nodes are tender) or lymphoma, both of which lupus patients may be predisposed to.

- **Other inflammatory diseases**: Lymphadenopathy may be a feature of sarcoidosis, eosinophilic granulomatosis with polyangiitis (of Churg–Strauss), rheumatoid arthritis and adult Still's disease.

- **Drugs**: For example, phenytoin.

Clinical Approach

Workup proceeds based on clinical suspicion.

- **For infection**: Inflammatory markers, viral serology (EBV IgM, CMV IgM, rubella), HIV testing, syphilis serology (venereal disease research laboratory [VDRL], rapid plasma reagin [RPR]) and CXR for miliary TB.

- **Autoimmune**: Start with a sensitive test, for example, antinuclear antibody (ANA). Proceed with specific testing based on clinical suspicion.

- **Biopsy**: If a viral illness is probable and the patient is well, observation is fair. If suspecting lymphoma or lymphadenopathy is persistent, biopsy should be performed.

Again, excision biopsy is ideal, especially for suspected lymphoma; FNAC does not allow examination of lymph node architecture, risks false negative results due to sampling error, and yields insufficient material for additional staining and genetic analyses. Beware a report of 'atypical lymphoid hyperplasia'—this sounds innocent but must be taken as cancer until proven otherwise.

 Using what you have learnt, **pen down your approach** to the Clinical Case at the start of the chapter **BEFORE reading the discussion** below.

Case Discussion

This young lady has progressively enlarging localised cervical lymphadenopathy. The main considerations are (a) tuberculosis, (b) lymphoma and (c) head and neck cancer. A bacterial or acute viral infection is less likely given the subacute time course.

(a) and (b) may present only with lymphadenopathy and no other symptoms. Alternatively, there may be fever, night sweats and weight loss. She may also have chronic cough, and a contact or family history of TB—as a foreign domestic worker, she is likely from a high-incidence origin country. Evaluation of (c) should begin with a careful clinical history for any neck lump, skin lump, blood-stained saliva or hearing loss. Examine skin and scalp for a skin cancer, look into the oral, nasal and ear cavities. Palpate for a goitre.

For this lady, initial investigations should include a blood count, chest X-ray (for concomitant pulmonary tuberculosis) and HIV test. The lymph node should be biopsied, and sent for gram stain and culture, TB PCR, acid-fast bacilli stain and culture and histology.

Key Lessons	1. Patients with localised lymphadenopathy should be worked up for an infection (including tuberculosis) or cancer in the anatomical region that the lymph node drains.
	2. Generalised lymphadenopathy may be due to infective (including HIV), malignant (lymphoma, metastatic) and inflammatory causes.
	3. Lymph node biopsy should be considered in most cases of persistent lymphadenopathy.
Common Pitfalls	1. Fine needle aspiration cytology often provides insufficient diagnostic material, and may be falsely negative in cases of lymphoma.
	2. Primary HIV infection is a cause of generalised lymphadenopathy.
Questions	1. **DISCUSS!** In some resource-limited developing countries, patients who present with lymphadenopathy are empirically treated for tuberculosis, without undergoing further investigations or biopsy. What are your thoughts on this approach?
	2. **EXPLORE!** Compare and contrast lymphoma vs. leukaemia, in terms of pathophysiology, clinical presentation and diagnostic approach.

Chapter

46 An Approach to Lower Limb Pain and Ulcers

Clinical Case

A 65-year-old gentleman with diabetes mellitus presents with 2 months of right foot pain at rest. On examination, he has a deep 3 cm × 3 cm ulcer under the first metatarsal head, which is sloughy with a foul-smelling discharge. The fourth and fifth toes are dusky, and the entire right foot appears pale. Dorsalis pedis and posterior tibial pulses are not palpable; capillary refill is 4 sec. Initial laboratory investigations reveal a creatinine of 150 μmol/L and HbA1c of 11%. What are the next steps?

Non-traumatic lower limb pain or ulceration may be due to arterial, venous, neurological or musculoskeletal disease. Four clinical pictures can be identified (Table 46.1):

1. Severe acute limb pain.
2. Chronic episodic pain on walking.
3. Chronic rest pain ± swelling (lower limb swelling alone is discussed in Chapter 47).
4. Tissue loss, for example, ulceration or gangrene.

Table 46.1. Clinical Presentations of Lower Limb Pain and Ulcers

	Arterial disease	Venous disease	Musculoskeletal/other
Severe acute pain	Acute limb ischaemia	Deep vein thrombosis	Infection Musculoskeletal injury
Chronic episodic pain	Vascular claudication		Neurogenic claudication Musculoskeletal pain
Chronic rest pain	Critical limb ischaemia	Varicose veins	Myalgia Inflammatory arthritis Musculoskeletal tumour
Tissue loss	Critical limb ischaemia	Venous ulceration	Neuropathic ulceration

Understand that these clinical pictures represent different points on the natural history of disease. For instance, atherosclerosis builds up over decades, initially silently. As it progresses, blood flow becomes insufficient to meet tissue demands during exercise, so patients experience episodic pain on walking (claudication). At a critical level of occlusion, blood flow cannot even meet tissue demands at rest, causing rest pain and tissue loss (critical limb ischaemia). By a separate mechanism, limb ischaemia can develop when an embolus from the heart (e.g., in atrial fibrillation) or aorta (e.g., from an atherosclerotic plaque or aortic aneurysm) occludes the iliac or femoral artery; this occurs suddenly without time for collateral circulation to develop, resulting in the clinical picture of acute limb ischaemia.

1. Severe Acute Pain

The few aetiologies of an acutely painful limb can be identified on clinical history and examination.

Workup

- **Acute limb ischaemia** (the six 'P's): The ischaemic limb is *p*ainful, *p*ale, *p*erishingly cold and *p*ulseless. *P*araesthesia and *p*aralysis are late signs; profound numbness, paralysis or rigor (stiffness) and fixed staining indicate a non-viable limb.

  - Intra-operative arteriography (if limb is viable and patient is operated on emergently)
  - CT angiogram

- **Deep vein thrombosis** (DVT): A swollen, tense and tender limb. Unlike an ischaemic limb, this limb is warm and pulses are palpable. Swelling can be objectively demonstrated by measuring calf diameter. The patient is likely to have risk factors, for example, immobility, active cancer or pregnancy.

  - Compression duplex ultrasound (see Chapter 47)

- **Infection**: In cellulitis, the limb is warm, with a well-demarcated area of skin erythema (more distinct than in DVT). Pulses are present unless there is underlying peripheral arterial disease (which predisposes to infection). Have a high index of suspicion for necrotising fasciitis—especially if pain is unusually severe or the patient is toxic. In doubt, mark out the erythema and review early; erythema, swelling and gangrene progresses over hours in necrotising fasciitis.

  - Blood cultures and inflammatory markers
  - Assess for an underlying cause, for example, arterial insufficiency
  - Necrotising fasciitis prompts emergent operation, not MRI!

- **Musculoskeletal injury**: Consider trauma (fractures, dislocations, etc.). If pain worsens in an injured limb, consider compartment syndrome, which presents as a disproportionately painful and tense limb, exacerbated by passive muscle stretch (e.g., toe dorsiflexion).

  - X-rays to exclude fractures if there is a history of trauma
  - Surgical decompression for compartment syndrome

2. Chronic Episodic Pain on Walking

Clinical features distinguish between (a) claudication vs. musculoskeletal pain, and (b) neurogenic vs. vascular claudication.

a. Claudication vs. Musculoskeletal Pain

- **Claudication**: Episodic lower limb muscle pain precipitated by exercise and relieved by rest. Pain is felt in the muscles and takes some time to come on with exercise.

- **Musculoskeletal pain** may be due to disease in the hip or knee joints and their surrounding structures. Pain is best felt in the joints or on specific movements, and may be present with the first step (see Chapter 50).

b. Neurogenic vs. Vascular Claudication

- **Vascular claudication**: The pain of arterial insufficiency starts after walking a fixed, reproducible distance and is relieved by rest. Pulses are diminished (Table 46.2).

- **Neurogenic claudication**: Neuropathic pain from lumbar spinal stenosis mimics vascular claudication. Characteristically, pain arises after walking a variable distance, and spine flexion (or walking uphill) relieves pain by opening up the nerve root space (Table 46.2).

Table 46.2. Differentiating Vascular vs. Neurogenic Claudication

	Vascular claudication	Neurogenic claudication
Claudication distance	Fixed. Claudication distance may decrease as arterial occlusion worsens with time	Variable
Nature of pain	Cramping, worst in the muscles distal to the diseased artery, e.g., calf pain in superficial femoral artery disease, and thigh/gluteal pain in aortoiliac disease	Shooting from proximal to distal, or cramping
Precipitating and relieving factors	Worse walking uphill Relieved by rest	Worse walking downhill Relieved by spine flexion
Associations	Diminished lower limb pulses Vascular risk factors	Back pain Lower limb numbness

Confirmatory Investigations

Vascular claudication:

- **Ankle-brachial pressure index** (ABPI): This is the ratio of ankle to brachial blood pressure, and is easy to do with a handheld Doppler. ABPI of 0.9 to 1.0 is normal. ABPI < 0.9 suggests arterial disease diminishing flow to the ankles, and values < 0.5 suggest critical stenosis. Readings are falsely high if vessels are calcified (e.g., in diabetics); therefore 'normal' ABPI may not rule out peripheral vascular disease.

- **Doppler ultrasound**: This directly visualises arterial blood flow, assessing the severity and distribution of arterial occlusion.

- **CT Angiography**: This is usually employed if aortoiliac disease is suspected (e.g., gluteal/thigh pain), as Doppler ultrasound is unable to assess the iliac vessels. Unfortunately many patients with vascular disease also have renal impairment; the risk of contrast nephropathy is often a relative contraindication.

- Search for vascular risk factors (e.g., diabetes, hypertension, hyperlipidaemia, smoking) and comorbids (e.g., ischaemic heart disease) as these are very common and should be addressed.

Neurogenic claudication: MRI spine—see Chapter 51.

3. Chronic Rest Pain

The causes of chronic lower limb pain can be identified clinically:

Workup

- **Critical limb ischaemia**: Usually an unrepentant vasculopath whose claudication has worsened over years, and now complains of rest pain in the foot, often worse at night and relieved on hanging the foot out of bed. The limb is pulseless, with a prolonged capillary refill time, and cutaneous signs of poor perfusion (pale, shiny, atrophic). Concomitant diabetic neuropathy may make this condition painless, but no less risky.

  – ABPI
  – Doppler ultrasound

- **Chronic venous insufficiency**: Aching, heaviness and swelling, worse after standing all day. Varicose veins, pitting oedema and skin changes (hyperpigmentation, lipodermatosclerosis, venous eczema) may be seen. Venous insufficiency is the result of valvular incompetency in superficial veins, causing reflux (i.e., retrograde blood flow). It may also arise after deep venous thrombosis (DVT) due to damage to vein segments and valves.

  – Venous duplex ultrasound excludes DVT and confirms reflux (retrograde blood flow when proximal tissue is squeezed)

- **Musculoskeletal disease**: Apart from vascular pathology, chronic limb pain can be the result of myalgia (polymyalgia rheumatica, statins), inflammatory joint pain and musculoskeletal tumours (see Chapter 48).

4. Ulceration

There are a number of causes of lower limb ulcers:

- **Critical limb ischaemia**: When arterial perfusion can no longer support tissue survival, tissue loss occurs, in the form of ulcers and gangrene.

- **Severe venous insufficiency**: Chronic venous stasis and venous hypertension leads to skin necrosis.

- **Peripheral neuropathy**: Accumulated unrecognised (painless) trauma, due to peripheral neuropathy, most often from diabetes. Examine for 'glove and stocking' sensory loss and Charcot joints.

- **Malignant ulcers**: Basal cell carcinoma (BCC) is an irregular rodent ulcer with a central scab and pearly rolled margin. Squamous cell carcinoma (SCC) appears fleshy and exophytic. SCC can develop in a longstanding venous or burn ulcer (a 'Marjolin ulcer').

- **Autoimmune**: For example, pyoderma gangrenosum in patients with inflammatory bowel disease, rheumatoid arthritis or vasculitis.

- **Chronic infection**: Tuberculous or fungal—especially in tropical rural areas.

- **Pressure sores**: On the back of heel or sacrum in bed-bound patients.

These can generally be differentiated clinically (Table 46.3).

Table 46.3. Differentiating Lower Limb Ulcers

	Arterial	Venous	Neuropathic	Malignant
Classic location	Toes, metatarsal heads and heel	Gaiter region, over malleoli, may be circumferential	Beneath pressure points of sole or bony prominences	Any location
Base	Dry, pale, covered with slough or necrotic tissue	Pink granulation tissue	Slough	Dried serum (BCC), necrotic (SCC)
Edge	Punched out or sloping if healing	Sloping	Punched out or sloping if healing	Irregular. Rolled (BCC), everted (SCC)
Depth	Shallow to deep	Shallow and flat	Deep	Deep if tissue invaded
Discharge	Thin serous exudate, or purulent	Seropurulent or bloody	Skin weeps plasma	Nil or foul discharge (SCC)
Pain	Severe pain	Mild pain	Insensate	Painless
Pulses	Pulseless, prolonged capillary refill time	Present, if no concomitant arterial disease	Present, if no concomitant arterial disease	Present
Surrounding skin	Pale, cold, atrophic	Hyperpigmentation, lipodermatosclerosis, venous eczema	Normal or callus formation	Surrounding tissue normal
Other signs	Gangrene	Varicosities, oedema	Charcot's foot	Lymphadenopathy

BCC, basal cell carcinoma; SCC, squamous cell carcinoma.

Additional Considerations

- Ulcers are often multifactorial, and may not fall neatly into the above categories.
- **Superimposed infection**: Look out for an infective component (e.g., pus, discharge). If present, send wound cultures from deep tissue (i.e., during debridement); avoid superficial wound swabs as these often pick up skin contaminants. A deep ulcer with exposed bone should elicit suspicion of osteomyelitis until proven otherwise; consider X-ray to look for bony erosions.

Workup for arterial and venous disease should proceed as discussed in the previous sections.

 Using what you have learnt, **pen down your approach** to the Clinical Case at the start of the chapter **BEFORE reading the discussion** below.

Case Discussion

This gentleman with poorly controlled diabetes has critical limb ischaemia, as evidenced by rest pain, pulselessness, prolonged capillary refill, ulceration and gangrene. His ulcer is likely mixed ischaemic and neuropathic; its location is classic for a neuropathic ulcer and he also has nephropathy (another microvascular complication of diabetes). The ulcer also appears infected, with a foul-smelling discharge.

He will require wound debridement with deep tissue cultures, plus an arterial Doppler ultrasound to establish the diagnosis of arterial insufficiency. Apart from treatment of infection and improving diabetic control, he is likely to require revascularisation ± amputation of the non-viable toes.

Key Lessons	
	1. In an acutely painful limb, exclude trauma and consider: (1) the pale, cold and pulseless ischaemic limb, (2) the swollen and tense limb of DVT and (3) the limb with a demarcated area of cellulitis.
	2. Claudication is a symptom of episodic pain precipitated by exercise and relieved by rest. It may be due to vascular insufficiency or lumbar spinal stenosis.
	3. Critical limb ischaemia presents with rest pain and tissue loss.
	4. Lower limb ulcers are commonly due to a combination of ischaemia, venous stasis, neuropathy ± superimposed infection. Atypical features may suggest malignancy or autoimmune disease.
Common Pitfalls	1. Typical venous skin changes do not rule out concomitant arterial disease. A third of patients have mixed arterial and venous disease; this affects management (e.g., if there is arterial disease, compression stockings worsen ischaemia and are contraindicated).

Questions

1. **EXPLORE!** Compare and contrast the pathophysiology, clinical presentation and management of arterial occlusion (atherosclerotic and embolic) in the (i) coronary arteries, (ii) carotid arteries, (iii) femoral arteries and (iv) mesenteric artery.

2. **DISCUSS!** In pairs or small groups, look up pictures of leg ulcers online, and practice describing them out loud. See if you can decide on the likely cause (or causes) of each ulcer simply on inspection.

3. **GO FURTHER!** Various tourniquet tests can be performed to demonstrate venous incompetence. While these are diagnostically obsolete in an age of ultrasound scans, they remain nifty bedside tricks. What is the principle of a tourniquet test, and how would you use it to demonstrate venous incompetence?

Chapter **An Approach to**
47 **Lower Limb Swelling**

Clinical Case

A 33-year-old Australian lawyer presents with a 2-day history of right lower limb pain and swelling, which started soon after a London to Melbourne flight. She has no past medical history and is on no medications, except for an oral contraceptive pill. On examination, her temperature is 37.8°C, BP 138/82, HR 117, SpO2 98% on room air. Her right thigh is swollen and tender, with a diameter of 40 cm measured 5 cm above the lateral malleolus (vs. 33 cm for the left thigh). How would you approach her case?

Lower limb swelling may reflect vascular or soft tissue disease in the leg, or systemic organ dysfunction with fluid overload or low albumin. Some of these conditions require urgent treatment, while others are mainly nuisances. A reasoned clinical approach is key (Figure 47.1).

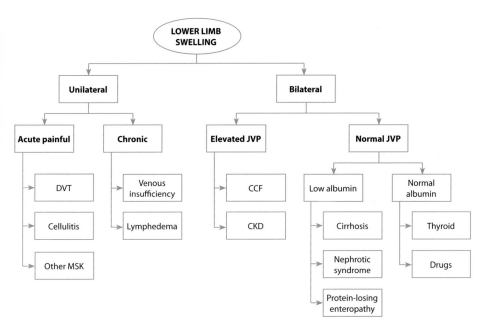

CCF, congestive cardiac failure; CKD, chronic kidney disease; JVP, jugular venous pressure; MSK, musculoskeletal.

Figure 47.1. Approach to lower limb swelling.

Unilateral Leg Swelling

Unilateral leg swelling suggests a local pathology in the vessels or soft tissues of the swollen leg. Asymmetry of swelling may be demonstrated by comparing bilateral leg or calf circumference, carefully measured at fixed distances from bony prominences. The first step is to ask if the swelling is acute and painful (< 1 week), or chronic.

Acute Painful Unilateral Leg Swelling

- **Deep vein thrombosis (DVT)**: A diffusely swollen, warm, erythematous and tender leg. There may be low-grade fever. Patients often have risk factors including immobility, active malignancy or pregnancy. Clinical prediction scores (e.g., Wells' score) are available to assess the pre-test probability of DVT (Table 47.1). An approach to DVT is presented later.

- **Cellulitis**: An erythematous, warm and tender limb, often associated with fever and raised inflammatory markers. Compared to DVT, the demarcation between erythematous (infected) and normal skin is usually more distinct, and swelling is less marked. It can be difficult to confidently distinguish cellulitis from DVT—in these cases, it may be necessary to workup for both differentials. Consider necrotising fasciitis if pain is out of proportion (see Chapter 46).

- **Ruptured Baker's (popliteal) cyst**: A Baker's cyst may rupture into the posterior calf muscles, causing swelling and pain, which mimics DVT. These cysts are more common in patients with underlying knee osteoarthritis.

- **Musculoskeletal trauma**: For example, soft tissue injury, calf haematoma (especially in patients on anticoagulation).

- **Thrombophlebitis**: Tender, palpable superficial veins, often at the site of former IV cannulae.

Table 47.1. Well's Score: Pre-Test Probability of DVT

	Factor	Points
Risk factors	Active cancer (or treated within 6 months)	+1
	Paralysis or recent lower limb immobilisation	+1
	Bedridden > 3 days or surgery within 4 weeks	+1
Physical findings	Swelling of entire leg	+1
	Calf swelling > 3 cm, compared to the normal leg	+1
	Pitting oedema, greater than the normal leg	+1
	Localised tenderness along the deep venous system	+1
	Collateral superficial veins (not varicose veins)	+1
Differential	Alternative differential as likely or more likely than DVT	−2

Interpretation: ≥ **3** High probability; **1–2** Moderate probability; ≤ **0** Low probability

Clinical Approach to Suspected DVT

1. **Confirm the diagnosis of DVT**: Choice of test depends on the degree of clinical suspicion of DVT.

   - **Compression duplex ultrasound** should be pursued if there is moderate to high pre-test probability. A vein that is not compressible, or that has abnormal flow on colour Doppler, is likely to be thrombosed.

   - **D-dimer**: This is a sensitive test that may be pursued in patients with low pre-test probability, if negative, it rules out DVT. A positive D-dimer is not specific for the diagnosis of DVT, and will require confirmation with ultrasound—ordering D-dimer is a commitment to pursue ultrasound, if D-dimer returns positive.

2. **Establish the risk of pulmonary embolism**: Not all DVT require anticoagulation. The risk of embolism determines whether treatment is necessary, or whether the patient can be monitored with follow-up scans.

   - **Superficial vs. deep**: Superficial vein thrombosis is not DVT and anticoagulation is often unnecessary (caution: the *superficial* femoral vein is a misnomer—it is actually a *deep* vein).

   - **Proximal vs. distal**: Asymptomatic below-knee DVT may not require treatment[1] as the risk of pulmonary embolism is low. Above-knee (popliteal, femoral, iliac) DVT carries a much higher embolic risk and should be treated (anticoagulation).

   - **Symptomatic vs. asymptomatic**: Symptoms (swelling, pain, heaviness) is itself an indication for treatment.

3. **Why is this patient getting DVT?** Evaluate for any provoking or predisposing factors:

   (a) **Is there an obvious cause**:

   - **Provoked DVT**: Recent immobility (major surgery, trauma, hospitalisation, orthopaedic casting), air travel > 6 hr, active cancer, pregnancy or contraceptive pills.

   - **Systemic disorders**: Pro-thrombotic disorders, for example, malignancy, lupus, nephrotic syndrome, liver cirrhosis.

   (b) **Do I need to workup for other predisposing factors?** The majority of patients with a first unprovoked DVT will not benefit from extensive workup beyond clinical history and examination, basic blood tests (full blood count, PT/aPTT, renal and liver panels) and age-appropriate cancer screening. Any abnormalities on these tests should be pursued. Patients with young DVT, recurrent miscarriages, recurrent venous thromboembolism, strong family history or unusual site thrombosis should receive further workup.

---

[1] If treatment is not given, a follow-up ultrasound should be performed 1 week later, to ensure that DVT has not progressed above the knee.

- **Prothrombotic disorders**: Pay heed to the population prevalence of specific prothrombotic disorders, before deciding what test to order. In Singaporean Chinese and Malays, test for protein C or S deficiency, antithrombin III mutation and anti-phospholipid syndrome (an unexpectedly prolonged aPTT, in the presence of thrombosis, suggests lupus anticoagulant). Factor V Leiden and prothrombin gene mutation are uncommon in Singaporean Chinese and Malays, but should be tested for in Caucasians and Indians.

- **Unusual site thrombosis** (e.g., cerebral, hepatic, mesenteric veins): In addition to prothrombotic disorders, consider workup for haematologic disease such as a myeloproliferative disease or paroxysmal nocturnal haemoglobinuria (page 318). In portal or mesenteric vein thrombosis, also consider evaluation for liver cirrhosis.

- **Occult malignancy**: Consider workup in older patients with recurrent DVT, or other suggestion of malignancy, for example, weight loss.

Chronic Unilateral Leg Swelling

This is usually more benign. Differentials include:

- **Chronic venous insufficiency**: An aching, swollen leg worse at the end of the day, with varicose veins and venous skin changes (see Chapter 46).

- **Lymphoedema**: Classically, there is cutaneous and subcutaneous thickening. Aetiologies include lymphatic damage after inguinal lymph node dissection, and filariasis (usually in patients from developing countries).

Bilateral Leg Swelling

Bilateral symmetrical leg swelling suggests systemic disease rather than local leg pathology. This may be obvious from the patient's medical history, or it may not. Look for other third-space oedema (e.g., pleural effusion, ascites, pulmonary oedema), and for an elevated jugular venous pressure (JVP).

Bilateral Leg Swelling + Elevated JVP

This points to intravascular hypervolaemia, which may be of cardiac or renal origin, or both. Patients may have exertional dyspnoea and pulmonary crackles or frank pulmonary oedema.

- **Congestive heart failure**: Symptoms include exertional dyspnoea, orthopnoea and paroxysmal nocturnal dyspnoea. CXR may show cardiomegaly ± pulmonary oedema (Figure 4.2a) and an ECG may suggest prior infarction (e.g., q waves, poor R wave progression). The diagnosis is made in the presence of compatible signs and symptoms, especially if the patient has known ischaemic heart disease or heart failure. Elevated NT-proBNP levels and echocardiographic evidence of reduced ejection fraction are supportive. Look for an acute precipitant of worsening fluid overload—

for example, new myocardial ischaemia, uncontrolled arrhythmia, noncompliance to fluid restriction or intercurrent infection.

- **Renal disease**: Renal disease is easy to identify from its raised urea and creatinine. Significant fluid overload tends not to occur until GFR $\leq$ 30 mL/min. Fluid overload in renal disease carries different implications, depending on context

  - **Acute kidney injury**: Search for a cause (see Chapter 18). Fluid overload makes management of volume status trickier in these patients.

  - **Known chronic kidney disease, not on dialysis**: Leg swelling results from an imbalance of fluid intake and output—for example, noncompliance to fluid restriction, acute kidney injury or inadequate dosing of diuretics. Look for any concomitant cardiac dysfunction.

  - **Patient on dialysis**: Leg swelling occurs due to noncompliance to fluid restriction, missed dialysis, dry weight set too high or technical issues (e.g., vascular access issues in haemodialysis, outflow issues in peritoneal dialysis).

Bilateral Leg Swelling + Normal JVP

Low albumin: Hypoalbuminaemia reduces capillary oncotic pressure, leading to accumulation of fluid in third-spaces, even as intravascular volume remains relatively normal (hence JVP is not elevated).

- **Nephrotic syndrome**: Heavy proteinuria > 3 g/day leads to hypoalbuminaemia and lower limb and periorbital oedema. Renal protein loss can be established by testing urine protein (spot or 24-hr); creatinine may be normal or abnormal (see Chapter 20).

- **Hepatic cirrhosis**: Fluid overload appears in decompensated cirrhosis. In addition to leg swelling, these patients tend to have marked ascites, jaundice, splenomegaly and cutaneous stigmata of chronic liver disease (see Chapter 10).

- **Gastrointestinal**: A protein-losing enteropathy (e.g., inflammatory bowel disease) or malnutrition can lead to hypoalbuminaemia. This should be apparent from other gastrointestinal symptoms.

Normal albumin:

- Bilateral venous insufficiency or bilateral lymphoedema (see earlier in this chapter).

- **Thyroid**: The oedema of thyroid disease is uniquely non-pitting, as it arises not from excess interstitial water, but from hyaluronic acid deposition. This can be seen in hypothyroidism (myxoedema) and Graves' disease (pretibial myxoedema) (see Chapter 36).

- **Pregnancy**: Oedema is common. Consider pre-eclampsia if there is also hypertension and proteinuria.

- **Drug induced**: In the absence of any other cause of oedema, pedal oedema may be ascribed to medications, for example, peripheral vasodilation (calcium channel blockers—common, hydralazine), renal vasoconstriction (NSAIDs, cyclosporine), and drugs causing fluid reabsorption (fludrocortisone, steroids and oestrogens).

Using what you have learnt, **pen down your approach** to the Clinical Case at the start of the chapter **BEFORE reading the discussion** below.

Case Discussion

This lady presents with acute painful unilateral lower limb swelling which began after a long flight. This is suspicious for deep vein thrombosis (DVT), with a differential of cellulitis. Low-grade fever does not discriminate between DVT and cellulitis. Obtain compression ultrasound to confirm DVT, and identify if above or below knee (the clinical suspicion is of above-knee DVT, given the thigh swelling). D-dimer is inappropriate in this patient as the clinical probability of DVT is moderate to high. If DVT is confirmed, it would be a provoked DVT (due to the long flight + contraceptive pills); workup for a prothrombotic disorder or occult malignancy is not indicated.

Key Lessons	1. Acute painful lower limb swelling is due to local leg pathology—deep vein thrombosis, cellulitis and other musculoskeletal causes. Patients with a high clinical probability of DVT should undergo compression ultrasound instead of D-dimer testing.
	2. Bilateral lower limb swelling is due to systemic disease—fluid overload (cardiac vs. renal), hypoalbuminaemia (cirrhosis, nephrotic syndrome) and by other mechanisms (thyroid disease, pregnancy, drugs).
Common Pitfalls	1. The *superficial* femoral vein is actually a *deep* vein; thrombosis in this vein is DVT.
	2. Think before ordering D-dimer. It is non-specific and often unexpectedly positive, which obliges you to do compression ultrasound. **Lesson**: do not order D-dimer if not suspecting DVT/PE, or if there is no intention to treat any DVT/PE (e.g., absolute contraindication to anticoagulation).
Questions	1. **REFLECT!** Have you ever encountered a patient with acute painful lower limb swelling? What are some of the challenges in distinguishing DVT vs. cellulitis?
	2. **DISCUSS!** We discussed D-dimer as a sensitive but non-specific test. What are some other tests (for any condition) that are (i) sensitive but not specific, (ii) specific but not sensitive, (ii) sensitive and specific? When might each type of test be useful in clinical diagnosis?
	3. **GO FURTHER!** Many patients have concomitant cardiac and renal disease. How might cardiac disease contribute to renal impairment, and renal impairment lead to cardiac disease? (cardiorenal syndrome).

Joints and Muscles

An Approach to
Joint Pain (General)

Clinical Case

A 30-year-old lady presents with joint pain. For the last 3 months, she has had pain and stiffness in her right wrist and the small joints of bilateral hands. This is worst when she gets up in the morning, and gets better during the day. She has noticed bilateral knee pain in the last 2 weeks, worse on the left. She has no back pain. Examination is remarkable for boggy swelling and tenderness over bilateral wrists and all metacarpal-phalangeal joints; there are no deformities. What is the likely diagnosis, and what workup would you perform?

A long list of conditions present with joint pain. Some are emergencies, which cause rapid joint destruction, others are nuisances without lasting harm. A number of key differentiators allow clear differentiation of the causes of joint pain. This chapter discusses a general approach to joint pain, especially polyarticular joint pain. Chapters 49–51 detail a more specific approach to pain in particular joints.

Initial Approach

Articular vs. non-articular: Begin by verifying that 'joint pain' truly comes from the joint. This is more likely if the joint is swollen, erythematous, tender on palpation of the joint line, or has restricted motion. Always consider non-articular causes:

- **Referred visceral pain:** 'Shoulder pain' may be a myocardial infarction in disguise. With a high index of suspicion, workup becomes obvious (e.g., ECG, troponin, etc.).

- **Tissue pain:** Patients may complain of joint pain instead of limb pain. Some of these conditions are emergencies—necrotising fasciitis, deep vein thrombosis, acute limb ischaemia (see Chapter 46).

- **Neuropathic pain:** Pain from a prolapsed intervertebral disc may radiate to the limb, and misleadingly present as 'joint pain' (see Chapter 51).

- **Periarticular musculoskeletal pain:** Due to ligaments, muscles and tendons. Diagnostic clues include: (1) on palpation, the point of maximal tenderness is not at the joint line, (2) pain on passive movement is less than on active movement and (3) pain is maximal in certain lines of muscle pull (this is the basis of various special tests). Ask about any trauma or inciting event (see Chapters 49–51).

- **Bone pain:** For example, fractures and dislocations due to trauma or injury.

Distribution and time course: Next, identify the distribution and time course of joint pain (Figure 48.1). Two key differentiators are (1) acute (hours to days) vs. chronic (weeks to months) joint pain, and (2) monoarticular vs. polyarticular involvement.

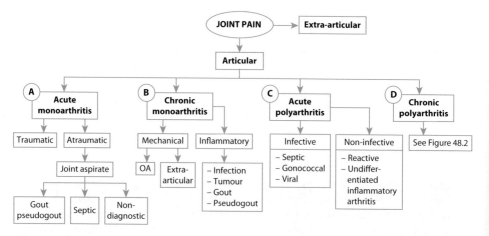

OA, osteoarthritis.

Figure 48.1. Approach to joint pain.

A. Acute Monoarthritis

Consider these differentials:

- **Trauma**: May result in acute haemarthrosis, periarticular fractures or dislocations. Always ask for a history of trauma or a precipitating event (e.g., sports injury, fall). Examine limb posture and range of motion. In any trauma, do not be fixated on the limb; resuscitate and look for any more pressing visceral injury.

- **Septic arthritis**: This must be considered in any acute monoarthritis, especially if there are predisposing factors, for example, joint surgery or prosthesis, joint disease (rheumatoid arthritis [RA], osteoarthritis [OA]), diabetes or IV drug use. Patients may be febrile and toxic, but on the other hand may look deceptively well.

- **Gout or pseudogout**: The typical history is of intermittent episodes of acute monoarthritis, with no pain between episodes. Certain joints are more classic for gout (e.g., podagra—first metatarsal phalangeal joint), and the same joint is often repeatedly affected. Examination may reveal tophi. In acute attacks, look for a precipitating factor, for example, purine-rich foods (beer, animal organs, red meats, sardines) or thiazide diuretics.

- **First presentation of a polyarthritis**: The causes of polyarthritis may present initially as a monoarthritis. Workup for such causes (see page 437) if the above differentials are unrewarding.

Approach and Workup

Exclude trauma on history and X-ray. Except in a long-standing history of intermittent gouty flares, or a clear-cut toxic patient, it is difficult to distinguish between gout and septic arthritis. Neither the nature of pain, presence or absence of fever, or examination findings is unique to either disease. Furthermore, known gout does not exclude septic arthritis. Joint aspiration is recommended in all acute monoarthritis (especially if first presentation), unless confident that septic arthritis is excluded.

Investigations for acute monoarthritis:

- **Joint X-ray:** Look for fractures or dislocations. This may not always be straightforward (Figures 48.2–48.4). If fractures are seen, exclude a pathological cause, for example, lytic lesions suggestive of metastases or myeloma. Gout may appear as punched-out erosions or lytic areas with overhanging edges, but these appear late. Chondrocalcinosis may be seen as calcification of articular cartilage or menisci in the wrists, knees and ankles.

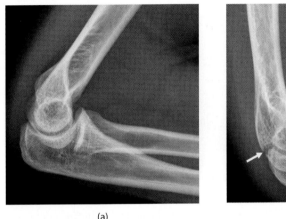
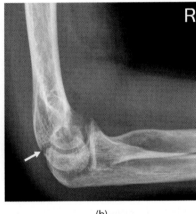

(a)   (b)

Figure 48.2. A 40-year-old man complained of right elbow pain after a fall. The initial elbow X-ray (a) showed no fracture, but a posterior fat pad is seen. A cast was prescribed, which he refused. He returned a week later with persistent elbow pain. Repeat X-ray (b) now shows the olecranon fracture.

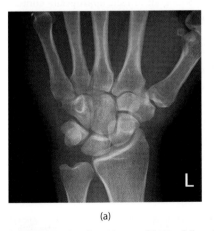
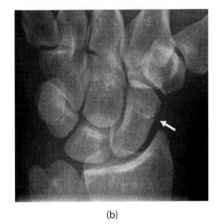

(a)   (b)

Figure 48.3. Another 40-year-old man fell on his outstretched left hand. A wrist X-ray (a) was reported as normal, but careful clinical examination found anatomical snuffbox tenderness. A scaphoid series (b) revealed an undisplaced scaphoid fracture.

(a)

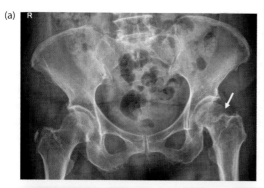

(b)

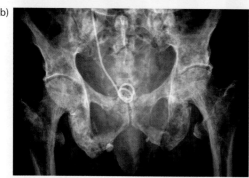

Figure 48.4. Two 70-year-old patients complained of left hip pain after minor trauma. (a) had an incomplete, undisplaced neck of femur fracture. These subtle neck of femur fractures are easy to miss—pay attention to the cortical irregularity. (b) had no fracture, but multiple sclerotic lesions from metastatic cancer. A right ureteric stent had previously been inserted for metastatic ureteric compression.

- **Joint aspiration**: This may be done at bedside or under image guidance (necessary in the hip joint). Examine the aspirate for blood (haemarthrosis) and turbidity (inflammation); normal joint fluid is straw-coloured. Send for microscopy (neutrophilic infiltrate seen in both infection and gout), gram stain, culture and crystal microscopy (negatively birefringent needle-shaped crystals in gout, and positively birefringent rhomboid-shaped crystals in pseudogout). In the appropriate context, consider TB PCR and cultures, fungal stains and cultures, as well as gonococcal cultures and PCR.

- **Inflammatory markers**: White blood cell (WBC) count, C-reactive protein (CRP) and procalcitonin are generally higher in septic arthritis than in gout, but there is no good cut-off to distinguish between the two; low values do not rule out septic arthritis.

- **Blood cultures**: Positive in 50% of septic arthritis and should be done.

- **Uric acid—not helpful in acute monoarthritis**: Elevated uric acid does not diagnose gout, and normal uric acid does not rule it out (levels may be falsely low during attacks). The only role of uric acid here is to establish a baseline for initiation of uric acid lowering therapy.

B. Chronic Monoarthritis

The first dichotomy is between mechanical and inflammatory pain:

- **Mechanical pain**: Exacerbated by movement or weight-bearing and relieved by rest. Any morning stiffness is < 15 min. Crepitus is often present, and there may be mild swelling but usually not gross swelling or erythema. Mechanical pain suggests an anatomical problem, for example, fractures, OA and periarticular causes of pain.

- **Inflammatory pain**: Rest pain exacerbated by immobility and relieved by motion. Night pain is a worrying feature. There may be morning stiffness (> 60 min), boggy synovitis and signs of inflammation (erythema, warmth, swelling, tenderness) and systemic response (e.g., fever).

Mechanical Chronic Monoarthritis

	Workup
- **Osteoarthritis (OA)**: A long history of slowly progressive joint pain, often symmetrical, associated with crepitus and reduced range of motion.	− Weightbearing X-ray of the joint
- **Other structural abnormalities**: For example, avascular necrosis of hip, undiagnosed stress fractures.	− X-ray
- Consider referred and periarticular causes.	

Inflammatory Chronic Monoarthritis

	Workup
- **Chronic infection**: Osteomyelitis, tuberculosis (TB) or fungal infection. There may be systemic features of infection (fever, chills, malaise). Look for a history of immunocompromise.	− Joint fluid: TB-PCR, TB and fungal stains and cultures − X-ray: bony erosions in osteomyelitis
- **Tumour**: Usually bony metastases or myeloma; primary bone tumours are rare. Look for constitutional symptoms, signs and symptoms of a primary tumour, as well as the hyper*c*alcaemia, *r*enal insufficiency and *a*naemia that suggests myeloma (together with *b*one pain, these make up the 'CRAB' features).	− X-ray or MRI: lytic lesions − Myeloma: screen full blood count (FBC), calcium, creatinine. If suspecting, do serum and urine protein electrophoresis and serum free light chains
- **Gout and pseudogout**: Episodic recurrences, often affecting the same joint (see earlier).	
- Spondyloarthropathy with asymmetrical peripheral oligoarthritis: Look for other features of spondyloarthropathy (see page 440).	

C. Acute Polyarthritis

Acute polyarthritis (≤ 6 weeks) may be infective or non-infective. In general, if the patient is unwell or if joints are hot and swollen, first consider bacterial sepsis (septic arthritis and disseminated gonococcal infection). If patients are relatively well and joint swelling less marked, consider viral polyarthritis (in the presence of infective symptoms), reactive arthritis (with a history of antecedent infection) and undifferentiated inflammatory arthritis (no prior infective symptoms).

Infective Causes

Workup

- **Polyarticular septic arthritis**: Septic arthritis tends to affect a single joint, but the same processes (e.g., haematogenous spread) may also lead to polyarticular infection.

  – Joint aspirate and culture
  – Blood culture

- **Disseminated gonococcal infection (DGI)**: Gonorrhoea causes two clinical pictures—(1) mono-articular septic arthritis, and (2) DGI, with migratory polyarthritis, tenosynovitis (tendon inflammation in wrist, fingers, ankles, toes ± dactylitis), a rash (painless vesiculopustular or pustular lesions) ± fever. Be suspicious in the presence of risk factors; note that simultaneous genitourinary symptoms are rare.

  – Joint aspirate and culture (in special gonococcal medium)
  – Blood culture (in special transport medium)
  – Urine gonococcal PCR

- **Viral polyarthritis**: Acute viral infections can cause prominent arthritis, with or without other symptoms. This list includes parvovirus, chikungunya, dengue (with low platelets, rash), HIV, hepatitis (with elevated liver enzymes), rubella, Epstein–Barr virus (EBV), enterovirus or adenovirus (with fever and/or respiratory or gastrointestinal symptoms). Joint pain is usually relatively symmetrical, and self-limiting.

  – FBC and liver enzymes
  – HIV; hepatitis B/C if liver enzymes abnormal
  – Other viruses: serology or observe (aetiological diagnosis usually not critical)

Non-Infective Causes

- **Reactive arthritis**: Asymmetrical oligoarthritis predominantly affecting large joints, several days to weeks *after* a diarrhoeal infection or urethritis (i.e., distinct from viral polyarthritis in time course). However, the classic triad of Reiter's syndrome (arthritis, urethritis, conjunctivitis) is rare. This is a spondyloarthritis; there may be features of spondyloarthritis (e.g., enthesitis, dactylitis) and positive HLA-B27. Diagnosis is clinical; there are no specific tests. Reactive arthritis usually settles by 6 months to 1 year.

- **Undifferentiated (early) inflammatory arthritis**: Some patients present with acute polyarthritis, without preceding infective symptoms, and go on to develop inflammatory arthritis. There is at least one swollen joint on examination, and there may be morning stiffness. The distribution of affected joints may be symmetrical and peripheral (resembling RA) or asymmetrical and appendicular (resembling spondyloarthritis), but does not always fall neatly into one type of inflammatory arthritis. Additional features develop with time. Consider serological investigations (start with FBC, electrolytes, liver enzymes, CRP/erythrocyte sedimentation rate (ESR), antinuclear antibody (ANA), rheumatoid factor, anti-cyclic citrullinated peptide antibody [anti-CCP]), these are helpful if positive, but may be negative when done early.

D. Chronic Polyarthritis

The aetiologies of chronic (> 6 weeks) polyarthritis can generally be classified into five groups: OA, RA, the spondyloarthropathies (SpA), polyarticular gout and other rheumatologic disease (e.g., lupus and scleroderma) with joint involvement.

A number of questions differentiate between these groups (Figure 48.5). Arthritis may be undifferentiated early on, or at the other extreme, 'burnt out', that is, grossly deformed joints which are no longer painful or swollen.[1]

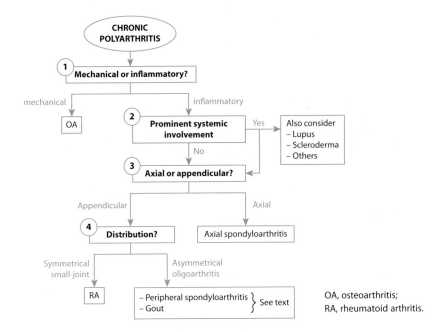

Figure 48.5. Approach to chronic polyarthritis.

---

[1] Usually burnt out rheumatoid arthritis, arthritis mutilans subtype of psoriatic arthropathy or mixed connective tissue disease.

1. Is Pain Mechanical or Inflammatory?

Mechanical pain—OA. Pain worse on movement or weight-bearing, relieved by rest, with minimal morning stiffness (<15 min) suggests OA. Weight-bearing X-rays may show loss of joint space, osteophyte formation, subchondral sclerosis and subchondral cysts (Figure 50.2), but the severity of X-ray changes do not always correlate with clinical symptoms. OA is common and two clinical pictures are seen:

- **Idiopathic OA:** Usually an elderly patient with longstanding symmetrical mechanical joint pain, commonly in knee (Asians), hip (Caucasians), spine or hands. OA may be limited to a few joints or be more extensive. In the hands, OA tends to affect the interphalangeal joints (Heberden's and Bouchard's nodes), while RA tends to affect the metacarpal-phalangeal joints.

- **Secondary OA:** Prior joint damage (e.g., trauma, other inflammatory arthritis, gout, septic arthritis) increases the risk of OA. Secondary OA may present younger and more atypically than idiopathic OA.

Inflammatory pain, on the other hand, is worse at rest, relieved by motion and associated with prolonged morning stiffness (often 30 min or more). This is more typical of RA, SpA, gout and other rheumatologic disease.

2. Is There Prominent Systemic Involvement?

In patients with multi-organ involvement, in addition to joint disease, other rheumatologic diseases like lupus and scleroderma enter the differential (Table 48.1). RA and SpA may have systemic features, but these are different from those of lupus and scleroderma, and joint disease tends to be more marked.

Table 48.1. Extra-Articular Manifestations of Inflammatory Arthritis

	RA	SpA	SLE	Scleroderma
Patient profile	Female > Male (3:1)	Male > Female (3:1) in AS Often (not always) HLA-B27 +ve	Female > Male (9:1)	Female > Male (3:1)
Joint pain	Symmetrical polyarthritis affecting small joints of hands and wrists	Inflammatory back pain Asymmetrical peripheral oligoarthritis	Any pattern, usually symmetric appendicular oligoarthritis	Pain, immobility due to fibrosis
Deformity	Hands: ulnar deviation, subluxation, swan neck, boutonniere, Z-thumb	Question-mark posture, decreased spine movements (in AS)		Microstomia

(Cont'd)

	RA	SpA	SLE	Scleroderma
Skin	Rheumatoid nodules Vasculitis Pyoderma gangrenosum	Psoriatic plaques (in PsA) Onycholysis, nail pitting (in PsA) Dactylitis	Rash: malar, discoid Alopecia Raynaud's phenomenon	Sclerodactyly Digital pitting, pulp atrophy Calcinosis Raynaud's phenomenon Telangiectasia
Soft tissues	Tendon rupture	Enthesitis, e.g., Achilles tendinitis		Digital gangrene Oral ulcers
Eyes	Episcleritis, scleritis	Anterior uveitis	Dry eyes (secondary Sjogren's)	
Heart	Accelerated atherosclerosis	Aortic regurgitation Arrhythmias	Constrictive pericarditis Pericardial effusion	Pericarditis, effusion Myocardial fibrosis, dysfunction
Lungs	Interstitial lung disease Rheumatoid pleural effusion Rheumatoid nodules Bronchiectasis	Interstitial lung disease	Pleura: pleurisy, effusion Pulmonary haemorrhage Interstitial lung disease	Interstitial lung disease Pulmonary hypertension
Gastro-intestinal		Inflammatory bowel disease (IBD-arthritis)	Gut vasculitis	Dysmotility: dysphagia, GERD, constipation
Blood	Neutropenia, splenomegaly (Felty's syndrome)		Cytopenias Antiphospholipid syndrome: foetal loss, DVT/PE	
Renal	Amyloidosis	Amyloidosis IgA nephropathy Nephrolithiasis	Lupus nephritis Chronic kidney disease	Scleroderma renal crisis: acute renal failure
Neuro-logical	Entrapment neuropathy, e.g., carpel tunnel syndrome Atlantoaxial subluxation, cervical myelopathy	Atlantoaxial subluxation Spinal arachnoiditis	Cerebral lupus: psychosis, delirium, cognitive difficulty	Cranial neuropathy Nerve entrapment Peripheral polyneuropathy Autonomic neuropathy

AS, ankylosing spondylitis; DVT/PE: deep vein thrombosis/pulmonary embolism; GERD, gastroesophageal reflux disease; IBD-arthritis, inflammatory bowel disease associated arthritis; PsA, psoriatic arthritis; RA, rheumatoid arthritis; SLE, systemic lupus erythematosus; SpA, spondyloarthritis.

3. Is Joint Involvement Axial or Peripheral?

Axial—SpA: Prominent axial (spine and sacroiliac joint) pain suggests SpA. There are a number of subtypes including psoriatic arthritis, inflammatory bowel disease associated arthritis, reactive arthritis (see page 436) and undifferentiated spondyloarthritis.

- **Ankylosing spondylitis:** The prototype is a young man with inflammatory back pain, enthesitis and uveitis. A gradual reduction in spine movements culminates in a classic 'question mark' posture. MRI may demonstrate sacroiliitis early on, and X-rays show a 'bamboo spine' in late disease.

- **Psoriatic arthritis:** Associated with psoriatic plaques and psoriatic nail changes (onycholysis, pitting).

- **Inflammatory bowel disease associated arthritis:** With flares of abdominal colic, bloody diarrhoea, malabsorption, and perianal skin tags (see page 130).

Peripheral: This may be RA, gout or a peripheral SpA (these may be predominantly axial or peripheral).

4. In Peripheral Inflammatory Arthritis, What is the Distribution of Joint Involvement?

The distribution of joint involvement (Table 48.2)—symmetry, number of joints affected, size of joints affected—and time course distinguishes between RA, peripheral SpA and polyarticular gout (80% of gout present as monoarthritis, but up to 20% are polyarticular).

5. Supportive Workup

The basis of rheumatologic diagnosis is clinical history and examination, not blood tests. Autoantibodies can be helpful, but have limited sensitivity and specificity, and come with many caveats. For example, rheumatoid factor is positive in 70% to 80% of RA but also 20% to 30% of lupus, and 5% to 10% of healthy individuals. A negative test does not rule out RA, and the extent to which a positive test confirms RA depends on the pre-test probability. Of note, blood tests *can be entirely normal* in inflammatory arthritis.

Supportive investigations are ordered based on the clinical differentials. This may include:

- **X-rays:** There may be supportive features—see sections earlier.

- **Inflammatory markers:** ESR, CRP may correlate with activity in peripheral arthritis.

- **Joint aspiration:** If there is a dominant swollen joint—look for gout as well as septic arthritis, which may complicate any of the chronic inflammatory arthritis.

- **In RA:** Rheumatoid factor, Anti-CCP.

- **In SpA:** HLA-B27 is often, but not always positive.

- **In lupus**: ANA (sensitive, non-specific), Anti-dsDNA (specific, non-sensitive), Anti-Sm, complement levels (C3 and C4 are consumed in active lupus), anticardiolipin antibodies. Consider testing renal, liver and haematological function looking for multi-organ involvement.

- **In scleroderma**: Anti-centromere (limited SSc), Anti-topoisomerase, anti-Scl-70 (diffuse SSc).

- **In Sjogren's syndrome**: Anti-SSA (Ro), Anti-SSB (La).

- **In mixed connective tissue disease**: Anti-RNP.

In addition to making a diagnosis, assess disease activity (active inflammation e.g., boggy swelling, tenderness), and the patient's function.

Table 48.2. Distribution of Joint Involvement in Peripheral Inflammatory Arthritis

	RA	SpA	Polyarticular gout
Symmetry	Symmetrical	Asymmetrical	Asymmetrical
Distribution of joints	Polyarthritis affecting small joints of hands and wrists	Oligoarthritis affecting few (1–3) large joints (e.g., knees and ankles)	Oligoarthritis affecting few large joints (e.g., big toe and knee)
Time course	Chronic inflammatory pain ± acute flares	Chronic inflammatory pain ± acute flares	Intermittent episodic pain, pain free intervals
Examination	Active synovitis (boggy swelling, tenderness) Deformities (ulnar deviation, swan neck and boutonniere deformity, joint subluxation) Rheumatoid nodules	Enthesitis Dactylitis ('sausage digit') Psoriatic plaque, nail changes	Erythematous warm joint Gouty tophi
Joint X-ray	Erosions, deformities	Pencil-in-cup appearance (classic for psoriatic arthritis)	Punched-out erosions or lytic areas with overhanging edges (appear late)
Other features			Joint aspiration—crystals

RA, rheumatoid arthritis; SpA, spondyloarthritis.

Using what you have learnt, **pen down your approach** to the Clinical Case at the start of the chapter **BEFORE reading the discussion** below.

Case Discussion

This is a young lady with chronic inflammatory polyarthritis, affecting the small joints of the hands and wrists, and also both knees. This pattern is most consistent with rheumatoid arthritis. She is early in the course, so she has active disease and little deformity—the aim of treatment is to prevent deformity and loss of function.

Atypically, however, there is some asymmetry in the joint involvement; consider the differentials of spondyloarthritis and polyarticular gout. Look for psoriatic skin or nail changes, or history of bloody diarrhoea consistent with inflammatory bowel disease, which would favour a spondyloarthropathy. Ask for any history of acute joint swelling which completely resolves (if such an episode is caught, the joint should be aspirated for crystal microscopy). Screen for other systemic involvement (e.g., rashes, haematuria, sclerodactyly) as that may suggest another rheumatologic disease (e.g., lupus) with articular involvement.

Other blood tests could include ESR, rheumatoid factor and anti-CCP antibody. If positive, these support a diagnosis of RA; negative tests do not rule it out. Do full blood count, renal and liver biochemistries to evaluate for other organ involvement and as part of pre-treatment evaluation.

Key Lessons	1. In patients presenting with joint pain, consider extra-articular causes, and classify articular joint pain as (i) acute or chronic, (ii) monoarthritis or polyarthritis.
	2. Most cases of acute monoarthritis should receive joint aspiration, for diagnosis of septic arthritis, gout and pseudogout.
	3. In chronic polyarthritis, key differentiators are (1) mechanical vs. inflammatory pain, (2) the distribution of joint pain (axial vs. appendicular, symmetrical vs. asymmetrical, small vs. large joint) and (3) extra-articular manifestations. These differentiate rheumatoid arthritis, osteoarthritis, spondyloarthropathy, polyarticular gout and other diseases.
Common Pitfalls	1. Delayed diagnosis of septic arthritis leads to joint destruction and systemic sepsis.
	2. Normal blood tests do not exclude inflammatory arthritis.
Questions	1. **REFLECT!** Have you ever seen a patient with rheumatoid arthritis? What did the patient first present with, and how was the diagnosis made?
	2. **EXPLORE!** Outline the technique of hand examination in a rheumatologic patient. What are your steps, and what do you look for?
	3. **DISCUSS!** To what extent do the *classification criteria* for rheumatoid arthritis, axial and appendicular spondyloarthropathy aid in diagnosis of these conditions?

4. **GO FURTHER!** Distinguishing septic arthritis from other causes of acute monoarthritis is challenging. Various authors have studied the extent to which specific clinical and laboratory features predict a diagnosis of septic arthritis. Look up Tables 2 and 3 in Carpenter, CR *et al.* (August 2011). Evidence-based diagnostics: adult septic arthritis. *Academic Emergency Medicine*, 18(8), 781–796. PMID: 21843213 (free access). Questions:

(a) What are likelihood ratios?

(b) Based on these tables, which clinical and laboratory features

(i) make septic arthritis very likely?

(ii) are unable to distinguish between septic arthritis and other diagnoses?

Chapter

49 An Approach to Shoulder Pain

Clinical Case

A 60-year-old man with a past medical history of diabetes and smoking presents with intermittent left shoulder pain. He has found it particularly difficult to carry heavy parcels to or from high shelves, which has been affecting his job as a warehouse assistant. He has no pain on off days, and no recent injury. How would you approach his complaint?

Shoulder pathology presents with pain, stiffness, weakness and instability. Pathology includes not only the glenohumeral joint, but also its surrounding muscles and tendons. This chapter builds on the general approach to joint pain (see Chapter 48), discussing aetiologies specific to the shoulder (Figure 49.1).

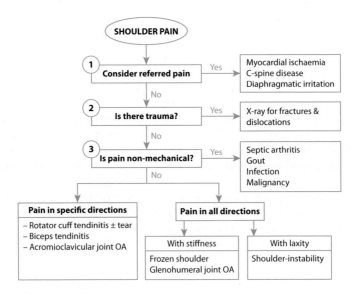

OA, Osteoarthritis.

Figure 49.1. Approach to shoulder pain.

Dangerous Causes

1. Consider Referred Pain

Consider referred pain, especially if pain is vague and diffuse, glenohumeral motion is painless, or there are non-musculoskeletal symptoms:

Workup

- **Myocardial ischaemia**: This may misleadingly present with shoulder pain, without classic chest pain. Watch out especially if there is diaphoresis, dyspnoea or the patient is high-risk (see Chapter 3).

  - ECG
  - Troponins

- **Cervical spine disease**: Radiculopathy may mimic shoulder pain. When asked to point to the site of maximal pain, these patients tend to point to the back of the shoulder or the trapezius muscle, rather than the anterior shoulder or laterally (at the deltoid insertion).

  - See Chapter 51

- **Diaphragmatic irritation** from lower lobe pneumonia or hepatobiliary disease may be referred to the shoulder via the phrenic nerve (C3–C5 roots).

  - As guided by further history and examination

2. Is There Trauma?

Any history of trauma, or an acute onset of pain, must prompt a search for fractures or dislocation. This may include clavicular or humeral fractures, acromioclavicular joint injury or glenohumeral dislocation. The first clue is usually an abnormal limb posture— for example, the patient carrying the affected arm with the other hand, squaring of the shoulders and 'Shirley's glenoid sign' in anterior shoulder dislocation. Be especially careful in the elderly, as minimal trauma may be enough to cause a proximal humeral fracture.

X-ray: Obtain shoulder X-rays in anterior–posterior, Y-scapula and axillary views (or Velpeau view, if the patient is in too much pain to tolerate the axillary view). Multiple views are important; dislocations are easily missed if only the anterior–posterior view is obtained (e.g., look for the light bulb sign of posterior dislocation). Ensure that in the Y-scapula view, the glenohumeral head sits on the junction of the 'Y'.

3. Is Pain Non-Mechanical?

- Acutely tender, swollen shoulder with restricted range of motion ± systemic features (e.g., fever)—suspect septic arthritis or gout. The joint should be tapped.
- Constant or night pain—worrying for infection, tumour and trauma.

- Significant morning stiffness, which gets better towards the end of the day—consider inflammatory disease, for example, rheumatoid arthritis (Note: patients with frozen shoulder also have significant stiffness, which does not usually get better towards the end of the day).

These conditions, and their workup, are discussed at length in Chapter 48.

Mechanical Shoulder Pain

Mechanical shoulder pain is triggered by exertion, and better at rest. As a general rule, pain triggered by movement in any direction points to a joint or capsular problem, while triggered by specific actions suggests that pain arises from the structures that are stressed by that particular action. By this principle, physical examination of the shoulder employs various provocative manoeuvres to stress its different structures.

Pain in Specific Directions

	Workup
• **Rotator cuff (supraspinatus) tendinitis ± tear**: This presents in a middle-aged to older patient with pain on abduction. This may be chronic or present acutely after unaccustomed shoulder activity. Pain is provoked by passive flexion in 30° abduction and internal rotation (Neer's sign), and internal rotation in 90° flexion of both elbow and shoulder (Hawkins test). In *tendinitis*, there is pain without weakness. With repetitive injury, the supraspinatus tendon may *tear partially*, causing pain and weakness in abduction (particularly in the first 15° of abduction before the deltoid muscle takes over). A *complete tear* results in dramatic weakness but relatively little pain. Passive range of movement remains full.	− Ultrasound: visualises tendon thickening (inflammation) and/or tear − Order X-ray with ultrasound to rule out missed fractures/ tumour − MRI shoulder if ultrasound non-diagnostic (and confirmation of diagnosis needed for management)
• **Biceps tendinitis**: Pain localised in the bicipital groove, exacerbated by carrying objects in the hand (uses the biceps). On examination, pain is provoked by resisted elbow flexion or supination.	
• **Acromioclavicular joint osteoarthritis**: Focal tenderness to palpation at the acromioclavicular joint (at the outer end of the clavicle), exacerbated by flexing the shoulder 90° and forcibly adducting it across the chest, like grasping a scarf on the opposite shoulder (scarf sign).	− X-ray to show osteoarthritic changes

Pain in All Directions + Stiffness

- **Frozen shoulder** (adhesive capsulitis): This classically goes through three phases. In the first phase, patients complain of diffuse shoulder pain. In the second phase, pain improves but severe stiffness develops, with loss of active and passive range of motion in all directions. Finally, after as long as 18 to 24 months, patients enter a recovery phase. Frozen shoulder is most common in the mid-50s age group, in whom it usually idiopathic or associated with diabetes or thyroid disease, but can occur at a younger age if there is a secondary cause (e.g., other shoulder pathology causing prolonged immobilisation).

  – Nil (clinical diagnosis), unless excluding other conditions
  – X-rays are normal

- **Glenohumeral osteoarthritis**: Chronic mechanical pain with restricted movements in all directions. This may be primary (usually in older patients, e.g., > 65 years old), or secondary to previous trauma, rotator cuff arthropathy, or rheumatologic disease.

  – X-ray may show narrowing of cartilage, osteophytes, sclerosis of humeral head

Pain in All Directions + Laxity

- **Shoulder instability**: These patients complain of shoulder pain, a 'loose shoulder' or one that 'comes out'. There may be a catching sensation or sudden weakness developing when the arm is overhead (e.g., throwing an object). Examination finds excessive ligamentous laxity and often a positive apprehension test. Shoulder instability occurs in: (1) young patients with poor muscular development or hypermobility syndromes, (2) after an injury in which the shoulder is forced into abduction, external rotation and extension or (3) older patients who tore their rotator cuff after a shoulder dislocation.[1]

  – Nil (clinical diagnosis)

Assess Function

In all cases do assess the effect of the shoulder pathology on the patient's daily activities, work, sport and hobbies.

---

[1] In older patients, shoulder dislocation without fracture may cause large rotator cuff tears. Younger patients have stronger rotator cuff muscles, so shoulder dislocation in younger patients tend to cause bony injuries (Bankart and Hill–Sachs lesions) rather than rotator cuff tears.

Using what you have learnt, **pen down your approach** to the Clinical Case at the start of the chapter **BEFORE reading the discussion** below.

Case Discussion

This gentleman presents with mechanical shoulder pain, worse on reaching above shoulder level, most likely due to rotator cuff tendinitis. Examine him to confirm pain in the impingement position (Neer's and Hawkin's tests) ± abduction weakness or difficulty initiating the abduction movement. Active range of motion may be limited if he has a partial supraspinatus tear, but he should have a full passive range of motion; if passive range of motion is impaired in all directions, frozen shoulder becomes more likely. If his shoulder examination is normal and pain is vague, consider angina, which could possibly present as exertion-induced shoulder pain.

Key Lessons	1. In all cases of shoulder pain, consider the causes of referred pain, exclude trauma and non-mechanical pain before proceeding to evaluate for mechanical shoulder pathology.
	2. Distinguish between mechanical shoulder pain provoked by certain actions, versus that occurring in all directions of movement. Pain provoked by specific actions is likely due to tendinitis (either of the rotator cuff or biceps tendon), while pain and stiffness in all directions suggests a joint (osteoarthritis) or capsular (frozen shoulder) problem. Pain and laxity occurs in shoulder instability.
Common Pitfalls	1. Myocardial ischaemia, presenting as shoulder pain, has been missed. Always look for the causes of referred pain.
Questions	1. **REFLECT!** Have you ever encountered patients with rotator cuff tendinitis or frozen shoulder? How do these diseases impact their daily function?
	2. **EXPLORE!** Shoulder examination employs a number of provocative tests. What are the key steps in examining the shoulder of a patient who presents with shoulder pain?
	3. **GO FURTHER!** Injection of local anaesthesia (lignocaine) into the shoulder joint can be used diagnostically (although this has been superseded by MRI in many centres where MRI is easily available). How would you interpret (i) a patient with apparent frozen shoulder whose range of movement improves markedly with lignocaine injection, and (ii) a patient with apparent rotator cuff tendinitis whose abduction weakness persists after lignocaine injection?

Chapter

50

An Approach to Knee Pain

Clinical Case

A 25-year-old man presents with severe left knee pain. Ever since he suffered a bad football tackle as a teenager, he has had left knee pain whenever he runs, associated with intermittent locking symptoms. In the last 2 days, however, his left knee pain was uncharacteristically severe, so much so that he was woken up from sleep by pain. There is no trauma. He has a past medical history of nephrotic syndrome on high-dose prednisolone. On examination, the left knee is warm and swollen; movements are limited by pain. How would you approach his complaint?

Knee disease may present with pain, swelling, stiffness, locking symptoms or instability. This chapter builds on the general approach to joint pain (see Chapter 48), discussing specific considerations in isolated knee pain (Figure 50.1).

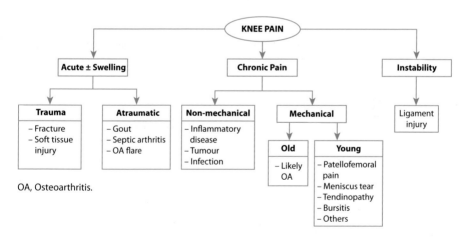

OA, Osteoarthritis.

Figure 50.1. Approach to knee pain.

Begin by screening the hip (e.g., osteoarthritis or fracture) and spine (e.g., lumbar radiculopathy) as pain in these joints may be referred to the knee.

Acute Knee Pain ± Swelling

Traumatic Knee Pain

Have a common-sense approach based on the severity of trauma. In high-energy trauma (e.g., road traffic accident), resuscitate according to the principles of advanced trauma life support; the knee is probably of lower priority. In low-energy trauma (e.g., twisting the knee while playing football), examine the tissues of the knee in turn:

- Examine neurovascular status of the lower limb (pedal pulses, power and reflexes and sensation)—major knee injury may disrupt the popliteal vessels and nerves supplying the foot.

- **X-ray**: Look for fractures and dislocations. A Segond fracture (bony avulsion of the lateral tibial plateau) implies a tear in the anterior cruciate ligament.

- Examine the joint for swelling, which is demonstrable by patella tap or a bulge test. Acute post-traumatic swelling is usually haemarthrosis, for which a ruptured anterior cruciate ligament is the most common cause. Medial joint line tenderness suggests a meniscus tear.

- Examine the ligaments (see knee instability, page 452).

- Examine active and passive movements.

- Remember to screen lumbar spine and hip joint to exclude referred pain.

Acute Atraumatic Knee Pain

- **Inflammatory causes**: Gout and septic arthritis commonly present in the knee. The latter is particularly important to look for, as it can rapidly destroy the knee. Known joint pathology (e.g., gout) does not exclude septic arthritis; a damaged joint is in fact *more* likely to turn septic. Joint aspiration should be performed. This is further discussed in Chapter 48.

- **Flare of chronic conditions**: Most commonly a flare of osteoarthritis, precipitated by activity. This is common, but it is a diagnosis of exclusion. Patients should receive joint aspiration if the diagnosis is in question.

Chronic Knee Pain

Exclude Non-Mechanical Pain

Distinguish between mechanical pain (worse on joint loading, better with rest) and non-mechanical pain (worse at rest, severe night pain). *Stiffness* is a common complaint in any knee disease; however, prolonged morning stiffness that becomes better with activity is worrisome for non-mechanical causes of pain. *Locking*, a sudden inability to flex or extend the knee, arises from a loose body (an avulsed osteophyte, bucket-handle meniscus tear or osteochondritis dissecans), which is consistent with mechanical pain.

Non-mechanical pain: If pain is non-mechanical, consider inflammatory causes of knee pain including tumour, inflammatory rheumatologic disease (e.g., spondyloarthropathy) and chronic infection (see Chapter 48).

Mechanical Pain: Older Patient

An elderly patient with chronic progressive mechanical knee pain on usual activities, occasional locking symptoms, and periodic flares of pain and swelling is most likely to have osteoarthritis. On examination, there may be bony enlargement, crepitus on active motion and restricted range of motion.

Approach:

- **X-ray**: *Weight bearing* AP, lateral and skyline views. Typical osteoarthritic changes include joint space narrowing, osteophytes, subchondral sclerosis and subchondral cysts (Figure 50.2).

- Look for underlying predispositions, for example, previous knee injury, varus deformity. Be especially wary of secondary osteoarthritis (e.g., due to previous trauma) in middle-aged patients who have premature osteoarthritis.

- Assess functional impairment: For example, wasting of the vastus muscles, impaired walking speed and distance, inability to squat and impact on activities of daily living and mobility.

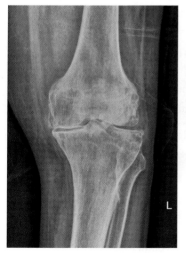
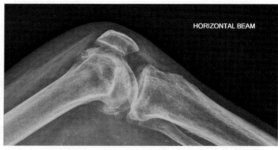

Figure 50.2. Knee osteoarthritis. A 70-year-old gentleman presented with longstanding bilateral mechanical knee pain. Anterior–posterior (left) and lateral (above) knee X-rays show joint space narrowing, osteophytes and subchondral sclerosis, typical for osteoarthritis.

Mechanical Pain: Younger Patient

Examine the tissues of the knee in turn, attempting to localise pain, identify any effusion. Ask if pain started after any specific activity (e.g., sport).

Localised pain: Causes with point tenderness on examination:

- **Meniscus tear**: Knee pain, swelling and/or locking symptoms, which typically began after a sports injury. Examination reveals medial or lateral joint line tenderness, and a positive McMurray stress test.

- **Osgood–Schlatter disease**: Apophysitis at the site of insertion of the patella tendon, causing pain localised to the tibial tuberosity, worse on knee flexion.

- **Quadriceps or patella tendinopathy**: Pain localised to the quadriceps or patella tendon, worse on knee flexion.

- **Bursitis**: Prolonged kneeling may result in suprapatella or infrapatella bursitis. This presents as a localised tenderness and swelling superficial to the patella.

Generalised pain:

- **Patellofemoral pain syndrome** (chondromalacia patellae). Patella maltracking and/or articular damage causing diffuse anterior knee pain, worse on stair climbing or prolonged sitting, with anterior crepitus on knee movements and a positive patella grind test. The pain characteristics and examination findings resemble that of osteoarthritis, except that X-rays are normal.

- **Articular cartilage injuries** (including osteochondritis dissecans): Diffuse knee pain, swelling and locking, worse after activity.

- **Recurrent patella dislocation**: This usually occurs in adolescents, who complain of discomfort and a sensation of the knee giving way when flexed. The patella apprehension test is positive. Palpate the medial patellofemoral ligament for tenderness (suggesting a tear, which predisposes to lateral patella dislocation), and look for generalised ligamentous laxity (e.g., Beighton score).

Workup: The initial management of these conditions is generally conservative (physiotherapy, analgesia).

- **X-rays**: To exclude a fracture (especially if pain came on suddenly during activity).

- **MRI knee**: Can be used to confirm clinical findings before surgery, or to reevaluate the diagnosis if the patient fails to improve with physiotherapy.

Knee Instability

Some patients complain predominantly of a sensation of the knee 'giving way', associated with discomfort and apprehension on weight bearing. The majority of these patients have ligamentous injuries, usually associated with prior sport injury (patients may remember a 'pop' sound, after which they could not continue playing).

    Clinical examination can localise the culprit ligament (combination injuries are possible).

- **Anterior cruciate ligament (ACL)**: Positive anterior drawer (or Lachman) test—that is, the endpoint is 'boggy' (be sure to exclude false-positive anterior drawer test by first ruling out a posterior sag).

- **Posterior cruciate ligament**: Posterior sag visible in flexion, loss of tibial step-off on palpation and a positive posterior drawer test.

- **Medial/lateral ligament tears**: Tenderness on palpation of the medial/lateral cruciate ligament, and valrus/varus deviation on application of a varus/valgus stress in 30° flexion.

Workup: MRI knee best visualises ligamentous and meniscus injuries. A torn ACL appears disrupted and white (oedema) on T2.

 Using what you have learnt, **pen down your approach** to the Clinical Case at the start of the chapter **BEFORE reading the discussion** below.

Case Discussion

This young gentleman has acute atraumatic inflammatory knee pain, on a background of chronic mechanical pain after a sporting injury (e.g., a meniscus tear). Recognise immediately that his acute presentation is quite different from the chronic pain, and must not be dismissed. The most important consideration here is septic arthritis, especially when he has a history of immunocompromise (high dose steroids). Joint aspiration should be performed urgently, with fluid sent for cytology, gram stain, culture and crystal microscopy. Blood cultures and inflammatory markers should be taken concurrently.

Key Lessons	1. In acute traumatic knee pain, obtain X-rays and examine each tissue of the knee (nerves, vessels, joint, ligaments and muscles) for injury. If there is no trauma, consider gout, septic arthritis and an osteoarthritis flare.
	2. Chronic non-mechanical knee pain may be due to rheumatologic disease, chronic infection or malignancy, and should be investigated.
	3. Chronic mechanical knee pain in an elderly patient is most likely osteoarthritis. In a younger patient, common causes include meniscus tear, patellofemoral pain syndrome and articular cartilage injuries. These causes can be identified based on history and examination.
Common Pitfalls	1. X-ray changes consistent with osteoarthritis are common; they do not necessarily mean that the patient has osteoarthritis, or that his/her symptoms are due to osteoarthritis.
Questions	1. **EXPLORE!** Read up on the technique of performing a knee aspiration. How would you take consent for this procedure?
	2. **DISCUSS!** Try drawing up an approach to hip pain. It is quite similar as that to knee pain, except that (i) greater emphasis must be placed on excluding hip fracture, given how common it is; (ii) avascular necrosis of the hip must be considered in the differential.
	3. **GO FURTHER!** A patient presents with acute left knee pain and was found to have a femoral shaft fracture. Unusually, he did not fall or sustain any trauma. Why might he have sustained an atraumatic fracture, and what workup should be performed?

Chapter

51

An Approach to
Back and Neck Pain

Clinical Case

Three 40-year-old taxi drivers present with lower back pain:

- *Patient A presents with a 1-day history of severe lower back pain after helping a passenger unload an overweight suitcase. On examination, he has bilateral foot drop and a palpable bladder.*

- *Patient B presents with a 3-month history of tiresome back pain, worst at the end of each shift. This is much relieved once he lounges in front of the television.*

- *Patient C presents with a 3-month history of progressively worsening back pain, worst at night and in the early morning, associated with low-grade fever and night sweats.*

For each patient, what is the most likely diagnosis, and what would you do next?

Back or neck pain is frustratingly common. It is often minor, not warranting further investigation, but occasionally heralds a serious condition. A robust clinical approach is essential so as not to miss dangerous conditions, yet not over-investigate (Figure 51.1).

Exclude trauma: Begin by excluding trauma (including road traffic accidents, falls from height, etc.)—significant trauma would require a systematic approach emphasising prioritisation of the greatest threats to life, with clinical evaluation and emergent treatment carried out concurrently. This is well taught in the Advanced Trauma Life Support framework (not covered here).

Neurology: Next, look for neurologic deficits including limb weakness or numbness, bladder/bowel dysfunction and anal tone laxity. Pain radiating from neck/back into the limbs in a dermatomal distribution (*radiculopathy*, previously termed *sciatica* in the sciatic nerve distribution) suggests nerve root irritation. Some patients may also experience episodic lower limb pain after walking a variable distance—neurogenic claudication (see page 418).

With Neurological Symptoms/Deficit

Acute-Onset

Clinical syndromes: It is important to recognise the differences between symptoms of radiculopathy, and the cauda equina syndrome (Table 51.1). For example, patients with L5 radiculopathy complain of pain shooting from the buttock, down the lateral leg, into the dorsum of the foot ('*sciatica*'), and may have numbness on the dorsum of the foot

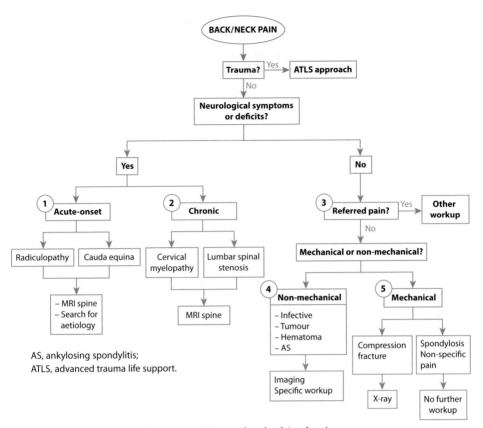

Figure 51.1. Approach to back/neck pain.

Table 51.1. Clinical Syndromes of Acute Back Pain with Neurological Symptoms

	Radiculopathy	Cauda equina syndrome
Pathophysiology	Compression of single nerve root	Compression of cauda equina (the *bundle* of nerve roots below the spinal cord's termination at L2)
Pain	Pain radiates from neck/back into the limbs down a dermatomal distribution. Straight leg raise (stretches sciatic nerve roots) replicates pain	Severe low back pain with bilateral radicular pain
Weakness and areflexia	Absent or limited to specific myotome	Severe, bilateral, affecting multiple nerve roots
Numbness	Absent or limited to specific dermatome	Severe, bilateral, affecting multiple nerve roots
Bladder and bowel	Normal	Bladder/bowel dysfunction (incontinence, urinary retention), lax anal tone, perineal anaesthesia

(L5 dermatome) and foot drop (L5 myotome). On the other hand, suspect cauda equina syndrome if weakness or numbness affects >1 nerve root, digital rectal examination finds a lax anal tone, or there is any urinary dysfunction (e.g., palpable bladder, overflow incontinence, elevated post-void residual urine).

Aetiologies:

- **Prolapsed intervertebral disc**: This is the most common cause, and usually presents in young to middle-aged patients with a history of straining (e.g., carrying a heavy load). A prolapsed disc may impinge laterally on a nerve root, causing radiculopathy (e.g., L4/5 prolapse compresses the exiting L4 nerve root or the transversing L5 nerve root). In contrast, a large central prolapse in the lumbar spine can compress the cauda equina, causing severe neurologic dysfunction—the cauda equina syndrome.

- **Serious aetiologies**: Occasionally, radicular symptoms or the cauda equina syndrome may be the first presentation of serious aetiologies including malignancy and infection (epidural abscess).

- If symptoms of weakness and areflexia predominate, with only mild back/neck pain, consider other disorders causing weakness (see Chapter 25).

Workup: MRI spine is the evaluation of choice, and will visualise prolapsed discs (Figure 51.2) and other lesions. It would be urgent in patients with cauda equina syndrome, as irreversible neurologic deficits may ensue without urgent intervention.

Chronic, in Middle-Aged to Elderly Patients

With age, degenerative changes cause spinal canal narrowing. These are gradual changes and nerves have time to adapt; hence, unlike acute disc prolapse, symptoms of acute irritation (e.g., radiculopathy) are absent.

- In the cervical spine—**Cervical myelopathy**: An elderly patient with gait disturbance, frequent falls, loss of hand dexterity (e.g., difficulty buttoning clothes, inability to use chopsticks), and variable weakness. Neck pain may or may not be present. Urinary symptoms develop late in the disease. The natural history is stepwise deterioration of function; many patients have subtle symptoms and learn to cope, while others present acutely after a fall. Examination reveals gait ataxia, upper motor neuron signs in the lower limbs (bilateral upgoing plantars, hyperreflexia) and variable upper-limb lower motor neuron signs. Hoffmann's sign may be positive. Myelopathy is notorious for giving varied signs; other differentials for weakness should be considered (see Chapter 25).

- In the lumbar spine—**Lumbar spinal stenosis**: Intermittent lower limb pain, weakness, numbness or paresthesia, exacerbated by walking but relieved on rest or spine flexion. There may be concomitant radicular symptoms if degenerative changes (e.g., osteophytes) also result in nerve root impingement. Examination is usually normal, with no upper motor neuron signs (as the spinal cord has ended at L2), and a negative straight leg raise.

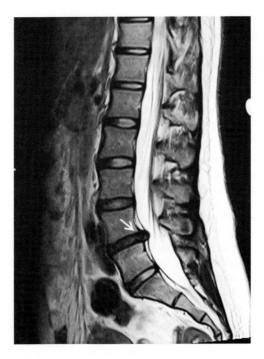

Figure 51.2. A 25-year-old nurse presented with sudden-onset severe back pain after lifting a heavy patient. His pain radiated down the right leg into the foot. Straight leg raise reproduced the pain, at an angle of 40°. MRI was performed, showing a prolapsed L4/L5 intervertebral disc.

Workup: MRI spine is the best modality to visualise degenerative bony and ligamentous changes, and spinal canal narrowing. Please only order MRI for symptomatic patients; abnormal MRI findings are common in asymptomatic people.

Without Neurological Symptoms

Consider Referred Pain

Consider the causes of referred pain, which can be life threatening.

- **Referred back pain**: Retroperitoneal abdominal pain is referred to the back. Emergent causes include an expanding abdominal aortic aneurysm or dissection, ectopic pregnancy and perforated gastric ulcer. Other causes include pancreatitis, urolithiasis and endometriosis (see Chapter 9). Always ask for other abdominal symptoms, and examine abdomen and lower limb pulses.
- **Referred neck pain**: Neck pain can be a manifestation of meningeal irritation (as in meningitis and subarachnoid haemorrhage), or tension headache. Consider the approach to headache (see Chapter 22).

Next, decide if pain is mechanical or non-mechanical.

Non-Mechanical Spine Pain

Pain worse on rest and relieved by movement, which wakes the patient up at night, or associated with fever, weight loss or significant morning stiffness is inconsistent with a degenerative structural lesion. Well-localised vertebral tenderness on examination is suspicious. Consider:

Workup

- **Infective**: Vertebral osteomyelitis or discitis. Be particularly suspicious in patients with diabetes, immunocompromise, a recent history of infection known to seed to the spine (e.g., *Staphylococcus aureus* bacteraemia) or intravenous drug abuse, or who are institutionalised. Fever and raised inflammatory markers may be present, but their absence does not exclude the diagnosis. The presentation may be acute in bacterial infection, or subacute to chronic in tuberculous infection (especially in patients with risk factors).

  − Inflammatory markers
  − Blood cultures
  − MRI spine directly if high clinical suspicion (can await inflammatory markers if low suspicion)

- **Tumour**: Suspicious features include weight loss, constitutional symptoms, relentlessly worsening rest pain and a history of malignancy. This is most commonly metastases from a solid organ tumour (especially breast, prostate, lung, kidneys and thyroid) or multiple myeloma (look out for hypercalcaemia, anaemia and renal impairment—page 311). Primary bone or spinal cord tumours are uncommon.

  − X-rays: look for bony destruction (may be subtle, e.g., missing pedicles on AP view—winking owl sign)
  − MRI spine

- **Hematoma**: Be especially suspicious if there has been recent spinal procedures, for example, lumbar puncture, epidural anaesthesia or spine instrumentation.

  − MRI spine

- **Axial spondyloarthropathy, for example, ankylosing spondylitis (AS)**: Patients are typically young (under 40) and may be male or female (3:1 ratio). AS presents with back pain worse on rest, with prominent morning stiffness. Refer these patients early—the development of marked impairment in back flexion (Schober's test) or a characteristic 'question mark' posture comes late (also see Chapter 48).

  − X-ray: marginal syndesmophyte formation (bamboo spine) in late AS
  − Possible role for MRI if high clinical suspicion but normal X-rays

Mechanical Spine Pain

Mechanical pain is worse on exertion and relieved by rest. This characteristic of pain is more consistent with degenerative structural disease.

Sudden-Onset or Severe Pain

- **Compression fracture**: The vertebrae is a common site for osteoporotic fractures, which may occur with very little trauma. Pain can be severe, or at times deceptively mild or even asymptomatic. Do also consider other causes of pathological fracture such as tumour.

Mild Episodic Mechanical Pain

- **Spondylosis**: With age, degenerative changes in the spine develop—intervertebral discs degenerate, its ligaments thicken and facet joints become osteoarthritic. Discogenic pain is worse on flexion (which stresses the anterior discs), while facet joint osteoarthritis causes pain worse on extension (which stresses posterior structures).
- **Developmental abnormalities**: Back pain is associated with scoliosis and other developmental spinal abnormalities.
- **Nonspecific musculoskeletal back pain**: The vast majority of patients have nonspecific musculoskeletal back pain. It is very common and usually of no great consequence.

What is the role of imaging studies? Spine X-rays (AP and lateral views) are helpful in sudden-onset or severe pain to look for any compression fracture (Figure 51.3a). Pay attention to height of each vertebrae and the bony alignment of the four columns (see discussion question at the end). Consider adding flexion/extension views, in the absence of recent trauma or known fracture, to assess instability (Figure 51.3c). Conversely, routine imaging in mild episodic mechanical pain, without red flags, is unwarranted and can lead to inappropriate tests and interventions. Many people will have degenerative findings on radiology but only a minority are symptomatic (Figure 51.3b). It is far more important to do a thorough neurological examination, including assessment of anal tone, to rule out radiculopathy from a prolapsed intervertebral disk or cauda equina syndrome—which an X-ray will miss.

Figure 51.3. X-rays in back pain. Three 70-year-old ladies present with back pain.

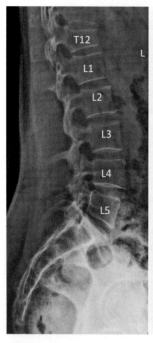 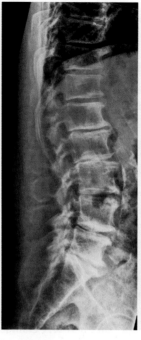 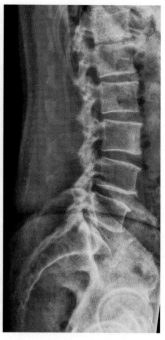

(a) **Compression fracture**: Note the loss of vertebral height implying a T12 wedge compression fracture.

(b) **Spondylosis**: Degenerative changes include disc space narrowing and osteophyte formation. These changes are common; patients may be asymptomatic, have back pain or neurogenic claudication.

(c) **Spondylolisthesis**: Observe anterior displacement of L5 over S1. In this case, it is relatively mild. Spondylolisthesis may be asymptomatic or symptomatic (back pain, neurogenic claudication).

 Using what you have learnt, **pen down your approach** to the Clinical Case at the start of the chapter **BEFORE reading the discussion** below.

Case Discussion

Patient A has acute-onset, severe back pain with bilateral neurological deficits and bladder dysfunction. This is the cauda equina syndrome, most likely from a large central disc prolapse precipitated by unloading the heavy suitcase. He will require an urgent MRI spine and surgical intervention.

Patient B has mechanical back pain, most likely posture-related while in the taxi. This is particularly common among taxi drivers. If further history and examination finds no red flags (see discussion question below), there is little role for further imaging studies.

Patient C has non-mechanical pain and fever. This is worrisome for infection (e.g., TB) or malignancy. He should receive an MRI spine, in addition to a clinical evaluation for these causes.

Key Lessons	1. Syndromes of back/neck pain plus abnormal neurology include the cauda equina syndrome, radiculopathy, cervical myelopathy and lumbar spinal stenosis. Each has a distinct presentation and unique clinical features.
	2. Apart from neurological abnormalities, worrisome features in back/neck pain include—non-mechanical pain, morning stiffness, fever or weight loss.
	3. Routine imaging studies are unwarranted in patients with mild episodic mechanical spine pain, with normal neurology and no trauma.
Common Pitfalls	1. Cases of aortic dissection, presenting as lower back pain, have been missed—at times with disastrous consequences. Always consider the causes of referred pain.
	2. A digital rectal examination is warranted in all patients with acute-onset back/neck pain.
Questions	1. **DISCUSS!** In a patient presenting to primary care with low back pain, what are the key red flags on history and examination that you would look for?
	2. **EXPLORE!** Read up on spine X-rays: (a) what are the normal features, (b) what are the abnormalities to look for and (c) what are the limitations of plain X-rays (i.e., what can it not see?)
	3. **GO FURTHER!** What are the key principles of advanced trauma life support? Summarise its key steps, beginning with the moment a trauma patient arrives in the emergency department.

Female
Genital Tract

Chapter

52   An Approach to Vaginal Bleeding (Non-Pregnant)

Clinical Case

An 18-year-old student is referred for a long history of heavy painless menstrual bleeding. She first presented 1 month ago, after fainting during a school excursion. Her GP found her pale and checked her haemoglobin, which was 7.8 mg/dL. She walks into your clinic, accompanied by her anxious 53-year-old mother. Her mother casually mentions that she used to have heavy periods her entire life. She underwent menopause 4 years ago but has recently started to get vaginal spotting again. How would you counsel mother and child?

Normal menstruation is <80 mL, lasts ~5 days and recurs in 21 to 35 day cycles. Patients present when vaginal bleeding deviates from what they know to be 'normal', causes anaemia, or is otherwise bothersome.

Always rule out pregnancy with a urine pregnancy test or serum beta-hCG, unless the patient is obviously menopausal (for vaginal bleeding in pregnancy, see Chapter 53). Verify that bleeding is vaginal, not rectal or urinary (haematuria). Next, elicit the relationship of symptoms to menstrual cycles and coitus, and identify the presenting syndrome (Figure 52.1):

1. **Heavy menstrual bleeding** (formerly known as menorrhagia): Cyclical menstrual bleeding but with increased volume (>80 mL) or duration (>7 days).

2. **Post-menopausal bleeding**: Bleeding after onset of menopause (defined as 12 months of amenorrhoea).

3. **Inter-menstrual bleeding**: Bleeding occurring between cyclically normal periods.

4. **Post-coital bleeding**: Bleeding after penetrative vaginal intercourse, unrelated to menstruation.

1. Heavy Menstrual Bleeding

Heavy menstrual bleeding is by definition cyclical; this excludes most cancers, which will not respect regular hormonal cycles. Heavy menstrual bleeding may cause symptomatic anaemia, presenting as fatigue, giddiness or dyspnoea.

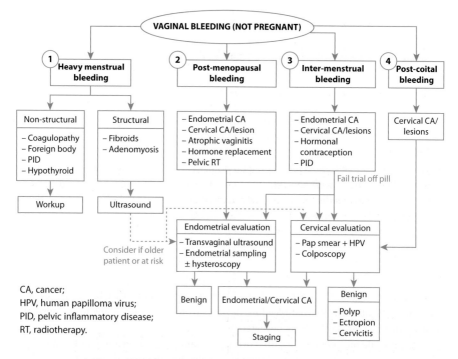

Figure 52.1. Approach to vaginal bleeding (non-pregnant).

Any Suggestion of Non-Structural Cause?

Take a history to elicit the non-structural causes:

- **Coagulopathy**: Heavy menstrual bleeding is a common presentation of a bleeding diathesis such as Von Willebrand's disease (N.B. haemophilia is X-linked recessive and presents in males). One would expect to also find easy bruising, and they may be a positive family history (see Chapter 33).

- **Foreign body**: Copper intra-uterine contraceptive devices, retained tampons or other foreign bodies.

- **Pelvic inflammatory disease**: Gonococcal or chlamydial infection can present as heavy menstrual bleeding, lower abdominal pain, vaginal discharge, ± fever. Examine for a friable cervix, purulent discharge, cervical excitation, adnexal and pelvic tenderness.

- **Hypothyroidism**: Lethargy, cold intolerance, weight gain and so forth (see Chapter 36). Heavy menstrual bleeding is unlikely a sole feature.

Workup

- Platelets, PT/PTT
- For Von Willebrand's: VWF antigen, ristocetin cofactor activity, factor 8

- Inflammatory markers
- High vaginal and endocervical swabs
- Urine for gonococcal and chlamydial PCR

- Thyroid function test

Workup for Structural Causes

After excluding non-structural causes, consider the structural causes of heavy menstrual bleeding:

Workup

- **Uterine fibroids and adenomyosis**: Heavy menstrual bleeding with dysmenorrhea. A pelvic mass may occasionally be palpable. Huge fibroids can cause mass symptoms, for example, urinary frequency or constipation, but this is rare.

    − Gynaecological ultrasound

- **Sinister causes**: Polyps, endometrial hyperplasia or malignancies more commonly present as inter-menstrual bleeding than as heavy menstrual bleeding. However, it would be wise to exclude sinister conditions in older patients (>45 years) or those with other risk factors.

    − Consider endometrial and cervical evaluation in the following sections

2. Post-Menopausal Bleeding

Post-menopausal bleeding is always abnormal. Some menstrual irregularity and spotting is common during the perimenopausal phase, but once menopause is firmly established, any bleeding is non-physiological. The key task is to exclude a malignancy—endometrial, cervical or (less commonly) vulval or vaginal cancer—via both endometrial and cervical evaluation. If both are negative for malignancy, consider various benign aetiologies.

Endometrial Evaluation

Except in very advanced uterine malignancy, most patients are asymptomatic apart from bleeding. Risk factors include unopposed oestrogen exposure (obesity, nulliparity), tamoxifen use and genetic predisposition (e.g., hereditary non-polyposis colorectal cancer). Workup begins with transvaginal ultrasound.

- **Transvaginal ultrasound**: Endometrial thickness risk-stratifies for endometrial cancer. Endometrial thickness <5 mm in post-menopausal women (not on tamoxifen or hormone replacement) is lower-risk, although a thin endometrium does not completely exclude cancer. Conversely, a thick endometrium (>5 mm) is more worrisome for endometrial cancer.[1]

- **Endometrial sampling** (e.g., Pipelle): Proceed to endometrial sampling unless endometrial thickness is low-risk. This provides a histological screen of malignancy.

- **Diagnostic hysteroscopy**: In selected cases, if symptoms are persistent and there is worry about false negative endometrial sampling.

---

[1] Rarely, it can also be a presenting feature of a hormone-secreting ovarian cancer (e.g., granulosa cell cancer).

Cervical Evaluation

- **Pap smear ± Human papilloma virus (HPV) testing**: Perform a pap smear, visually inspecting the vagina, vulva and cervix while performing the procedure. The pap smear samples cervical cells for histological analysis. A normal result is reassuring. Any dyskaryosis (low or high-grade squamous intraepithelial lesion) should be followed up by colposcopy. Atypical squamous cells of uncertain significance (ASCUS) is in itself ambiguous; HPV testing can clarify such results—if negative for high-risk strains of HPV, ASCUS is not relevant.

- **Colposcopy**: Proceed to colposcopy if pap smear is abnormal. On colposcopy, identify abnormal areas as acetowhite lesions that do not stain brown with iodine, or with vascular abnormalities (e.g., punctuations or mosaic patterns). Biopsy any abnormality.

Negative for Malignancy—Consider Benign Aetiologies

If endometrial and cervical evaluation is negative for malignancy, and there are no other structural abnormalities (e.g., polyps), consider the benign causes of post-menopausal bleed:

- **Atrophic vaginitis**: Common and often underdiagnosed. On examination, the vagina is pale, dry and shiny; it may also be erythematous.

- **Hormone replacement therapy**: May cause irregular bleeding.

- **Previous pelvic radiation therapy**: Can cause late vaginal bleeding due to tissue necrosis.

If there are any gastrointestinal symptoms, also consider colonoscopy. Fistulation from colon cancer or diverticular disease can rarely present as bloody or feculent vaginal discharge.

3. Inter-Menstrual Bleeding

Unlike heavy menstrual bleeding, inter-menstrual bleeding does not respect regular hormonal cycles and is therefore more worrisome. Aetiologies include:

- **Hormonal contraception**: Irregular bleeding is a common feature of progesterone-only pills, depot injections and implantable devices (e.g., implanon). Inter-menstrual bleeding may also be present in the initial use of combined oral contraceptive pills and hormonal intrauterine contraceptive devices.

- **Endometrial hyperplasia and cancer**.

- **Cervical cancer and other lesions** (see the following).

- **Pelvic inflammatory disease** (page 466).

Approach: Offer endometrial and cervical evaluation for malignancy (page 467). Alternatively, if there is a clear link to hormonal contraception, consider a trial off contraception, with a view towards endometrial and cervical evaluation if inter-menstrual bleeding persists.

4. Post-Coital Bleeding

During penetrative vaginal intercourse, the penis comes into contact with the cervix, causing contact bleeding if there is a friable cervical lesion. Therefore, post-coital bleeding suggests cervical pathology. This may include:

- **Cervical cancer**: This is the sinister cause to exclude. It may even be visible on speculum examination.

- **Cervical polyp**.

- **Cervical ectropion**: Endocervical eversion exposes columnar epithelium to the vagina, which appears as a raw area.

- **Cervicitis**: Usually due to a sexually transmitted infection such as Chlamydia. There may be vaginal discharge and a history of risky sexual behaviour.

- **Idiopathic**: Investigations may find no cervical abnormality. This is a diagnosis of exclusion.

Workup: This entails pap smear, HPV testing, followed by colposcopy if the pap smear is abnormal (see page 468).

 Using what you have learnt, **pen down your approach** to the Clinical Case at the start of the chapter **BEFORE reading the discussion** below.

Case Discussion

The young lady has heavy menstrual bleeding. The commonest cause in this age group is fibroids and adenomyosis. Atypically, she has no dysmenorrhoea. Coupled with the mother's history of 'heavy periods her entire life', this should prompt consideration of Von Willebrand's disease, an inherited coagulopathy. Further history may reveal easy bruising. Investigations for a bleeding diathesis should be pursued over gynaecologic scans. A pap smear can be offered if she is sexually active, as per screening recommendations.

Her mother has post-menopausal bleeding—worrisome for endometrial or cervical cancer. She will require transvaginal ultrasound, endometrial sampling and pap smear.

Key Lessons	
	1. Heavy menstrual bleeding may be due to structural (e.g., fibroids) and non-structural (e.g., coagulopathy) causes, but rarely malignancy.
	2. In contrast, inter-menstrual bleeding and post-menopausal bleeding are worrisome for a malignancy—pursue pap smear, transvaginal ultrasound and endometrial sampling.
	3. Post-coital bleeding suggests a cervical pathology, including cervical cancer.

Common Pitfalls	1. Post-menopausal bleeding is never normal and should not be dismissed.
Questions	1. **REFLECT!** Have you ever encountered a lady with a bleeding diathesis? Was vaginal bleeding part of her presentation, and at the initial presentation was it clear that she had a systemic disease rather than a local gynaecological problem?
	2. **DISCUSS!** In what situation would you *not* offer further investigation (ultrasound and endometrial sampling) to an elderly lady with post-menopausal bleeding?
	3. **GO FURTHER!** The International federation of obstetrics and gynaecology has a classification system for abnormal uterine bleeding (PALM-COEIN). Do you find this useful?

Chapter
An Approach to
53 Vaginal Bleeding (Pregnant)

Clinical Case

A 26-year-old foreign domestic helper presents with a 1-day history of profuse vaginal bleeding. She had thought that it was a heavier-than-expected period. You ask for a urine pregnancy test and it unexpectedly returns positive. Informed of this result, she asks to terminate the consultation and leave your clinic immediately. How would you handle the situation?

Vaginal bleeding is distressing to any pregnant lady. While not uncommon, it may indicate miscarriage or other life-threatening pathology. This chapter presents an approach to vaginal bleeding in pregnancy (excluding obstetric complications during delivery) (Figure 53.1). For vaginal bleeding in the non-pregnant, see Chapter 52.

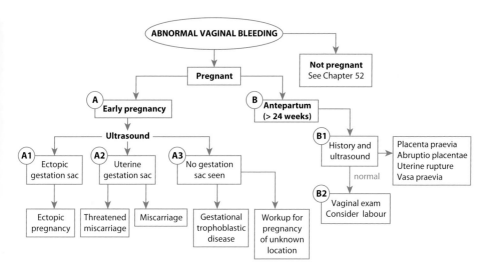

Figure 53.1. Approach to vaginal bleeding in pregnancy.

A. Early Pregnancy Bleeding

Vaginal bleeding is common in early pregnancy (up to 20 weeks), at times even before the patient realises that she is pregnant. This is a circumstance where history and examination is unable to reliably distinguish normal pregnancy from life-threatening causes of bleeding. Begin with a transvaginal ultrasound (US) and determine if the gestation sac is uterine, ectopic or not visible.

A1. Ectopic Gestation Sac

An extra-uterine gestation sac (usually in the fallopian tube) is an ectopic pregnancy. Non-ruptured ectopic pregnancies may have only mild bleeding and adnexal tenderness, while rupture presents with severe abdominal pain, guarding and hypotension. Ectopic pregnancy carries a risk of catastrophic rupture and requires urgent referral to a gynaecology or early pregnancy unit. It often requires surgery.

A2. Uterine Gestation Sac

Mild symptoms: In a patient with only mild vaginal bleeding, no uterine contractions, and a uterine gestation sac on ultrasound, consider:

- **Threatened miscarriage:**[1] US reveals a viable foetus (visible yolk sac, foetal heartbeat seen). This is quite common in early pregnancy.

- **Missed miscarriage**: US reveals no viable foetus, that is, no foetal heartbeat despite crown rump length > 7 mm, or absence of yolk sac despite gestation sac > 25 mm.

- **Indeterminate**: If pregnancy is too early (crown rump length < 7 mm or gestation sac < 25 mm), US may not identify a yolk sac or foetal heartbeat even if one is present. In such situations US is inconclusive and should be repeated in a week. Increase in gestation sac length, or appearance of foetal heartbeat suggests a viable pregnancy, that is, the vaginal bleeding was a threatened miscarriage.

Symptomatic: If the patient has severe vaginal bleeding and/or painful contractions, consider:

- **Inevitable miscarriage**: Patient has painful uterine contractions and a dilated cervical os. Miscarriage is likely, regardless of US findings.

- **Incomplete miscarriage**: Products of conception remaining in utero after a miscarriage can lead to continued and possibly severe bleeding. US reveals no viable foetus.

A3. No Gestation Sac Seen

- **Pregnancy of unknown location**: The possibilities are:
  - **Normal** pregnancy, but too early to visualise a gestation sac on US.
  - **Ectopic** pregnancy, but not visualised on US.
  - **Complete miscarriage**: No gestation sac is visible because the products of conception have already passed out, with or without the patient's knowledge. Symptoms diminish with time.

---

[1] An intrauterine gestation sac does not *always* rule out ectopic pregnancy. Heterotopic pregnancy (simultaneous uterine and ectopic pregnancy) can occur, especially with a history of in-vitro fertilisation, previous ectopic pregnancy, damaged fallopian tubes (e.g., pelvic inflammatory disease, tubal surgery) or an intra-uterine contraceptive device.

- **Gestational trophoblastic disease**: Hydatidiform mole or its malignant counterpart, choriocarcinoma. In additional to vaginal bleeding, these present with an unusually large uterus and unusually high beta-hCG. US reveals a 'snowstorm' pattern with absent foetal heartbeat.

- **False-positive β-hCG**: For example, granulosa cell tumour, hCG injections for fertility treatment and drugs (e.g., chlorpromazine and phenothiazine).

Workup for pregnancy of unknown location: The first aim is to exclude ectopic pregnancy.

- **Quantitative serum β-hCG**: β-hCG levels rise with gestation. In a normal pregnancy, one would expect to visualise an intrauterine gestational sac above a certain β-hCG level (the 'discriminatory zone'). The exact level varies by institution but is generally around 1500 IU/L.

  - β-hCG > **discriminatory zone**: High β-hCG with no intrauterine gestational sac strongly suggests ectopic pregnancy.

  - β-hCG < **discriminatory zone**: This suggests very early pregnancy, so it may be too early to visualise an intrauterine gestational sac. Provided that the patient is stable, proceed to trend β-hCG. If levels double in 48 hr, a normal pregnancy is likely. If levels halve, miscarriage is likely. Levels in between are indeterminate and do not exclude ectopic pregnancy—these patients should be managed by a specialist.

- **Adjunct: Progesterone levels**. This is produced by the corpus luteum to sustain an early pregnancy. Hence, high levels suggest a normal pregnancy, and low levels suggest either a failing or an ectopic pregnancy.

B. Antepartum Bleeding

Antepartum bleeding refers to vaginal bleeding after 24 weeks' gestation (i.e., after foetal viability), unrelated to labour and delivery. Vaginal examination can cause severe haemorrhage and is *contraindicated* until placenta praevia has been excluded.

B1. Initial Approach

Start with a history, US and foetal monitoring (cardiotocogram). This may reveal:

- **Placenta praevia**: While the classic presentation is painless vaginal bleeding, pain or contractions is present in 20% of cases. US will visualise a low-lying placenta.

- **Abruptio placentae**: Vaginal bleeding with painful contractions, foetal distress and a 'woody hard' uterus on abdominal palpation. The patient is usually distressed and in shock (although this can also occur in pre-eclampsia). Abruptio is a clinical diagnosis with high maternal and perinatal mortality, and requires urgent management and resuscitation. US is poorly sensitive.

- **Uterine rupture**: Sudden onset of intense pain ± bleeding. Foetal monitoring will be abnormal and foetal parts may even be palpable abdominally. The mother will be distressed with an acute abdomen, tachycardia and hypotension. A high index of suspicion is required, especially if there are risk factors (e.g., previous fibroid surgery, previous caesarean section) or trauma.

- **Vasa praevia**: In this condition, foetal vessels abnormally transverse the membranes covering the cervical os. These vessels can bleed, leading to foetal blood loss, rapid exsanguination and foetal death. Doppler US visualises blood vessels with foetal arterial/venous waveforms passing over the internal cervical os.

B2. Vaginal Examination

Once placenta praevia has been ruled out on US, proceed with vaginal exam (speculum and digital examination). This may reveal:

- **Labour**: If the cervical os is dilated, suspect onset of labour with a bloody show.
- **Conditions unrelated to pregnancy**: For example, cervical cancer and polyps (see Chapter 52).
- Otherwise normal finding.

 Using what you have learnt, **pen down your approach** to the Clinical Case at the start of the chapter **BEFORE reading the discussion** below.

Case Discussion

This is a dicey situation for the patient in more than one way. Indeed, the unexpected pregnancy has ramifications on the patient's employment and residency status. More importantly, it is a dicey situation because the most dangerous differential here is an ectopic pregnancy, which may rupture with life-threatening haemorrhage. You should make every effort to coax her from leaving. She will require pelvic ultrasound to look for an ectopic gestation sac, and urgent gynaecologic consultation.

Key Lessons	1. The most important differential of early pregnancy bleeding is ectopic pregnancy. Ultrasound is the key to reveal an ectopic pregnancy, a miscarriage or a viable intra-uterine pregnancy.
	2. Antepartum bleeding has a number of dangerous causes, including placenta praevia, abruption placentae and uterine rupture.
Common Pitfalls	1. Vaginal examination is contraindicated in antepartum bleeding, until placenta praevia has been ruled out.
Questions	1. **REFLECT!** Have you ever seen a patient with an ectopic pregnancy or placenta praevia? Why are these conditions so dangerous?
	2. **DISCUSS!** In the scenario that a pregnant lady is unable to tell you her gestational age, what would suggest that she is more than 24 weeks pregnant?

Chapter

54 An Approach to Amenorrhoea and Virilisation

Clinical Case

A 34-year-old lady presents with irregular periods. She has only had two light periods in the last 6 months. She is otherwise well with no other symptoms. On examination, she is obese with a BMI of 37. She has severe acne and is growing a moustache. Investigations reveal normal FSH, LH and oestrogen, as well as mildly raised testosterone and normal dehydro-epiandrosterone (DHEA). Thyroid function tests and prolactin are normal. What is the most likely diagnosis?

Amenorrhoea, the absence of menstruation, may be primary or secondary. A girl who fails to undergo menarche has primary amenorrhoea—this presents in adolescents and will not be covered here. Secondary amenorrhoea describes a lady who has previously had normal periods but misses three cycles or ≥ 6 months; this may be due to dysfunction in any component of the hypothalamic–pituitary–ovarian–uterine axis. **Oligomenorrhoea** is infrequent menstruation (> 35 days apart), often irregularly so, in a woman who has previously had regular periods. Its differentials and approach is as for secondary amenorrhoea.

Virilisation is the development of male physical characteristics in a female. This includes hirsutism (excessive male-pattern hair growth in androgen-dependent areas, for example, moustache, chest hair, genital hair), deepening of voice, increased muscle bulk, acne, male-pattern hair loss, oligomenorrhoea and amenorrhoea. Virilisation indicates androgen excess.

Secondary Amenorrhoea and Oligomenorrhoea

1. Exclude Pregnancy and Exogenous Hormones

The most common cause of amenorrhoea is pregnancy, as well as the use (or recent discontinuation) of hormonal contraception (oral pills, implantable device, etc.). These should be excluded—get a urine pregnancy test or serum beta-hCG. Spotting or oligomenorrhoea does not rule out pregnancy as first-trimester bleeding is common.

2. Localise the Defect

The clinical history may immediately suggest an aetiology. Failing which, a hormonal profile (FSH, LH, oestrogen, testosterone and prolactin) localises the lesion on the

Table 54.1. Hormone Levels in Amenorrhoea

Defect	FSH and LH	Oestrogen	Testosterone	Prolactin
Hypothalamic	Low or inappropriately normal	Low or inappropriately normal[a]	Normal	Normal
Pituitary	Low or inappropriately normal	Low or inappropriately normal[a]	Normal	Usually raised
PCOS	Normal or LH slightly high	Normal to slightly high	Mildly raised	Normal
Ovarian failure	Markedly raised	Low[a]	Normal	Normal
Uterine	Normal	Normal	Normal	Normal
Adrenal tumour[b]	Low	Low[a]	Markedly raised	Normal

[a]Understand the mechanism of derangement. Oestrogen is low in hypothalamic/pituitary disorders, as it is not stimulated by FSH/LH. It is low in ovarian failure because the ovaries do not produce oestrogen. It is suppressed by elevated testosterone in androgen-secreting adrenal tumours.

[b]See page 478.

PCOS, polycystic ovary syndrome.

hypothalamic–pituitary–ovarian–uterine axis (Table 54.1), and suggests specific aetiologies to pursue.

Additional Workup

(a) **Hypothalamic dysfunction** results in inadequate GnRH (not directly measured), and in turn inadequate stimulation of FSH, LH and oestrogen. Therefore, the biochemical picture is one of low or inappropriately normal[1] FSH, LH and oestrogen, with normal testosterone and prolactin.

- **Functional hypothalamic amenorrhoea**: Reflects energy conservation in a nutritionally scarce state—major illnesses, weight loss from anorexia or malabsorption, intense exercise, for example, competitive sports, or severe psychological stressors. The clinical history may be apparent or subtle (e.g., psychological stressors). Many patients with 'idiopathic' amenorrhoea have a functional hypothalamic aetiology.

- **Structural hypothalamic disorder**: For example, tumours, infiltration (e.g., sarcoidosis, Langerhans cell histiocytosis). These are rare; consider these if there are other signs of neurological dysfunction

− MRI hypothalamus

---

[1] Understand the concept of 'inappropriately normal'—in a hypo-estrogenic state, the appropriate physiological response is stimulation of FSH and LH, hence 'normal' FSH/LH is actually low.

(e.g., marked mood and personality changes, focal neurologic deficit) or severe headache.

(b) Pituitary dysfunction

- **Adenoma and other structural lesions**: In addition to amenorrhoea, there may be dysfunction of other pituitary hormone axes, with hypothyroidism (lethargy, cold intolerance, weight gain), hypocortisolism (postural hypotension, hypoglycaemia) and so forth. Hyperprolactinaemia is common and may lead to galactorrhoea; it may be due to a prolactin-producing adenoma or compression of the pituitary stalk (prolactin is inhibited by hypothalamic dopamine; stalk compression removes this inhibition). Structural pituitary lesions include:

    - **Pituitary adenomas**: Examine visual fields; a large adenoma may also cause bi-temporal hemianopia.

    - **Iatrogenic**: Previous surgery, cranial radiation.

    - **Sheehan syndrome**: In major obstetric haemorrhage.

    - **Infiltration**: Hemochromatosis, sarcoidosis or Langerhans cell histiocytosis.

  — Test thyroid, cortisol and growth hormone axes
  — Pituitary MRI looking for an adenoma

- **Drugs**: Hyperprolactinaemia due to dopamine antagonists, for example, haloperidol, metoclopramide.

- **Thyroid disease**: May interfere with sex hormone function.

  — Thyroid function test

(c) Ovarian dysfunction

- **Polycystic ovary syndrome (PCOS)**: Presents with oligomenorrhoea, mild hyper-androgenism (acne, hirsutism, male-pattern hair loss) and polycystic ovaries. Patients often have the metabolic syndrome (e.g., obesity and diabetes). The biochemical picture shows mildly elevated testosterone, slightly elevated LH/FSH and oestrogen, and a normal prolactin. This is a diagnosis of exclusion and differentials (e.g., Cushing's syndrome and adrenal tumour) should be considered—in particular, severe hyper-androgenism is more suggestive of an adrenal tumour than of PCOS.

  — Pelvic ultrasound for polycystic ovaries
  — Metabolic screen for diabetes, lipids and so forth

- **Ovarian failure**: In these disorders, the ovaries fail to produce oestrogen. Patients experience menopausal symptoms, for example, hot flushes, vaginal dryness, sleep disorders and decreased libido. Biochemically, low oestrogen causes marked stimulation

  — Screen for complications, for example, osteoporosis

of FSH and LH by a normal pituitary. Testosterone and prolactin are normal.

- **Menopause**: Occurring after 40 years.

- **Premature ovarian failure**: Oocyte depletion before 40 years. This may be idiopathic or secondary to chemotherapy, radiation or autoimmune disease.

- **Surgical oophorectomy**.

- **Turner's syndrome**: A young patient with primary or secondary amenorrhoea, short stature, dysmorphisms, but normal secondary sexual characteristics. The biochemical picture (high LH/FSH, low oestrogen) resembles ovarian failure (the mechanism appears to be early follicular depletion).

  − Karyotype

(d) **Uterine dysfunction**: All hormones are normal but the target organ (uterus) fails to respond to hormones. For example:

  − Ultrasound may be suggestive but is not definitive
  − Hysteroscopy

- **Asherman's syndrome**: Intrauterine adhesions due to repeated instrumentation (e.g., previous gynaecological procedures) or genital TB.

- **Surgical hysterectomy**.

(e) **Adrenal disorders**: See the following section.

Virilisation and Hirsutism

The presentation of androgen excess varies by patient group. In females, it presents as virilisation. In pre-pubertal males, it presents as precocious puberty. In post-pubertal males, there are few clinical manifestations.

Clinical Presentation

In many instances, the clinical picture is strongly suggestive of an aetiology.

- **Androgen-secreting adrenal or ovarian tumour**: This presents as rapid-onset severe virilisation, especially in later life. It is most commonly due to an adrenal tumour—either carcinoma (often large by the time it is clinically symptomatic) or adenoma (less common). An androgen-secreting ovarian tumour may present in the same manner, and can be distinguished from an adrenal tumour by DHEA levels (see the following).

- **Polycystic ovarian syndrome (PCOS)**: Hirsutism (not severe virilisation) with oligo/amenorrhoea, infertility and obesity (page 477).

- **Cushing's syndrome**: Weight gain with Cushingoid features (central obesity, moon face, abdominal striae, thin skin), mild hirsutism and acne (see Chapter 38).

- **Non-classical congenital adrenal hyperplasia (CAH)**: CAH arises from a defect in the steroid metabolism pathway (defective 21-hydroxylation of 17-hydroxyprogesterone to 11-deoxycortisol). In classical CAH, a severe enzyme defect leads to inadequate glucocorticoid and mineralocorticoid production, presenting in infancy as adrenal insufficiency and salt wasting. In non-classical CAH, the enzyme defect is milder; sufficient glucocorticoid and mineralocorticoid production is maintained, albeit at elevated ACTH levels (stimulated in response to decreased cortisol), generating excess steroid precursors, which are shunted into the androgen-production pathway. Non-classical CAH presents as primary amenorrhoea, or in adulthood with signs of androgen excess, which can be indistinguishable from PCOS.

- **Androgen-containing drugs**: This features in some (often illicit) sports enhancing drugs.

Biochemical Differentiation

Measure FSH, LH, oestrogen, testosterone and dehydroepiandrosterone (DHEA). Further tests, which may be helpful to distinguish the causes of virilisation are given in Table 54.2.

Table 54.2. Hormone Levels in Virilisation

Aetiology	FSH, LH, oestrogen	Testosterone	DHEA	Other tests
Adrenal tumour	Low	**Markedly raised**	**High**[a]	
Androgen-secreting ovarian tumour	Low	**Markedly raised**	**Low**[a]	
Cushing's syndrome	Normal	Normal to mildly raised	Normal	**Dexamethasone suppression test**: failure to suppress cortisol
PCOS	Normal to slightly high	Mildly raised	Normal	**Ultrasound**: demonstrates ovarian cysts
Non-classical CAH	Normal	Mildly raised	Normal	**8 am 17-OHP**[b]: high **Short synacthen test**: exaggerated 17-OHP response

[a] DHEA is produced only by the adrenals. Therefore, while elevated testosterone may be found in all hyperandrogenic states, elevated DHEA strongly suggests an adrenal tumour, over another source of androgens.

[b] 17-OHP accumulates in CAH due to defective hydroxylation of 17-OHP to 11-deoxycortisol. Under ACTH stimulation (in the short synacthen test), far more 17-OHP is produced than can be hydroxylated, leading to an exaggerated rise in 17-OHP. This is helpful to differentiate non-classical CAH from polycystic ovary syndrome, in which a short synacthen test results in a less exaggerated 17-OHP rise.

Note: Specific cut-off values have been omitted, in favour of a focus on principles. There is significant overlap between 'mildly raised' and 'markedly raised' testosterone levels; interpretation can be controversial, and exact cut-offs depends on the literature quoted.

17-OHP, 17-hydroxyprogesterone; CAH, congenital adrenal hyperplasia; DHEA, dehydroepiandrosterone; PCOS, polycystic ovary syndrome.

Next Steps

- **Suspected adrenal tumours**: Adrenal CT or MRI should be ordered.
- **Cushing's syndrome**: Work up for an aetiology. See Chapter 38.

 Using what you have learnt, **pen down your approach** to the Clinical Case at the start of the chapter **BEFORE reading the discussion** below.

Case Discussion

This lady has obesity, oligomenorrhoea and mild hyper-androgenism. Biochemistry suggests a normal hypothalamic–pituitary–ovarian axis. Elevated testosterone with normal DHEA implies that the testosterone arises from an extra-adrenal cause (i.e., unlikely adrenal tumour). This picture fits best with polycystic ovary syndrome (PCOS). A gynaecological ultrasound may demonstrate ovarian cysts.

PCOS is a diagnosis of exclusion. If obesity is predominantly central, with Cushingoid features of moon face, abdominal striae and thin skin, a dexamethasone suppression test should be performed. If virilisation progress rapidly or become severe, there is an urgent need to exclude an androgen secreting tumour in the adrenal gland or ovary; the next test would be DHEA levels, which will be high in an adrenal source.

The metabolic implications of PCOS are significant. Screen for diabetes (fasting glucose), hyperlipidaemia (fasting lipids), obstructive sleep apnoea and fatty liver disease (liver enzymes). Weight loss and cardiovascular risk factor reduction must be pursued in tandem with addressing the menstrual abnormalities of PCOS.

Key Lessons	1. In the approach to a- or oligo-menorrhoea, think through the hypothalamic–pituitary–ovarian (PCOS, ovarian failure)–uterine axis. Dysfunction in each component results in a characteristic hormonal profile.
	2. Rapid onset severe virilisation with high DHEA suggests an adrenal tumour. Milder hirsutism may be due to Cushing's syndrome, polycystic ovary syndrome or non-classical congenital adrenal hyperplasia.
Common Pitfalls	1. Always exclude pregnancy and oral contraceptive pill use—these are the commonest causes of secondary amenorrhoea.
	2. Beware the inappropriately normal: In a hypo-estrogenic patient, 'normal' FSH/LH is not normal.
Questions	1. **DISCUSS!** Oligomenorrhoea is common and many patients are not bothered by it. When might oligomenorrhoea be a variation of normal, and what are some features on history or examination that would prompt you to urge further investigations?

2. **EXPLORE!** Pituitary tumours may present in many ways. Can you list some of these ways, and explain their pathophysiological basis?

3. **GO FURTHER!** Adrenal masses are frequent incidental findings ('incidentalomas') on abdominal CT scans performed for other reasons (i.e., no clinical suspicion of adrenal tumour). How would you approach an adrenal incidentaloma?

Index to Conditions